Artificial Intelligence and Data Science in Healthcare Applications

Artificial Intelligence and Data Science in Healthcare Applications provides a thorough in-depth examination of how AI and data science are transforming predictive analytics and outlier detection in every industry. With in-depth examinations of machine learning, neural networks, NLP, and ethics of AI, this book prepares readers with both theoretical principles and practical tools to create smart, scalable systems. Real-world healthcare, cybersecurity, and finance case studies exemplify real world applications, and tutorials with leading libraries serve as a starting point for implementation.

Features:

- Offers a broad overview of both foundational and advanced topics in artificial intelligence and data science, focusing particularly on their applications in prediction and detection.
- Addresses the ethical implications and social impact of artificial intelligence and data science, discussing topics such as algorithmic bias, privacy, and the ethical use of predictive technologies.
- Discusses enhanced deep learning model to detect lung diseases from Chest-Xray.
- Highlights lung cancer prediction using variational autoencoders and early stopping for neural network clustering and optimal tuning.
- Evaluates mental well-being through wearable sensors utilizing machine learning.

It will serve as an ideal text for senior undergraduates, graduate students, and academic researchers in electrical engineering, electronics and communications engineering, computer engineering, information technology, and biomedical engineering.

Computational and Intelligent Systems

Series Editor: Ramesh Chandra Poonia

CHRIST (Deemed to be University), Bangalore, Karnataka, INDIA - 560029

About the Series:

In todays' world, the systems that integrate intelligence into machine-based applications are known as intelligent systems. In order to simplify the man-machine interaction, intelligent systems play an important role. The books under the proposed series will explain the fundamentals of intelligent systems, reviews the computational techniques and also offers step-by-step solutions of the practical problems. Aimed at senior undergraduate students, graduate students, academic researchers and professionals, the proposed series will focus on broad topics including artificial intelligence, deep learning, Image processing, cyber physical systems, wireless security, mechatronics, cognitive computing, and industry 4.0.

Natural Language Processing and Information Retrieval
Principles and Applications
Edited By Muskan Garg, Sandeep Kumar, Abdul Khader Jilani Saudagar

Soft Robotics for Medical and Healthcare Applications
Edited by Shaik Himam Saheb, Tharakeshwar Appala and Mohammad S Khan

Smart Cyber Physical Systems
Innovations and Real-World Implications
Edited by Ramesh Chandra Poonia, Kamal Upreti and Mohammad S Khan

Cognitive Cloud Computing
Building Intelligent Systems for Tomorrow
Edited by Fr. Jossy George, Kamal Upreti, Ramesh Chandra Poonia, Ankit Gautam and Danish Nadeem

Computational Techniques in Precision Agriculture
Algorithms and Applications
Edited by Bhoomika Batra, Vinod Kumar Shukla and Vaibhav Bhatnagar

Artificial Intelligence and Data Science in Healthcare Applications
Edited by Ashwani Kumar, Gautam Srivastava, P. K. Gupta and Mohit Kumar

For more information on this series page, please visit our website link: https://www.routledge.com/Computational-and-Intelligent-Systems/book-series/CRCCIS

Artificial Intelligence and Data Science in Healthcare Applications

Edited by
Ashwani Kumar
Gautam Srivastava
P. K. Gupta
Mohit Kumar

CRC Press
Taylor & Francis Group
Boca Raton London New York

CRC Press is an imprint of the
Taylor & Francis Group, an **informa** business

Designed cover image: © Shutterstock Images

First edition published 2026
by CRC Press
2385 NW Executive Center Drive, Suite 320, Boca Raton FL 33431

and by CRC Press
4 Park Square, Milton Park, Abingdon, Oxon, OX14 4RN

CRC Press is an imprint of Taylor & Francis Group, LLC

ISBN: 978-1-041-06256-1 (hbk)
ISBN: 978-1-041-06257-8 (pbk)
ISBN: 978-1-003-63456-0 (ebk)

DOI: 10.1201/9781003634560

Typeset in Sabon
by SPi Technologies India Pvt Ltd (Straive)

Contents

About the editors

Ashwani Kumar (Senior Member, IEEE) is working as an professor, in the Department of Computer Science and Engineering, School of Engineering and Technology, at Bennett University, India. He has more than Fifteen years of teaching and research experience. He has published more than 80 research papers in internationally reputed journals indexed in SCI/SCIE Web of Science and Scopus. His research area includes image security, watermarking techniques, multimedia applications, security and privacy, cryptography, and network security. He is also a lifetime member of professional societies like IEEE, IACSIT, IAENG, and SDIWC.

Gautam Srivastava (Senior Member, IEEE) is currently a professor of Computer Science at Brandon University, Brandon, Canada. In his 10-year academic career, he has published a total of 400 papers in high-impact conferences in many countries and high-status journals (SCI and SCIE). He is an editor of several international scientific research journals, including *IEEE Transactions on Industrial Informatics*, *IEEE Transactions on Computational Social Systems*, and *IEEE Internet of Things Journal*.

P. K. Gupta is post doctorate from University of Pretoria, South Africa. He is currently working as a professor and Head – CSE(Core), in the Department of Computer Science and Engineering & IT, at Jaypee University of Information Technology (JUIT), Solan, India. He has more than twenty five years of extensive experience in the IT industry and Academics in India and abroad. He has research experience in the Internet of Things, Artificial Intelligence, Cloud Computing, and Fog Computing. He has authored more than a hundred research papers in referred journals and international conferences. He is currently serving as a Life Member of the Computer Society of India (CSI), a Life member of the Indian Science Congress Association (ISCA), a Member of IEEE, a Professional member of ACM, a Senior member of IACSIT, and a Member of the Indian Society for Technical Education (ISTE).

Mohit Kumar is presently working as an Associate Professor, in the Department of Computer Science & Engineering, at Amity University Jharkhand, Ranchi, India. He has authored/co-authored papers in reputed top-cited journals like IEEE Transaction in Industrial Informatics, IEEE Transaction on Network Science and Engineering, Journal of Information Science & Engineering, MDPI Sensors, Symmetry, Electronics, and many more with a cumulative impact factor of >50. His research interests include Wireless Sensor Networks, Internet of Things, Data Science, Machine Learning, and Deep Learning.

Contributors

Tanvir Ahmad
Department of Computer Engineering
Jamia Millia Islamia
New Delhi, India

A. Jyothi Babu
Department of CA
School of Computing
Mohan Babu University
Kotala, India

J. Sankar Babu
Department of CSE
Sri Venkateswara College of Engineering
Tirupathi, India

Latha Banda
JEMTEC
Greater Noida, India

Pallab Banerjee
Department of Computer Science Engineering
Amity University Jharkhand
Jharkhand, India

Rudraksh Singh Chandel
Department of Computer Science
SCSET
Bennett University
Greater Noida, India

Tanya Chauhan
Department of Computer Science and Engineering
Echelon Institute of Technology
Faridabad, India

Jason Das
Department of Computer Science and Engineering (AI & ML)
SIET
Hyderabad, India

Jaya Dash
School of Computer Science Engineering and Technology
Bennett University
Greater Noida, India

Harsh Davey
Department of Computer Science and Engineering (AI & ML)
SIET
Hyderabad, India

Umar Faaruk
Department of Computer Science and Engineering (AI & ML)
SIET
Hyderabad, India

Sadiya Faizan
Department of Computer Science
SCSET
Bennett University
Greater Noida, India

Ahmad Faraz
Department of Computer Science Engineering
Amity University Jharkhand
Jharkhand, India

Swathi Gowroju
Department of Computer Science and Engineering (AI & ML)
SIET
Hyderabad, India

Riwitika Gupta
School of Computer Science Engineering and Technology
Bennett University
Greater Noida, India

Suraj Gupta
Department of Computer Science and Engineering
Jaypee University of Information and Technology
Solan, India

Kota Harshitha
Department of Computer Science and Engineering (AI & ML)
SIET
Hyderabad, India

Dipika Jain
School of Computer Science Engineering and Technology
Bennett University
Greater Noida, India

Md Khalid Jamal
Department of Computer Science and Applications
Sharda University
Greater Noida, India

Sonia Juneja
Department of Computer Science and Engineering
IMS Engineering College
Ghaziabad, India

Takreem Fatima Khan
Department of Computer Science
Aligarh Muslim University
Aligarh, India

Shlok Kohli
School of Computer Science Engineering and Technology
Bennett University
Greater Noida, India

Ashwani Kumar
School of Computer Science Engineering and Technology
Bennett University
Greater Noida, India

Mohit Kumar
Department of Computer Science Engineering
Amity University Jharkhand
Jharkhand, India

M. Sirish Kumar
Department of CSE(DS)
School of Computing
Mohan Babu University
Kotala, India

G. Laasyapriya
Department of CA
School of Computing
Mohan Babu University
Kotala, India

Tanya Liyaqat
Department of Computer Science and Applications
Sharda University
Greater Noida, India

Yuvika Mishra
School of Computer Science Engineering and Technology
Bennett University
Greater Noida, India

Dipra Mitra
Department of Computer Science Engineering
Amity University Jharkhand
Jharkhand, India

Kajol Mittal
Department of Computer Science & Engineering
Galgotias College of Engineering & Technology
Greater Noida, India

Mohit Mittal
Department of Computer Science and Engineering
Galgotias College of Engineering and Technology
Greater Noida, India

Rajni Mohana
Department of Computer Science and Technology
Amity University
Mohali, India

Ramesh Chandra Poonia
Department of Computer Science and Engineering
CHRIST (Deemed To be University)
Delhi NCR, India

Pallavi Ranjan
School of IT
Murdoch University
Dubai, UAE

Pratyush Rathore
Department of Computer Science and Engineering
SCSET
Bennett University
Greater Noida, India

Garima Saini
IITM, Janakpuri
Sobhasaria Group of Institutions
Sikar, India

Mala Saraswat
Department of Computer Science and Engineering
SCSET
Bennett University
Greater Noida, India

Shitharth Selvarajan
School of Built Environment, Engineering and Computing
Leeds Beckett University
Leeds, UK

Aman Sharma
Department of Computer Science and Engineering
Jaypee University of Information and Technology
Solan, India

Umang Sharma
Department of Computer Science and Engineering
Jaypee University of Information and Technology
Solan, India

Raj Shekhar
School of Computer Science
Engineering and Technology
Bennett University
Greater Noida, India

Shiv Naresh Shivhare
School of Computer Science
Engineering and Technology
Bennett University
Greater Noida, India

Neelam Shrivastava
Department of Computer Science &
Engineering
Galgotias College of Engineering &
Technology
Greater Noida, India

Rashmi Singh
Department of Computer Science
and Engineering
IIMT University
Meerut, India

B. Spandana
Department of Computer Science
and Engineering (AI & ML)
SIET
Hyderabad, India

Richa Suryavanshi
Department of Computer Science
and Engineering
Echelon Institute of Technology
Faridabad, India

Tina Tomazic
Faculty of Electrical Engineering
and Computer Science
University of Maribor
Maribor, Slovenia

Ishaan Tripathi
Department of Computer Science
and Engineering
SCSET
Bennett University
Greater Noida, India

Priyanka Tyagi
Department of Computer
Science & Engineering
Galgotias College of
Engineering & Technology
Greater Noida, India

Swaleha Zubair
Department of Computer Science
Aligarh Muslim University
Aligarh, India

Preface

In the ever-evolving landscape of technology, the convergence of Artificial Intelligence (AI) and Data Science has emerged as a transformative force, shaping industries, economies, and societies worldwide. As we stand on the threshold of a new era defined by unprecedented connectivity and data abundance, the significance of harnessing AI and Data Science capabilities for prediction, detection, and envisioning future prospects cannot be overstated.

This book, titled *Artificial Intelligence and Data Science in Healthcare Applications*, is a comprehensive exploration into the multifaceted realm of AI and Data Science applications. It delves into the intricate mechanisms behind predictive modelling, anomaly detection, and the profound insights they offer for shaping tomorrow's realities. Within these pages, readers will embark on a journey through the intricacies of predictive analytics, uncovering the methodologies employed to forecast outcomes with remarkable precision. From predictive modelling techniques such as machine learning algorithms to advanced statistical analyses, this book elucidates the tools and techniques indispensable for making informed decisions in an uncertain world.

Moreover, the book delves into the vital role of detection methodologies in identifying anomalies, irregularities, and outliers within vast datasets. Through case studies and practical examples, readers will gain a deeper understanding of how AI and Data Science empower organizations to detect fraud, mitigate risks, and enhance security across various domains. Beyond prediction and detection, this book also casts a visionary gaze towards the future, exploring the transformative potential of AI and Data Science in shaping tomorrow's landscapes. From healthcare and finance to transportation and environmental sustainability, the implications of AI-driven insights are boundless, offering unprecedented opportunities for innovation and progress.

Importantly, this book is not merely a theoretical exploration but a practical guide for professionals, researchers, and enthusiasts alike. Through hands-on tutorials, real-world scenarios, and best practices, readers will acquire the skills and knowledge necessary to leverage AI and Data Science effectively in their respective domains. As editors of this volume, we have endeavored to assemble a diverse array of perspectives and expertise, ensuring a comprehensive examination of the subject matter. We extend our gratitude to the contributing authors whose insights and experiences enrich the discourse within these pages. A detailed overview of the content is given as follows:

Chapter 1 deals with the automated diagnosis of ADHD disease with a few state-of-the-art artificial intelligence algorithms. The experimental study and the results obtained after implementing advanced deep learning approaches to EEG signals specifically for the classification of ADHD. This research incorporates six models: Temporal Convolutional Network, Temporal Convolutional Network with Attention, Recurrent Neural Network, Graph Neural Network, CNN with GRU, and a hybrid model that has CNN, RNN, and Attention. Having a significant literature review of numerous relevant and recent research works along with the experimental details, this chapter can be a significant part of this book.

Chapter 2 states that health is very important for human life. In particular, the health of the brain, which is the executive of the vital resource, is very important. Diagnosis for human health is provided by magnetic resonance imaging (MRI) devices, which help health decision makers in critical organs such as brain health. Images from these devices are a source of big data for artificial intelligence. In this study, authors aim to classify brain tumors such as glioma, meningioma, and pituitary tumor from brain MR images. They provide a detailed study of related work and then implement CNN models and compare them on basis of their performance.

Chapter 3 explores how machine learning (ML) can forecast mental health treatment needs across the lifespan, from childhood to older adulthood. By examining supervised and unsupervised algorithms, it highlights practical methods—such as random forest and neural networks—while addressing ethical and interpretative challenges. In the broader context of the book, AI and Data Science in Healthcare Applications, this work exemplifies how data-driven insights can enhance clinical decision-making, offering earlier detection and more personalized intervention strategies. Ultimately, the chapter demonstrates how ML can optimize resource allocation and complement clinical expertise, signaling a significant stride toward transformative, patient-centered mental healthcare.

Chapter 4 focuses on leveraging machine learning-powered predictive analytics to transform healthcare by facilitating early disease identification, prevention, and individualized therapy. This study suggests a strong prediction framework that combines electronic health records (EHR), demographic information, and environmental factors to predict the onset and progression of diseases in order to address the growing burden of chronic disease and the need for proactive healthcare interventions.

Chapter 5 generates complex, interpretable models to better detect and treat neurological and mental health illnesses. It is bridging significant gaps in the application of artificial intelligence in neurology. The study guarantees a flawless integration into healthcare systems by using modern ethical ideas for data security and openness and a real-time data processing pipeline.

Chapter 6 explores the role of machine learning (ML) in the early detection and diagnosis of Parkinson's disease (PD), a neurodegenerative disorder with significant impacts on patients' quality of life. It highlights the challenges of current diagnostic methods and emphasizes the need for more accurate and objective tools. The chapter discusses how various ML techniques—such as support vector machines, random forests, neural networks, and deep learning—are applied to diverse data sources, including clinical assessments, neuroimaging, genetic data, and wearable devices, to develop predictive models for PD.

Chapters 7 focus of this investigation is on the ways in which artificial intelligence has the potential to transform wearable technology for the treatment of respiratory disorders, cardiovascular diseases, and chronic ailments such as diabetes. Because they collect and analyze physiological data in real time using artificial intelligence, these wearables significantly enhance patient outcomes.

Chapters 8 states that the worldwide healthcare industry Medical supplies and medications are in higher demand than ever. Costs of development, time to market, and earnings are all increasing. Millions of individuals throughout the world now have access to life-saving medications. To address these issues, tech-based methods of testing medical devices have been developed so that they do not need to be tested on humans during the development phase.

Chapter 9 proposed YOLOv11-based system for fire and smoke detection has exhibited exceptional results so far in terms of accuracy, precision, and recall. The findings indicate that it has the potential to be used as an excellent safety device in all controlled and complex environments. This system has a wide array of useful applications. It is best employed in high-risk environments such as forests, industrial sites, residential areas, and public spaces.

Chapter 10 provides and comprehensive analysis of the enabling technologies for Edge AI, with a focus on the latest advancements in Edge AI frameworks and devices. It explores recent developments in edge computing, highlighting new software and hardware innovations designed to address the limitations of traditional cloud computing. The current state of Edge AI devices and frameworks is evaluated based on key features in the context of Edge Computing research, providing a comparative assessment of their suitability for different applications.

Chapter 11 explores the application of Artificial Intelligence (AI) in lung cancer detection using Computed Tomography (CT) scans emphasizing the role of AI-driven frameworks in enhancing diagnostic accuracy and efficiency. The discussion aligns with the broader theme of Artificial Intelligence and Data Science in Healthcare Applications by showcasing how AI advancements can revolutionize lung cancer diagnosis, ultimately contributing to improved patient outcomes.

Chapter 12 discussed that the existing approaches to exercise prescription are ineffective and ignorant. Yoga and meditation, two forms of traditional Indian medicine, provide numerous benefits for both mental and physical health, such as boosting immunity, promoting sound sleep patterns, and reducing stress and sadness. By strengthening the immune system, regular exercise lowers the risk of cancer, type 2 diabetes, obesity, heart disease, and stroke.

Chapter 13 addresses underpinning data science and AI principles, the mainstay of what follows is also a description of how these influence changing traditional processes in medicine. Some of the main applications like natural language processing, computer visioning, predictive analytics, and decision support systems and their bearing on patient care and clinical decisions are discussed as well.

Chapter 14 examines that to meet medical needs, healthcare systems are continuously in need of a new medications. As a result, scientists discover new medicines through a multi stage process called the drug discovery and development process. But conventional experiments are time and money consuming. Hence, advancements in computer based technology have been heavily used to expedite this process and battle time and expense issues.

Chapter 15 investigates that Electroencephalogram (EEG) is a non-invasive test which records the electrical activity of the brain and collects the data which can be used for seizure detection. However, traditional diagnostic techniques, such as EEG analysis, are labor-intensive and reliant on the expertise of trained professionals. Machine learning (ML) provides a promising alternative, offering automated, reliable, and efficient methods for seizure detection. Machine learning is the process of teaching computers to perform tasks by gaining experience.

Chapter 16 addresses how getting data privacy in the world of centralized identification systems today is a myth because of its many problems, the primary one being data control by one single entity. Self-Sovereign Identity (SSI) is a model that allows its utilizers complete control over their data privacy and security. This paper gives an overview of developing such a model over a private blockchain network using several Hyperledger frameworks, which are majorly open source.

Through its detailed exploration of AIDS in Healthcare Applications, this book aims to provide readers with a nuanced understanding of how these systems address contemporary challenges and create opportunities for innovation. Each chapter integrates cutting-edge research with real-world applications, making this book a valuable guide for those seeking to harness the power of SCPS in their respective fields.

We hope this book catalysis further research and development, inspiring solutions that will shape the future of intelligent, interconnected systems and their implications for society.

Acknowledgments

The successful development of this book, *Artificial Intelligence and Data Science in Healthcare Applications*, is the result of collaborative effort, intellectual dedication, and a shared vision to explore the transformative potential of AI and data science in the healthcare domain.

First and foremost, we extend our deepest gratitude to all contributing authors and researchers who brought their expertise, time, and passion to this volume. Each chapter is a testament to their commitment to advancing the state of the art in predictive modeling, anomaly detection, and intelligent systems applied to real-world healthcare challenges. Their scholarly work has laid a strong foundation for this book's comprehensive and multidimensional approach.

We sincerely thank the reviewers and domain experts who provided valuable feedback throughout the development of this proposal. Their constructive suggestions ensured the technical rigor, clarity, and relevance of the content presented. Special appreciation goes to our academic institutions and research centers for offering unwavering support and an environment conducive to innovation and inquiry. Their encouragement was instrumental in enabling us to delve deeply into the intersections of technology, healthcare, and data science.

Special recognition is extended to my colleague, Dr. Mohit Kumar from Amity University, Ranchi, India, whose invaluable contributions have been instrumental in the compilation of this book. We are also deeply grateful to Prof. (Dr.) Ramesh Chandra Poonia of CHRIST University, Bangalore, Karnataka, India, for his significant input and insightful suggestions throughout this process. A heartfelt thanks goes to Gauravjeet Singh Reen, Senior Editor for Engineering, Ergonomics, Human Factors, Occupational Health, and Safety (India and Sub-Saharan Africa) at CRC Press, Taylor & Francis Group, for providing us with the opportunity to undertake this book project.

We also acknowledge the contributions of numerous data scientists, medical practitioners, and technology professionals whose insights, real-world experiences, and ongoing research have inspired many of the practical applications and case studies within these chapters. Finally, we are grateful to the editorial and publishing teams who believed in the vision of this book and supported us at every stage—from conceptualization to final proposal. Their guidance and dedication have been critical in shaping this work into a resource that we hope will empower students, researchers, and professionals to make meaningful advances in AI-driven healthcare solutions.

Chapter 1

Computer-aided ADHD diagnosis using EEG analysis

Yuvika Mishra, Shlok Kohli, Sadiya Faizan, Shiv Naresh Shivhare, and Tina Tomazic

1.1 INTRODUCTION

One of the most common development disorders is Attention Deficit Hyperactivity Disorder (ADHD), which hampers normal functioning through inattention, hyperactivity, and impulsivity [1]. ADHD is a condition that can occur in both adults and children and is usually diagnosed based on behavior and the patient's history, which can be inaccurate due to biases and inconsistencies [2]. Electroencephalography (EEG) is effective in providing real-time, non-invasive brain activity data, making it a useful tool in the diagnosis of ADHD [3]. Research indicates that those with ADHD exhibit distinct brain patterns that distinguish them from individuals without ADHD, such as changes in theta and beta wave ratios [3]. However, reliable signal analysis faces challenges, including the high dimensionality, noise, and variability between subjects found in EEG data. These challenges severely hinder the use of EEG in diagnosis. Sophisticated methods, often involving elaborate signal processing and machine learning (ML) techniques, are required to derive meaningful information from these signals [4].

The use of ML and deep learning (DL) to identify ADHD patterns in EEG data shows promise in overcoming these challenges through automated identification of relevant patterns [5]. Several studies have demonstrated the ability of models such as Convolutional Neural Networks (CNNs) and Long Short-Term Memory (LSTM) networks to classify ADHD and non-ADHD EEG data with high accuracy [6]. However, some research gaps persist despite these advances. One of the most significant gaps is the lack of well-defined preprocessing techniques for EEG data [4]. Different noise reduction research approaches can produce results that differ and affect the degree to which the findings can be applied [7]. Furthermore, feature extraction presents another difficulty, since deep learning techniques need large classified datasets, which are sometimes difficult to obtain, while conventional methods may not adequately capture the intricacy of EEG data. By applying an effective approach that uses deep learning techniques for

DOI: 10.1201/9781003634560-1

the identification of ADHD using EEG data, this study aims to close these gaps. Our main goals are:

1. We aim to improve ADHD detection through improved preprocessing of EEG data and robust deep learning models.
2. We applied multiple neural network architectures, including a hybrid model, to detect ADHD using EEG signals.
3. In this paper, we break down the details of various models and use various metrics to determine how effective each model is.

In this chapter, we intend to help create more accurate and effective ADHD diagnostic tools, which may eventually improve patient outcomes and clinical judgment.

1.2 RELATED WORKS

Numerous studies have explored understanding the neurobiological and ML-driven approaches to ADHD and other neurological disorders. Maiti et al. [8] emphasized the crucial role of dendritic spine dynamics in synaptic plasticity and neurological conditions, describing the complex signaling pathways that under-pin spine pathology and its restoration. In a similar vein, Eslami et al. [9] surveyed ML techniques for diagnosing Autism Spectrum Disorder (ASD) and ADHD using fMRI, highlighting deep learning models' capabilities and limitations, including generalization challenges (Table 1.1).

Uddin et al. [13] explored the potential of artificial intelligence in precision medicine for neurodevelopmental disorders, emphasizing the heterogeneity in genetic and phenotypic profiles that complicate predictive models. Their review pin-pointed AI's potential to harness genomic data for early interventions, although progress remains slow compared to advances in oncology and cardiology. Luo et al. [14] conducted an extensive review of the heterogeneity of ADHD, highlighting its multifactorial causes and wide-ranging clinical presentations, suggesting that customized research on etiological risk factors could facilitate targeted therapeutic interventions. Cao et al. [15] provided a narrative on ML's application in understanding ADHD, detailing studies utilizing behavioral, genetic, and neurobiological data. They noted that while ML can unravel complex variable interactions, interpretability and model reliability remain limitations. Mostert et al. [16] focused on functional connectivity in adults with ADHD through resting-state fMRI, identifying stronger connectivity in the anterior cingulate gyrus and cerebellum networks, though effect sizes were modest.

Hoekzema et al. [12] presented findings on neural dysregulation in adult ADHD, revealing increased coherence between the dorsolateral prefrontal cortex and the default mode network (DMN). This supports the idea that

Table 1.1 Summary of a few significant and relevant methods for fake news detection with their advantage and drawbacks

Author(s)	*Dataset*	*Advantage*	*Limitation*
Maiti et al. [8]	Data from animal models, especially transgenic mice related to neurodegenerative diseases.	Limited by model variability and challenges in human translation.	Findings may be limited by variability in experimental models and challenges in translating animal studies to humans.
Hoggman et al. [10]	Pooled structural MRI data from 23 international research groups, including thousands of participants.	Large international sample size boosts statistical power and generalizability of findings on brain structure in ADHD.	Data heterogeneity across sites and potential confounding factors may introduce variability.
Eslami et al. [9]	Uses multimodal neuroimaging datasets, including sMRI and fMRI, referencing "Biomarkers of Autism at 12 Months".	ML methods enhance diagnostic accuracy for ASD and ADHD by leveraging complex neuroimaging data.	Limitations include variability from multi-site datasets and challenges from cross-sectional designs.
Tang et al. [11]	Utilizes the ADHD-200 dataset with neuroimaging data from 973 individuals across multiple sites.	Achieves 99.6% classification accuracy using a novel auto-encoding neural network, enhancing ADHD diagnosis reliability.	Relies on the ADHD-200 dataset, limiting generalizability due to its small sample size and potential biases.
Hoekzema et al. [12]	Resting-state fMRI data from 22 medication-naïve males with ADHD and 23 neurotypical controls.	Uses independent components analysis to identify neural network dysregulation in adults with ADHD.	Small sample size and male-only focus may limit generalizability to the broader ADHD population.

ADHD is characterized by diffuse connectivity between functional networks, with insufficient suppression of the DMN during rest. Sethu and Vyas [17] discussed ML approaches for the prediction of ADHD, indicating that the SVM and ANN models are particularly effective, with genetic programming that improves diagnostic precision. Cervantes-Henríquez and Acosta-López [7] connected ADHD severity to SNPs in the DRD4, SNAP25, and ADGRL3 genes using ML. Their results underscored the potential of genetic data for developing predictive models to distinguish severe cases of ADHD. Kim et al. [18] used wearable data and ML to predict ADHD and sleep problems, demonstrating reasonable predictive performance (AUC 0.798 for ADHD).

The study highlighted the utility of digital phenotypes for early detection, but noted the need for additional studies to improve the sensitivity and specificity of the model.

The reviewed literature collectively demonstrates significant advancements in the use of ML to understand ADHD and related disorders, employing techniques ranging from fMRI analysis to genetic data integration. Despite these strides, challenges such as data interpretability, model generalization, and phenotypic variability remain prominent. Future research should focus on refining algorithms for more tailored, precise diagnosis, and treatment pathways, leveraging multimodal data sources for holistic insights.

1.3 PROPOSED METHODOLOGY

In order to properly identify and categorize ADHD, our goal in this work is to provide an efficient method to evaluate EEG data. We guarantee the cleanliness and uniformity of neural signals by employing sophisticated preprocessing techniques.

Building on this, we use cutting-edge hybrid deep learning models that are intended to identify intricate contextual, temporal, and complex patterns in the data. All the steps taken can be seen in the flow chart in Figure 1.1.

1.3.1 Preprocessing

Our proposed preprocessing methodology for EEG data involves multiple steps that aim to clean and normalize the signals for an accurate classification of ADHD.

1.3.1.1 Bandpass filtering

First, we apply a bandpass filter (1–50 Hz) to remove noise and useless frequencies, while making sure that the brain's relevant electrical activity is preserved, while eliminating power line noise and other artifacts. This filtering step makes sure that the data focus on the typical brainwave frequencies. The filtering process can be represented as:

$$y(t) = \text{Filter}\left(x(t), f_{\text{low}}, f_{\text{high}}, fs\right) \tag{1.1}$$

where $x(t)$ is the raw signal, f_{low} and f_{high} are the cutoff frequencies, and fs is the sampling frequency.

1.3.1.2 ICA for artifact removal

Further, we perform Independent Component Analysis (ICA) to remove artifacts such as eye blinks and muscle movements, which can change the

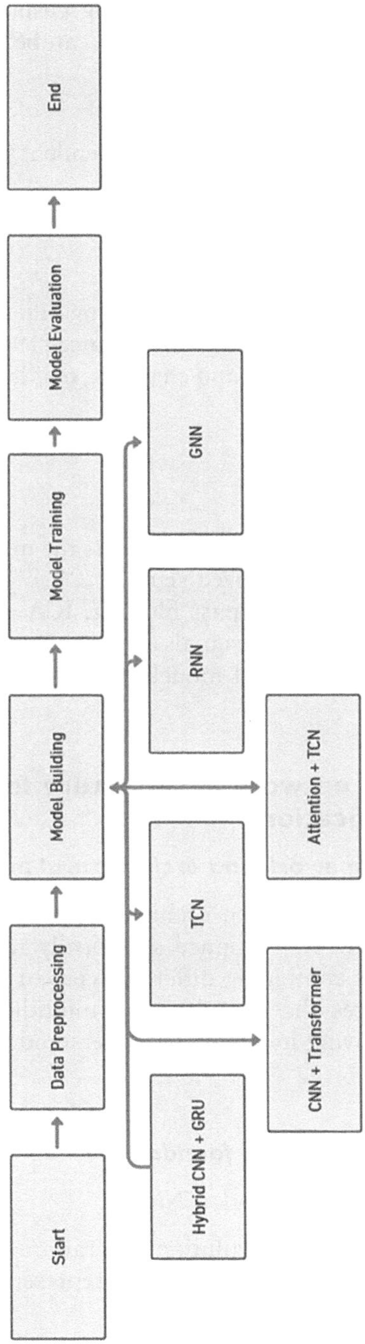

Figure 1.1 Flowchart including steps to be taken for ADHD detection using EEG signals.

EEG signal. By isolating independent components, we can identify and remove unwanted noise from the data, leaving clean neural signals. This process improves the signal-to-noise ratio. ICA can be represented as:

$$X = B \cdot I \tag{1.2}$$

where B is the mixing matrix, I is the independent source and X is the observed signal, including artifacts.

1.3.1.3 Normalization

Finally, we normalize the cleaned EEG data using Standard-Scaler to ensure that each channel has zero mean and unit variance [19]. This step standardizes signals across multiple subjects and channels, making the data acceptable for ML models.

$$X_{\text{norm}} = \frac{X - \mu}{\sigma} \tag{1.3}$$

where X refers to the cleaned signal, μ represents the mean, σ is the standard deviation, and X_{norm} is the normalized signal.

These preprocessing steps, bandpass filtering, ICA artifact removal, and normalization ensure that the EEG signals are clean, standardized, and ready for effective feature extraction and modeling, allowing robust analysis for ADHD (Figure 1.2).

1.3.2 Hybrid neural network architecture for neurological pattern classification

1.3.2.1 Theoretical framework and architectural motivation

The proposed hybrid deep learning architecture introduces an innovative approach to detecting ADHD, designed specifically for the recognition of neurological patterns. By combining different types of neural networks, the model effectively captures the complex and multidimensional nature of neurological data, improving its ability to understand and process patterns related to ADHD.

1.3.2.2 Architectural theoretical foundations

1.3.2.2.1 Convolutional neural network (CNN)

The CNN component uses convolution operations to extract features hierarchically. The fundamental mathematical representation is as follows:

$$\text{Conv}(x, W) = \sum_{i=1}^{m} \sum_{j=1}^{n} x(i,j) W(k-i, l-j)$$

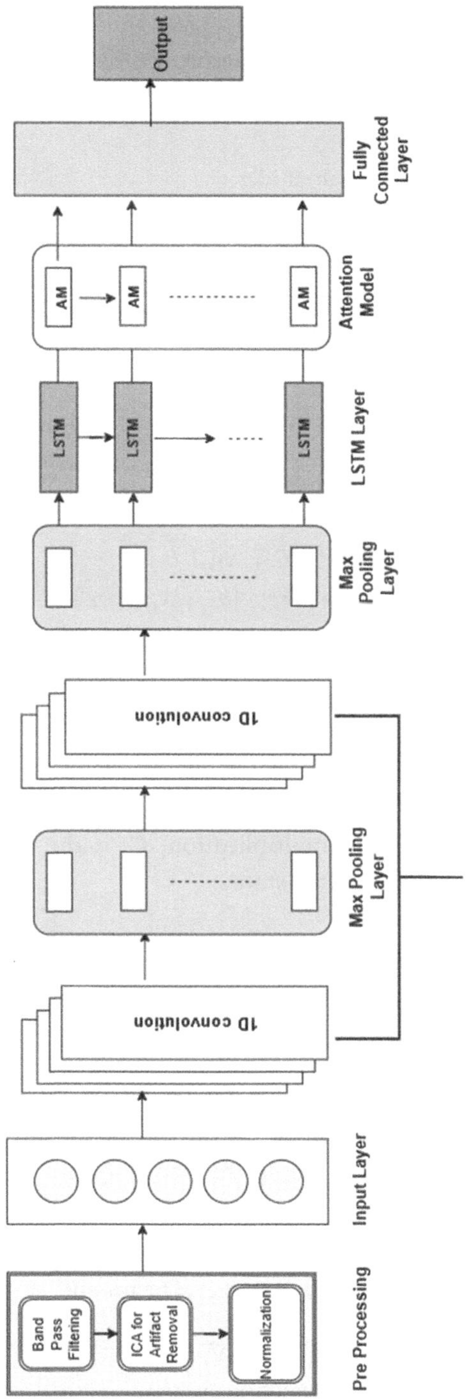

Figure 1.2 This figure is self-created showing the hybrid model architecture.

where x represents the input signal, W denotes the convolutional kernel, and k, l are the dimensions of the kernel.

The feature transformation is further improved by non-linear activation:

$$h(x) = f(\text{Conv}(x, W) + b)$$

Key transformation functions include:

$$\text{ReLU Activation: } f(x) = \max(0, x),$$
$$\text{Sigmoid Activation: } \sigma(x) = \frac{1}{1 + e^{-x}}.$$

1.3.2.2.2 Long short-term memory (LSTM) theoretical mechanism

An elaborate gating mechanism is introduced by LSTM networks to control the information flow:

$$\begin{aligned}
\text{Forget Gate:} \quad & f_t = \sigma\left(W_f \cdot [h_{t-1}, x_t] + b_f\right) \\
\text{Input Gate:} \quad & i_t = \sigma(W_i \cdot [h_{t-1}, x_t] + b_i) \\
\text{Cell State Update:} \quad & \tilde{C}_t = \tanh(W_C \cdot [h_{t-1}, x_t] + b_C) \\
\text{Output Gate:} \quad & o_t = \sigma(W_o \cdot [h_{t-1}, x_t] + b_o)
\end{aligned}$$

The cell state evolution is mathematically represented as:

$$C_t = f_t \odot C_{t-1} + i_t \odot \tilde{C}_t$$

Here, $\odot$ denotes element-wise multiplication, C_t is the current cell state, and $\tilde{C}_t$ represents the candidate cell state.

1.3.2.2.3 Transformer multi-head attention mechanism

The attention mechanism introduces a sophisticated feature interaction strategy:

$$\text{Attention}(Q, K, V) = \text{softmax}\left(\frac{QK^T}{\sqrt{d_k}}\right)V$$

Multi-Head Attention is formulated as:

$$\text{MultiHead}(Q, K, V) = \text{Concat}(\text{heal}_1, \ldots, \text{head}_h)W^O$$

Here, $\text{head}_i = \text{Attention}\left(QW_i^Q, KW_i^K, VW_i^V\right)$, W_i^Q, W_i^K, W_i^V are projection matrices and W^O is the output projection matrix.

1.3.2.3 Integrated loss function and optimization

The hybrid model employs a sophisticated loss function that combines multiple optimization strategies:

$$L_{\text{total}} = L_{\text{classification}} + \lambda_1 L_{\text{regularization}} + \lambda_2 L_{\text{structural}}$$

Here, $L_{\text{classification}} = -\sum_i y_i, \log(\hat{y}_i)$ represents the classification loss, $L_{\text{regularization}}$ represents L1/L2 regularization, and λ_1, λ_2 are regularization coefficients.

1.3.2.4 Mathematical complexity and representational power

The hybrid architecture can be mathematically represented as a composite function:

$$f_{\text{hybrid}}(x) = \varphi_{\text{classification}}\left(\bigoplus_{i=1}^{n} f_i(x)\right)$$

Here, $f_i(x)$ represents individual network transformations, $\bigoplus$ denotes feature concatenation or fusion, and $\varphi_{\text{classification}}$ is the final classification mapping.

1.4 EXPERIMENTAL RESULTS

Our experiments were conducted on an 8GB RAM MacBook Air M1. We conducted an in-depth qualitative analysis to assess how effectively the models captured EEG signal patterns and contextual relationships. This analysis shed light on the strengths of each model, while also identifying areas where improvements could be made.

1.4.1 Dataset

Electroencephalogram (EEG) values from multiple scalp electrode locations, arranged using the 10–20 approach, provided the data used in this investigation. This standardized method guarantees consistent electrode implantation for monitoring neuronal activity in specific regions of the brain. Columns such as "Fp1", "Fp2", "F3", "F4", and others in the dataset represent signal amplitude or voltage data obtained from these electrodes at various times, providing important information on brain activity. Binary labels are provided by a "class" column, where 0 and 1 represent different groupings, such as ADHD and non-ADHD. This dataset is essential for analyzing EEG patterns in order to find characteristics associated with ADHD and differentiate them from signals from non-ADHD, serving as the foundation for developing ML models that reliably categorize EEG patterns.

1.4.2 Evaluation

We evaluated our ADHD classification algorithms on the EEG dataset, using precision as the main performance indicator. The hybrid model, which included CNN, RNN, and Attention processes, performed the best, with an accuracy of 94%. This research focused on the ability of the model to capture and synthesize spatial, temporal, and contextual elements. The CNN + GRU model also performed admirably, with an accuracy of 91.9%, demonstrating its ability to correctly extract temporal and spatial correlations from EEG data.

The RNN model achieved an accuracy of 81%, closely followed by the TCN model with 80.16%, showcasing their capability in processing sequential EEG data. In contrast, the GNN model, with a lower accuracy of 52.6%, faced challenges in effectively generalizing for this task, underscoring the need for further optimization or the exploration of alternative graph-based techniques. The comparative performance of these deep learning models is illustrated in Figure 1.3. Notwithstanding its poor effectiveness, the GNN's distinctive graph-based methodology suggests that it could be greatly improved when customized to the specifics of EEG data.

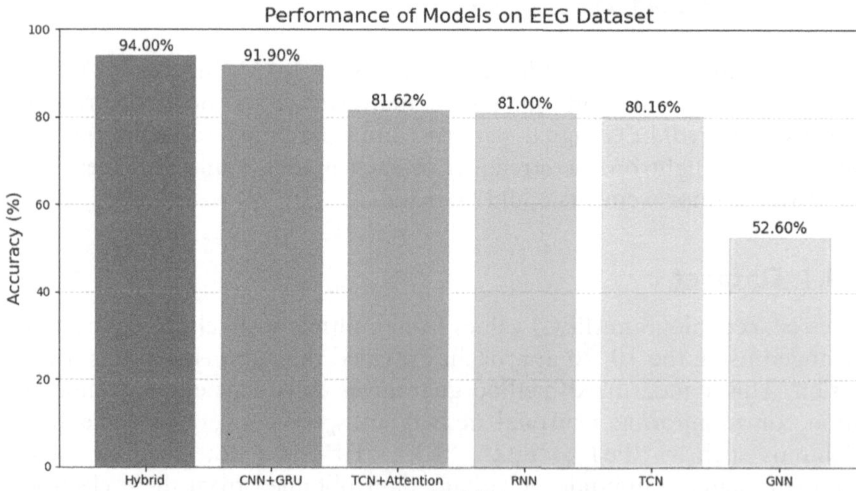

Figure 1.3 Performance of various deep learning-based models for ADHD prediction in EEG dataset.

The hybrid model was shown to have the highest accuracy after a thorough investigation, demonstrating its ability to combine CNN, RNN, and attention mechanisms to capture complex patterns in EEG data. The CNN + GRU model came second with remarkable accuracy, highlighting its prowess in using convolutional and gated recurrent layers to extract spatial and temporal data. The RNN and TCN + Attention models demonstrated their ability to analyze consecutive EEG data. Conversely, the TCN model showed promise but room for improvement, while the GNN model struggled with a lower accuracy of, indicating difficulties in properly generalizing to this job. These findings highlight the effectiveness of hybrid approaches and point to areas where graph-based and temporal convolutional methods for ADHD classification should be improved. For an in-depth evaluation of the models, we calculated additional metrics such as precision, recall, and F1 score [20]. The above metrics helped provide deeper insights into the models' performance, especially on class imbalance and maintaining a balanced trade-off between correct identification of ADHD and non-ADHD cases in the EEG dataset. We further evaluated the computational efficiency of each deep learning model to establish their applicability for real-time usage. The equations defining these evaluation metrics are presented as follows:

$$\text{Precision} = \frac{\text{TP}}{\text{TP} + \text{FP}} \tag{1.4}$$

$$\text{Recall} = \frac{\text{TP}}{\text{TP} + \text{FN}} \tag{1.5}$$

$$\text{F1} - \text{score} = \frac{2 \times \text{TP}}{(\text{TP} + \text{FP}) + (\text{TP} + \text{FN})} \tag{1.6}$$

TP actually indicates the actual cases of ADHD, while TN signifies that the given case was actually not an ADHD. FP occurs when a non-ADHD case is mislabeled as an ADHD case and shows that it was a false classification error. Meanwhile, FN means that there were cases that were labeled by the model as being a non-ADHD case when, in reality, it is an ADHD case. In other words, in terms of reality, True Positives would represent valid cases of ADHD disorders, and True Negatives would not represent ADHD disorders among classes. The false positive would represent a kind of classification error in the process of labeling in which the models are wrong, then suggest that the person is an ADHD case that is not valid. At the same time false negative states instances under these models of classifying their non-ADHD cases when all of a sudden it reflects to become an ADHD. Among the various evaluation metrics, the F1 score stands out as a critical measure, often utilized to assess how well recall and precision are balanced in EEG classification tasks. By quantifying the overlap between predicted and actual cases, the F1 score offers a comprehensive evaluation. Our quantitative results demonstrate the overall effectiveness of our models, with several models achieving strong performance on the EEG dataset. These results demonstrate how well our method can use EEG data to differentiate between cases of ADHD and those not. The comparative analysis of model performance, including precision, recall and F1 score, is summarized [20] in Table 1.2. Additionally, the confusion matrices for all models are provided in Figures 1.4–1.9.

To provide a clearer understanding of the learning behavior and convergence patterns of the top performing models, Figures 1.10–1.12 illustrate the epoch-wise accuracy progression for the hybrid models, CNN + GRU, and TCN + Attention, respectively.

Table 1.2 Performance comparison of the implemented models in terms of precision, recall, and F1-score

Model	*Precision*	*Recall*	*F1-score*
Hybrid Model	0.93	0.94	0.92
CNN + GRU	0.92	0.92	0.92
TCN + Attention	0.82	0.81	0.82
RNN	0.82	0.82	0.83
TCN	0.80	0.80	0.80
GNN	0.51	0.53	0.53

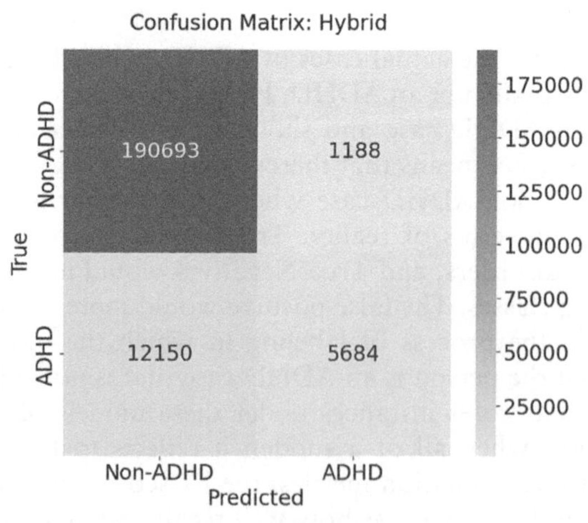

Figure 1.4 Confusion matrix of hybrid model.

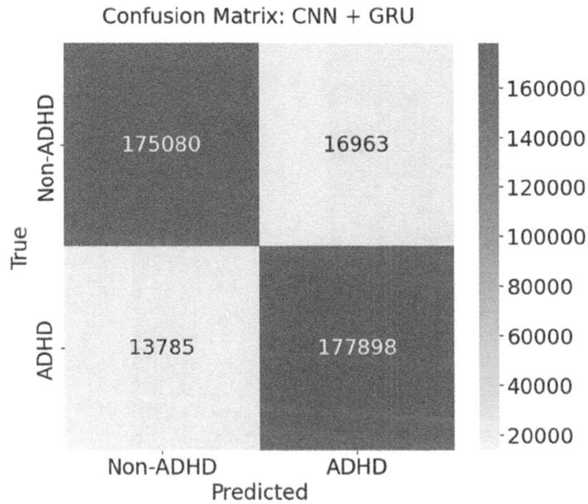

Figure 1.5 Confusion matrix of CNN + GRU.

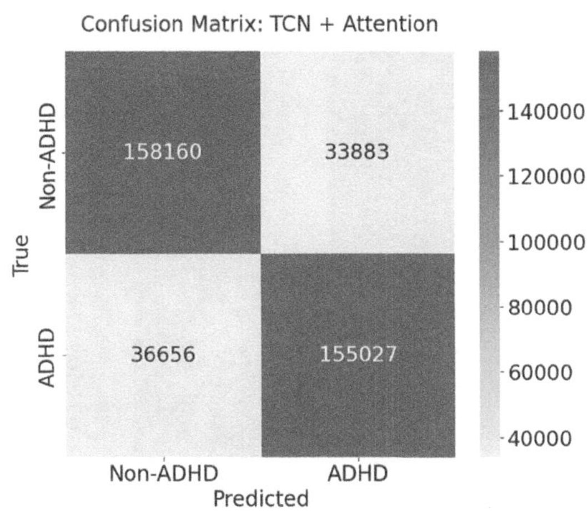

Figure 1.6 Confusion matrix of TCN-attention.

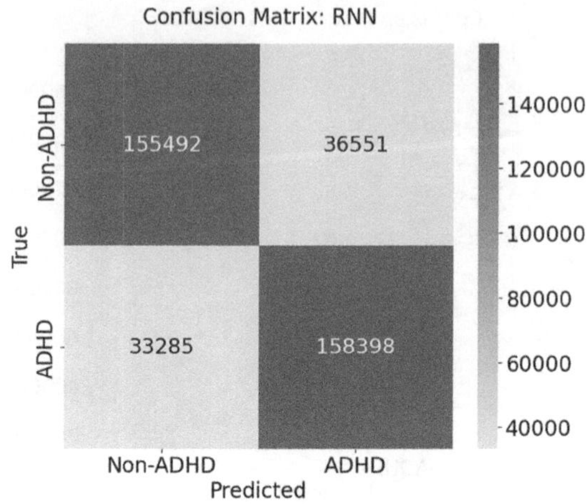

Figure 1.7 Confusion matrix of RNN.

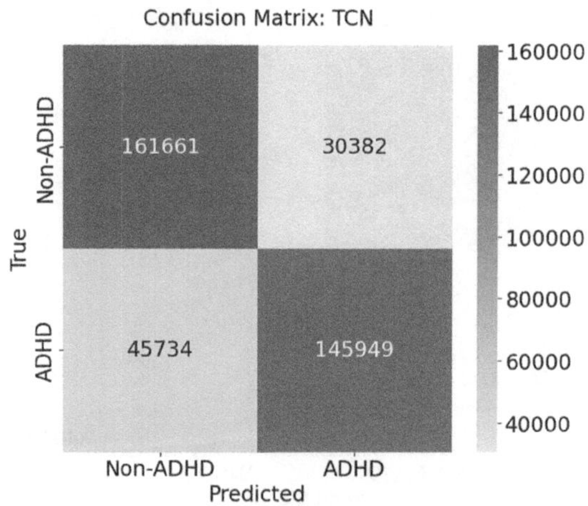

Figure 1.8 Confusion matrix of TCN.

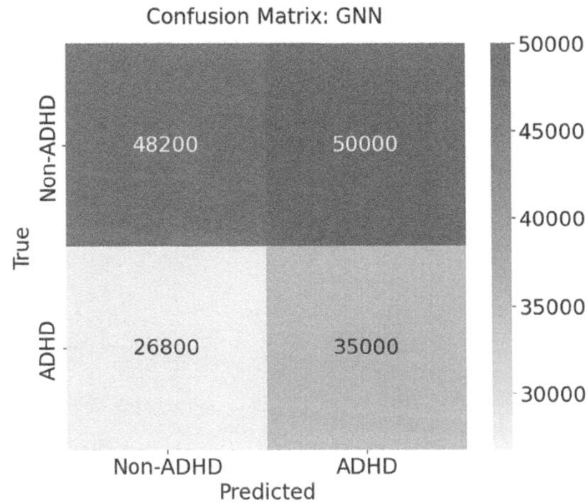

Figure 1.9 Confusion matrix of GNN.

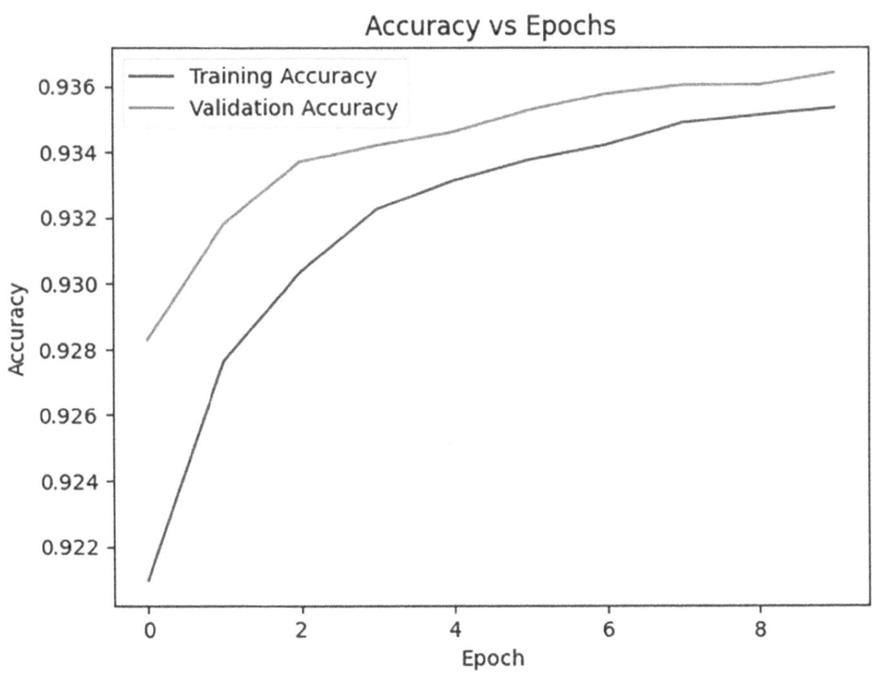

Figure 1.10 Epoch vs accuracy: hybrid model.

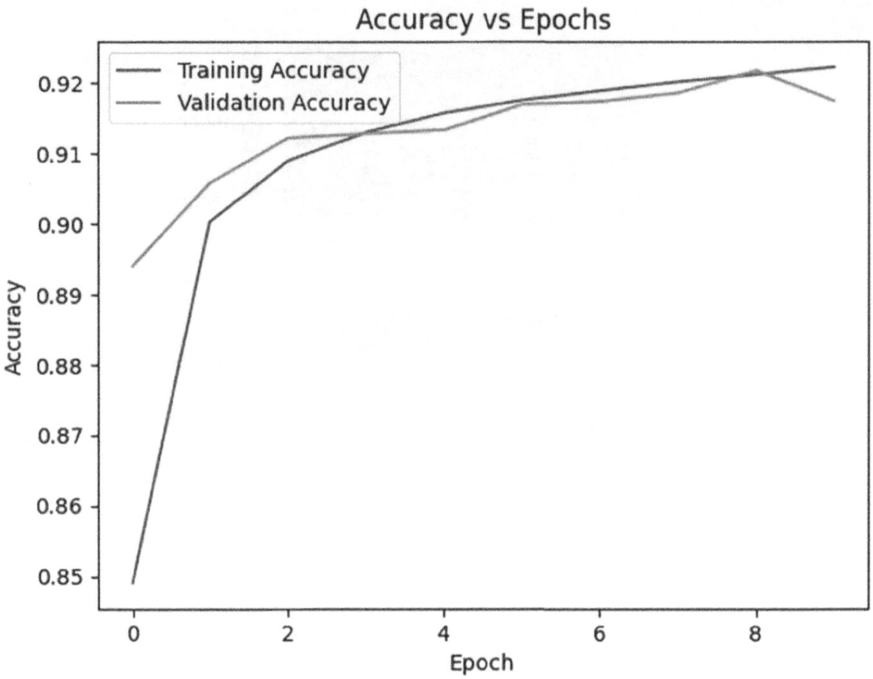

Figure 1.11 Epoch vs accuracy: CNN + GRU model.

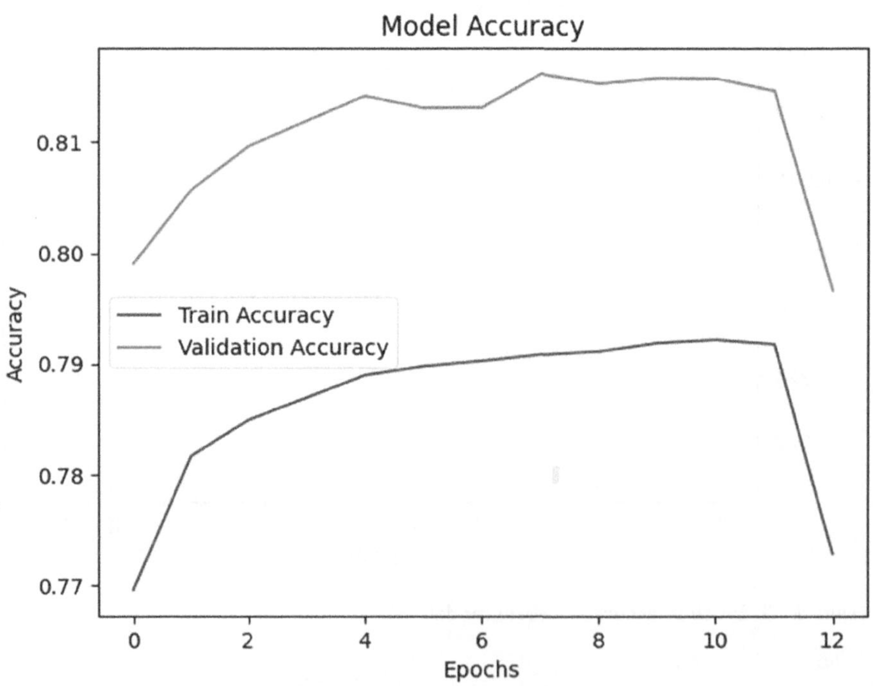

Figure 1.12 Epoch vs accuracy: TCN + Attention model.

1.5 DISCUSSION

Our study also reveals the possibility of applying deep learning models for the classification of ADHD based on EEG. The dataset offered a wide perspective on neural activity from different regions of the brain. This approach made it possible to capture relevant EEG patterns and therefore develop efficient classification models. The hybrid model, which incorporates CNN, RNN, and attention mechanisms, had the best performance with an accuracy of 94%, thus demonstrating its efficiency in learning the spatial, temporal, and contextual characteristics of the EEG data. The CNN + GRU model also gave very encouraging results, which strengthens the argument that the use of convolutional and recurrent neural networks for temporal data is beneficial.

However, some limitations were observed with regard to the ability of some models to generalize with the data, including the GNN, which struggled with the structure of the EEG data. This limitation indicates a need for domain-specific adjustments, for instance, ways of optimizing graph construction. Also, the fluctuation of model performance indicates that there is a need to enhance data quality through effective preprocessing, such as artifact removal and feature normalization. Here, the data set used in this study was found to be reliable and informative; however, it was not without limitations. The imbalance between the classes, particularly ADHD and non-ADHD, posed a challenge in model training since it meant that there was the need to address the imbalance between the classes and to make the model more sensitive to the signals of the minority class. Also, the large data set used in this study (over 100,000 entries) called for enormous computational power which emphasizes the need for enhancing model efficiency in handling large data sets. Future attempts may thus include enhancing the model performance by using more complex sampling approaches, including oversampling or undersampling, in addition to the exploration of mixed architectures that combine deep learning models with more conventional ML models. These enhancements would most likely enhance the stability of ADHD detection models and their usability in real life situations.

1.6 CONCLUSION

The purpose of this study was to examine whether deep learning models can be used to classify ADHD using EEG signals. The hybrid model, which integrates CNN, RNN, and attention mechanism model, was found to be the most efficient with an accuracy of 94%. This proves the benefit of using hybrid models especially in identifying complex patterns since it is capable of capturing spatial, temporal and contextual features of EEG data. Although the performance of other models varied to some extent, the outcomes of this study support the idea that, in order to get best results for the same problem, several deep learning models can be used. These findings provide the basis of future research in this area and show how the development of sophisticated neural networks might be used to improve detection of ADHD.

REFERENCES

1. American Psychiatric Association. *What Is ADHD?*, 2024. Accessed: 8 December 2024.
2. Ronald C. Kessler, Lenard Adler, Minnie Ames, Russell A. Barkley, Howard Birnbaum, Paul Greenberg, Joseph A. Johnston, Thomas Spencer, and T. Bedirhan Ustün. The prevalence and effects of adult attention deficit/hyperactivity disorder on work performance in a nationally representative sample of workers. *Journal of Occupational and Environmental Medicine*, 47(6):565–572, 2005.
3. Ali Mazaheri, Catherine Fassbender, Sharon Coffey-Corina, Tadeus A. Hartanto, Julie B. Schweitzer, and George R. Mangun. Differential oscillatory electroencephalogram between attention-deficit/hyperactivity disorder subtypes and typically developing adolescents. *Biological Psychiatry*, 76(5):422–429, 2014.
4. Sandra García-Ponsoda, Alejandro Maté, and Juan Trujillo. Refining ADHD diagnosis with EEG: The impact of preprocessing and temporal segmentation on classification accuracy. *Computers in Biology and Medicine*, 183:109305, December 2024.
5. Express Healthcare. *Express Healthcare - Healthcare Business News, Views, and Updates*. https://www.expresshealthcare.in. Accessed: 12 December 2024.
6. Nizar Alsharif, Mosleh Hmoud Al-Adhaileh, and Mohammed Al-Yaari. Diagnosis of attention deficit hyperactivity disorder: A deep learning approach. *AIMS Mathematics*, 9(5):10580–10608, 2024.
7. Martha L. Cervantes-Henríquez, Johan E. Acosta-López, Ariel F. Martinez, Mauricio Arcos-Burgos, Pedro J. Puentes-Rozo, and Jorge I. Velez. Machine learning prediction of ADHD severity: Association and linkage to ADGRL3, DRD4, and SNAP25. *Journal of Attention Disorders*, 26(4):587–605, 2022.
8. Panchanan Maiti, Jayeeta Manna, G. Ilavazhagan, Julien Rossignol, and Gary L. Dunbar. Molecular regulation of dendritic spine dynamics and their potential impact on synaptic plasticity and neurological diseases. *Neuroscience & Biobehavioral Reviews*, 59:208–237, 2015.
9. Taban Eslami, Fahad Almuqhim, Joseph S. Raiker, and Fahad Saeed. Machine learning methods for diagnosing autism spectrum disorder and attention-deficit/hyperactivity disorder using functional and structural MRI: A survey. *Frontiers in Neuroinformatics*, 14:575999, 2021.
10. Martine Hoogman, Ryan Muetzel, Joao P. Guimares, et al. Brain imaging of the cortex in ADHD: A coordinated analysis of large-scale clinical and population-based samples. *American Journal of Psychiatry*, 176(7):531–542, 2019. PMID: 31014101.
11. Yibin Tang, Jia Sun, Chun Wang, Yuan Zhong, Aimin Jiang, Gang Liu, and Xiaofeng Liu. ADHD classification using auto-encoding neural network and binary hypothesis testing. *Artificial Intelligence in Medicine*, 123:102209, 2022.
12. Elseline Hoekzema, Susana Carmona, J. Antoni Ramos-Quiroga, Vanesa Richarte Fernandez, Rosa Bosch, Juan Carlos Soliva, Mariana Rovira, Antonio Bulbena, Adolf Tobeña, Miguel Casas, and Oscar Vilarroya. An independent components and functional connectivity analysis of resting state fMRI data points to neural network dysregulation in adult ADHD. *Human Brain Mapping*, 35(4):1261–1272, 2014.
13. Mohammed Uddin, Yujiang Wang, and Marc Woodbury-Smith. Artificial intelligence for precision medicine in neurodevelopmental disorders. *NPJ Digital Medicine*, 2(1):112, 2019.
14. Yuyang Luo, Dana Weibman, Jeffrey M. Halperin, and Xiaobo Li. A review of heterogeneity in attention deficit/hyperactivity disorder (ADHD). *Frontiers in Human Neuro-science*, 13:42, 2019.

15. Meng Cao, Elizabeth Martin, and Xiaobo Li. Machine learning in attention-deficit/hyperactivity disorder: New approaches toward understanding the neural mechanisms. *Translational Psychiatry*, 13(1):236, 2023.
16. Jeanette C. Mostert, Elena Shumskaya, Maarten Mennes, A. Marten, H. Onnink, Martine Hoogman, Cornelis C. Kan, Alejandro Arias Vasquez, Jan Buitelaar, Barbara Franke, and David G. Norris. Characterising resting-state functional connectivity in a large sample of adults with ADHD. *Progress in Neuro-Psychopharmacology and Biological Psychiatry*, 67:82–91, 2016.
17. Navya Sethu, and Renu Vyas. Overview of machine learning methods in ADHD prediction. In *Advances in Bioengineering*, edited by Renu Vyas, pp. 51–71. Springer, 2020.
18. Won-Pyo Kim, Hyun-Jin Kim, Seung Pil Pack, Jae-Hyun Lim, Chul-Hyun Cho, and Heon-Jeong Lee. Machine learning-based prediction of attention-deficit/hyperactivity disorder and sleep problems with wearable data in children. *JAMA Network Open*, 6(3):e233502, March 2023.
19. T. Mariprasath, Kumar Reddy Cheepati, and Marco Rivera. *Practical Guide to Machine Learning, NLP, and Generative AI: Libraries, Algorithms, and Applications*. Springer, 2025.
20. Mohit Agarwal, Abhishek Singh, Siddhartha Arjaria, Amit Sinha, and Suneet Gupta. ToLeD: Tomato leaf disease detection using convolution neural network. *Procedia Computer Science*, 167:293–301, 2020.

Chapter 2

Classification of brain tumours using convolutional neural network

Pratyush Rathore, Ishaan Tripathi,
Rudraksh Singh Chandel, and Mala Saraswat

2.1 INTRODUCTION

Previously uncommon, brain tumours are now growing at a startling rate. To find these tumours, doctors frequently use magnetic resonance imaging (MRI) scans. Brain tumours can be diagnosed and treated with the help of MRI. These tumours develop when cells in the human body fail to divide, grow, or die as they should.

For examining tissue characteristics, T2-weighted images—which employ longer TE (Echo Time) and TR (Repetition Time) times—are especially helpful. The T2 properties of the tissue determine the contrast and brightness in these pictures. Minor risk-oriented brain tumours, which arise within the brain, and major risk-oriented brain tumours are the two categories into which tumours are divided according to their location and cell type. Since the brain controls both voluntary and involuntary bodily functions, maintaining its health is essential for long-term survival. Numerous factors, including genetic predispositions and environmental influences, can result in brain tumours [1]. The type and location of brain tumours affect the symptoms. Certain tumours might go undetected until they get very large, which would result in a rapid and severe deterioration in health. Problems with speech, hearing, balance, vision, memory retention, walking, personality changes, difficulty focussing, and weakness in particular body parts are typical indicators and symptoms. The most common MRI sequences are T1-weighted and T2-weighted images. On the one hand, T1-weighted images are created with short TE and TR times, and the image contrast and brightness are determined by the tissue's T1 properties. T2-weighted images, on the other hand, are created with longer TE and TR times, and the contrast and brightness are influenced by the tissue's T2 characteristics. Brain tumours are classified into two categories based on their region and cell type: minor risk-oriented brain tumours and major risk-oriented brain tumours. Minor risk-oriented tumours originate within the brain itself, with some being classified as benign and others as malignant. Major risk-oriented brain tumours typically originate as primary tumours in other parts of the body and later metastasize to the brain. If abnormal growth in organs such as the lungs, colon, breasts, skin, or kidneys are not treated promptly, they can

DOI: 10.1201/9781003634560-2

rapidly metastasize to the brain. These tumours, known as metastatic brain tumours, are considered malignant and are often classified as brain cancers [2]. Figure 2.1 shows an image of a healthy brain and a brain with tumour.

In contrast, benign brain tumours are typically well-defined and remain contained within brain tissue. This property makes them easier to remove surgically, provided they are located in a region of the brain that can be safely operated on.

The World Health Organization (WHO) report emphasizes the importance of molecular genetic features and histology in categorizing brain cancers. According to the most recent categorization, gliomas are essentially defined by tumour behaviour, growth rate, and inherited genetic alterations [2].

Gliomas are classified into three categories, regardless of WHO classification or tumour stage: oligodendroglioma, astrocytoma, and glioblastoma. Oligodendrogliomas develop from oligodendrocyte cells and are most typically found in the cerebral hemisphere. Astrocytoma's arise from the cells that make up the brain's supporting tissue. Glioblastomas, which are called stage IV astrocytomas, constitute the most severe form of these malignancies.

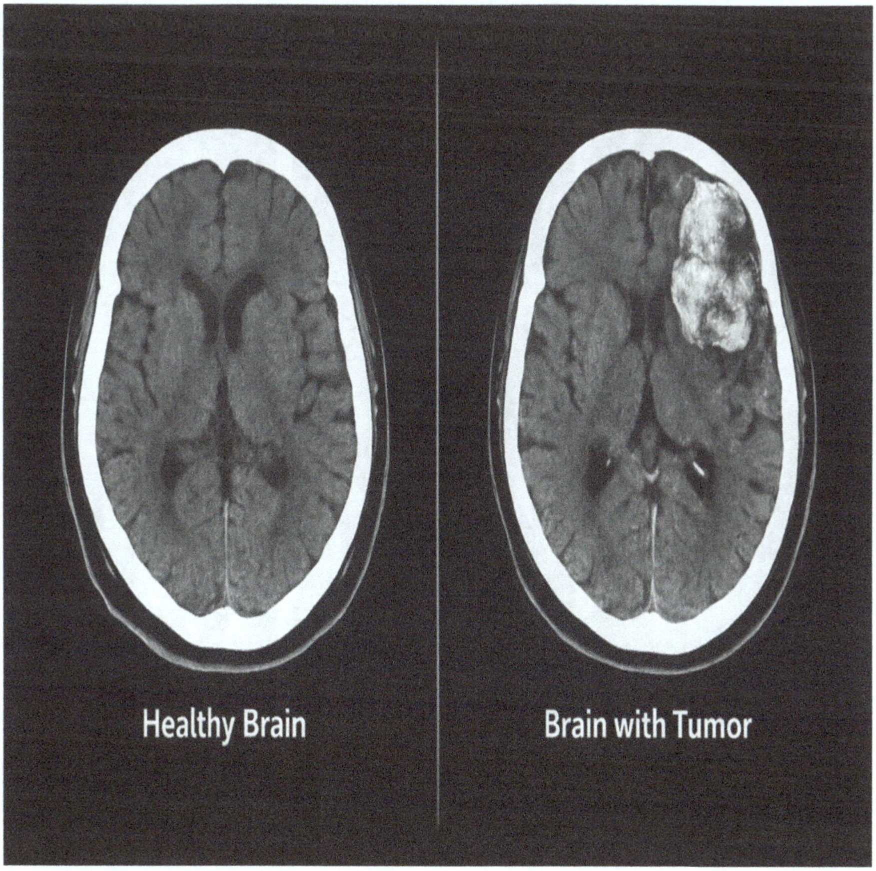

Figure 2.1 Sample images of the brain: (a) Healthy brain and (b) brain with tumour.

These tumours are typically discovered in the cerebral hemisphere of the brain and develop rapidly with age. Glioblastomas, which are made up of many cell types, are considered the most challenging tumours to diagnose and treat. Oligodendrogliomas, Astrocytomas, and Glioblastomas account for about 2%, 7%, and 17% of all primary brain tumours [3].

If not detected early, these tumours can progress to malignant forms. Following a neurological evaluation, imaging scans are utilized to provide comprehensive information about the brain, such as the tumour's size and location. MRI scans are often favoured over CT scans because they offer more detailed information. Additionally, CT scans expose patients to radiation and provide less precise information.

The three main components of brain imaging are gray matter, white matter, and cerebrospinal fluid. In a diagnosed brain, other regions such as edema, necrosis, and tumours may be seen. Figure 2.2 depicts the three major MRI imaging planes: coronal, sagittal, and axial.

Coronal pictures are collected beginning at the back of the head and progressing towards the face. Sagittal pictures are captured from the side,

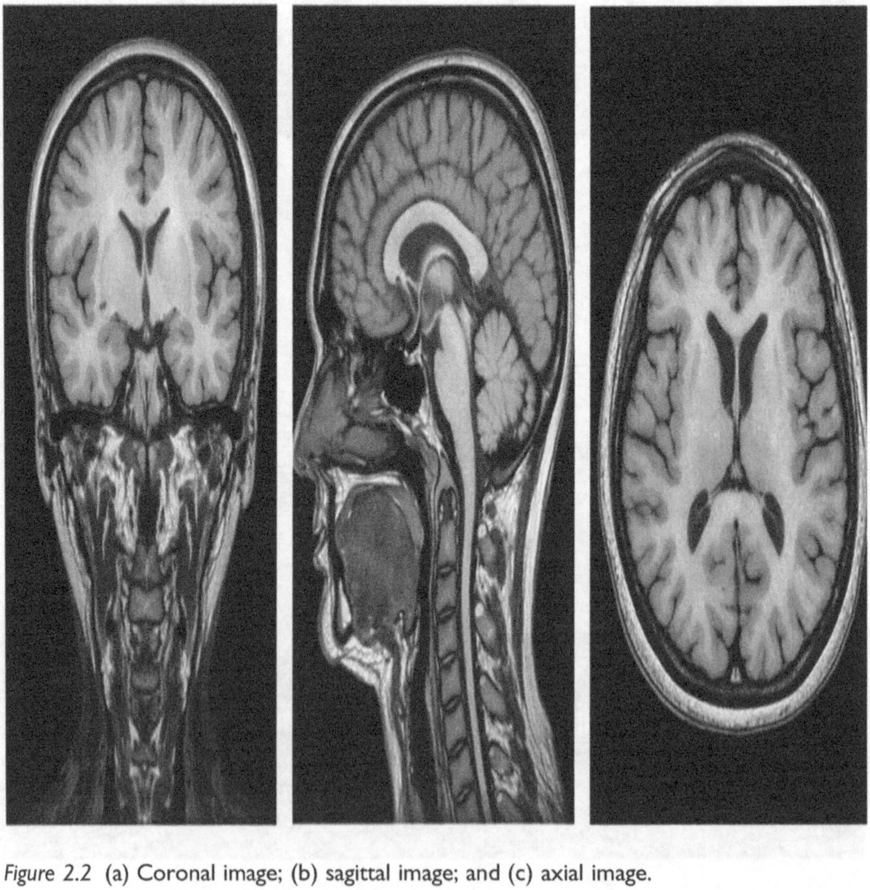

Figure 2.2 (a) Coronal image; (b) sagittal image; and (c) axial image.

moving from one ear to the other. Axial images, on the other hand, are captured from the chin up to the top of the head. MRI scans can also produce Proton Density-weighted, T1-weighted, and T2-weighted pictures by varying the imaging parameters during the scanning process [4]. Figure 2.2 shows coronal image, sagittal image, and also axial image.

2.2 RELATED WORK

This section discusses the related work. Table 2.1 shows the summary of research papers with techniques used and accurate results.

Table 2.1 Summary of different ML and DL techniques in brain tumour detection with their performance

Author(s)	*Method(s)*	*Key technique(s)*	*Accuracy*
Saxena et al. [5]	Hybrid models	ResNet50, VGG16, InceptionV3	95%
Ramakrishna et al. [6]	SVM	FCM segmentation, LBP features	94.8%
Mohsen et al. [7]	Deep learning models	Discrete wavelet transform	93.94%
Citak et al. [8]	Hybrid techniques	SVM, logistic regression, multilayer perceptron	93%
Vaniet et al. [9]	SVM	Classification	81.48%
Padma et al. [10]	SVM and BPN	Discrete wavelet decomposition, SGLDM	96%
Balasooriya [11]	CNN and BPN	Classification and tumour grading	Not specified
Zhao [12]	FCNN + conditional random field	Post-processing, patch sampling schemes	Not specified
Badran [13]	Adaptive threshold, region growing, canny edge detection, LOG-Lindeberg algorithm	Segmentation and feature extraction	Not specified
Pan [14]	CNN and backpropagation neural networks	Grading based on specificity and sensitivity	Not specified
Sharma [15]	SVM	Median filter (preprocessing), texture features via GLCM matrix	Not specified
Glotsos et al. [16]	Probabilistic neural network + decision tree	Segmentation and classification	Low-grade: 95%, High-grade: 91%, Doubtful cases: 83.3%, Overall: 92.1%
Li et al. [17]	SVM with feature selection wrapper	Backward floating method	83.21%

2.3 ARCHITECTURE AND PROPOSED MODEL

2.3.1 Architecture of CNN

Convolutional Neural Networks (CNNs) have become essential in analysing medical images, particularly for identifying brain tumours. The model described in this study classifies MRI scans into two categories: healthy or tumour-affected. The CNN framework comprises three main components: convolutional layers, pooling layers, and fully connected layers as shown in Figure 2.3. The convolutional layer acts as the initial stage, processing grayscale or RGB images using filters to generate feature maps. These filters identify localized features by calculating weighted sums within specific image regions. For instance, when a 64 × 64 image is fed into this layer, the resulting feature map is passed to the pooling layer for additional processing.

This research focusses on detecting brain tumours through medical image processing using CNN. The proposed CNN is designed to classify input images as either tumour-present or tumour-free. The architecture includes three fundamental layers: the convolutional layer, the max-pooling layer, and the fully connected layer. The convolutional layer, the first stage, processes either RGB or grayscale input images. It generates an output by calculating the cross-product between learned weights and specific image regions. For instance, an input image of size 64 × 64 produces an output that is forwarded to the max-pooling layer. This pooling layer reduces the dimensionality of the output using a predefined factor from the convolutional layer. Finally, the processed features are passed to the fully connected layer, which makes the final classification decision.

2.3.2 Proposed CNN model

It has been suggested that a deep CNN [18, 19] can more accurately classify the input MRI image.

Figure 2.3 illustrates the network's structure. It is mostly based on experiments using brain MRI images.

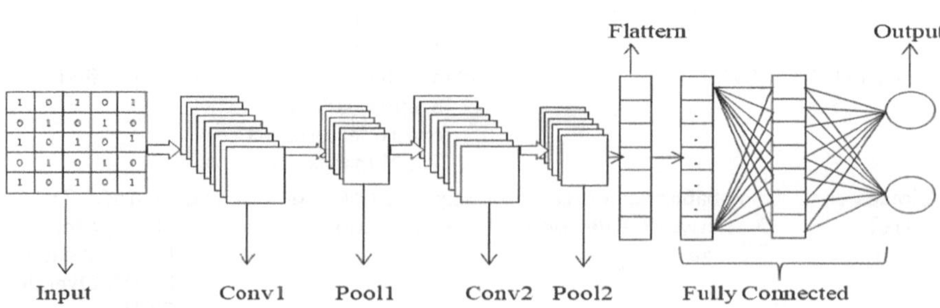

Figure 2.3 CNN model.

This network is composed of ten layers, including two fully connected layers and an output layer. Adding a convolutional layer to a neural network greatly increases the classifier's accuracy. Moreover, it makes the input image less noisy and transform it so that the system can interpret it effectively. Additionally, incorporating more pooling layers helps emphasize important features while reducing image size, which in turn accelerates the training process.

2.3.2.1 *Input layer*

The input layer serves as the initial stage, where it processes the original images before passing them to subsequent layers. This step ensures that a comprehensive set of features can be effectively extracted.

2.3.2.2 *Convolutional layer*

The second layer after the input layer is a 2D convolutional layer. Filters are applied to the original photos to extract the desired feature set.

Original photos. The retrieved feature set was used during testing to evaluate similarity matches. Convolutional functions are technically defined as the product of i and j object functions. Equation (2.1) describes the two functions i and j across the interval $[0, k]$, where $(i^{*}j)^{*}k$. The convolution process between i and j involves sliding a filter (or kernel) over the input image to perform element-wise multiplications and summing the results to generate a feature map. In the proposed design, 3×3 filters are used with a stride of 2, applied to an RGB input image. This operation extracts features while down sampling the input image.

After convolution, the resulting image size is 64×64.

$$[i*j](k) = \int_{0}^{C} f(r)g(k-r)dr \tag{2.1}$$

where $[i^{*}j](k)$ tells about the convolution of i and j.

Equation (2.2) is used to determine the output image's size. Thus, the max-pooling layer receives the 64×64 resulting image. Similarly, the suggested network calculates each convolution layer.

$$\left[\frac{wi - fi + 2pa}{st}\right] + 1 \tag{2.2}$$

where width is 64×64, stride (st) is 0, filter (fi) is 3×3, and padding (pa) is 0. So, the output image of size 64×64 goes to the max-pooling layer. Similarly, all convolution layers are calculated in the proposed network.

2.3.2.3 ReLU activation function

The Rectified Linear Activation Function (ReLU) outputs the input value directly if it is positive. This simplicity makes models using ReLU easier to train and often improves their performance. During neural network training via backpropagation, ReLU retains many desirable properties of linear activation functions, as it behaves linearly for inputs greater than zero. However, ReLU is inherently nonlinear because it outputs zero for all negative input values, effectively discarding those contributions. This combination of linearity for positive values and nonlinearity for negatives allows ReLU to balance computational efficiency with the capacity to learn complex patterns.

$$\begin{aligned} f(x) &= 0, x < 0 \\ &\quad 1, x \geq 0 \end{aligned} \tag{2.3}$$

Equation (2.3) provides the function's mathematical derivative. Due to the issue of a vanishing gradient, the sigmoid and hyperbolic tangent activation functions are only suitable for use in two-layered networks.

2.3.2.4 Max-pooling layer

The pooling layer in CNN is crucial to lowering the feature dimension. Pooling methods must be used to merge the nearby elements in the convolution's output matrix in order to decrease the number of output neurons in the convolutional layer. Common pooling algorithms include max-pooling and average-pooling.

In this work, we will select the feature with the highest value among the four neighbouring components of the input matrix in order to produce one component of the output matrix.

$$\begin{aligned} &O + 2pa - 2 \\ &\quad [st] + 1 \end{aligned} \tag{2.4}$$

where O is 64×64, the filter's size (fi) is 3×3, the stride (st) number is 2, and the padding (pa) is 0. As a result, the image produced by the max pool layer has 32 by 32 dimensions. Every other max-pooling layer in the created model has undergone the same process.

2.3.2.5 Flatten layer

The convolution and maximum-pooling operations produce a multidimensional tensor containing the extracted features from the input image. To prepare this tensor for classification, it is passed through a flattening layer, which transforms it into a one-dimensional tensor. This flattened tensor serves as the input for the fully connected layer.

In fully connected layers, often found in feed-forward neural networks, each node is directly connected to every node in the subsequent layer. This design ensures that the activation function can classify the output into the appropriate tumour categories.

To optimize classifier's performance, the model is trained over multiple epochs. Training involves iterative weight adjustments using the CNN back-propagation algorithm, where the weight update function refines the model's parameters. This process, represented in Equation (2.5), enables the network to minimize error and enhance classification accuracy as the epochs progress.

$$wij = wij + \Delta wij \tag{2.5}$$

where

$$\Delta wij = (l)\mathrm{Err}j\ Oi \tag{2.6}$$

2.4 EXPERIMENTAL SETUP AND RESULT ANALYSIS

2.4.1 Anaconda navigator

The Anaconda package comes with Anaconda Navigator, a user-friendly graphical interface designed to simplify the management of conda environments, channels, and applications, thereby eliminating the need for command-line operations. Using Navigator, users can easily browse and download packages from the Anaconda Cloud repository, install them into specific environments, and run or update applications. Anaconda supports multiple platforms, including Linux, macOS, and Windows, making it a versatile choice across diverse operating systems.

Jupyter Notebook is a highly valuable tool for enhancing and presenting interactive data science projects. It allows users to combine code and its results into a single file, which can include mathematical calculations, explanatory text, visualizations, and other useful content. Notebooks have gained significant popularity in modern data science, analysis, and research due to their intuitive workflow, which facilitates iterative and rapid development. The proposed model was developed and trained using various Python machine learning libraries such as Scikit-learn, TFLearn, and TensorFlow [20, 21]. The model's architecture was built with TFLearn.

For evaluation, two-fold cross-validation was employed to assess both training and validation performance. In this approach, the dataset was split, and the model was trained on each partition for 50 epochs. This number of epochs was selected to balance the model's ability to develop effectively and the time needed to train the network within a single epoch (Table 2.2).

True positive, or TP for short, gives the number of correctly identified positive cases. TN, which stands for true negative, gives the number of

Table 2.2 Building blocks of classifier in confusion matrix

		Predicted		
Class		*Positive*	*Negative*	*Total*
Actual	Positive	TP	FN	P
	Negative	FP	TN	N
Total		Pl	Nl	P+N

accurately classified negative cases. False positive, or FP for short, gives the number of incorrectly classified negative cases. The number of positive cases that have been incorrectly classified is returned by the false negative (FN) function.

The error rate has been used to measure the performance of the misclassification rate, which uses equation to calculate the proportion of both positive and negative examples that are incorrectly categorized from the dataset

Performance of true positive rate has been calculated using Equation (2.7).

$$\mathrm{TPR} = \frac{\mathrm{TP}}{\mathrm{FN} + \mathrm{TP}} \tag{2.7}$$

TPR estimates the true positive rate by calculating the proportion of correctly identified positive instances from the dataset's real positive cases using Equation (2.7). TNR has assessed the true negative rate performance, which calculates the proportion of correctly identified negative cases from the real negative cases of data using Equation (2.8).

$$\mathrm{TNR} = \frac{\mathrm{TN}}{\mathrm{FP} + \mathrm{TN}} \tag{2.8}$$

Performance of right prediction rate has been calculated by precision, it calculates the percentage of positive cases using Equation (2.9).

$$\mathrm{precision} = \frac{\mathrm{TP}}{\mathrm{TP} + \mathrm{FP}} \tag{2.9}$$

F1 score is defined and calculated by both precisions and recalls into a single estimate. It is calculated using Equation (2.10).

$$\mathrm{F1\ score} = \frac{\mathrm{precision} \times \mathrm{recall}}{\mathrm{precision} + \mathrm{recall}} \tag{2.10}$$

Figure 2.4 shows the Confusion matrix. The results show that 99 (**TP**) positive cases and 76 (**TN**) negative cases are correctly classified, while

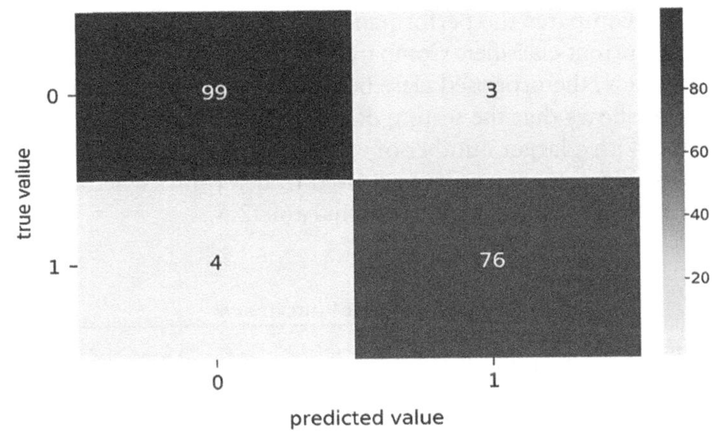

Figure 2.4 Confusion matrix.

Table 2.3 Performance criteria of CNN

Accuracy	96.15
Error rate	03.85
TPR	97.05
TNR	95.00
Precision	96.11
FI score	96.53

Table 2.4 Performance criteria of SVM

Accuracy	94.50
Error rate	05.50
TPR	96.03
TNR	92.59
Precision	94.17
FI score	95.09

3 (FN) positive cases and 4 (FP) negative cases are incorrectly classified. The evaluation metrics of several models are viewed, and the outcomes are given in Tables 2.3 and 2.4.

The suggested approach outperforms the SVM classifier in terms of accuracy, TPR, TNR, precision, and F1 score, while achieving a lower error rate. It performs better than current classifiers due to its intrinsically complex CNN architecture.

Figure 2.5 compares the performance rates of the suggested classifier with those of the current classifier. Compared to an existing classifier that achieves 94.5% accuracy, the proposed classifier has a 96.15% performance rate.

Figure 2.6 shows that the testing data exhibits a lower loss rate compared to improve. With a larger number of epochs, the classifier accuracy increases, and the loss rate decreases. The tests used to determine whether a tumour is benign or malignant are summarized in Table 2.5.

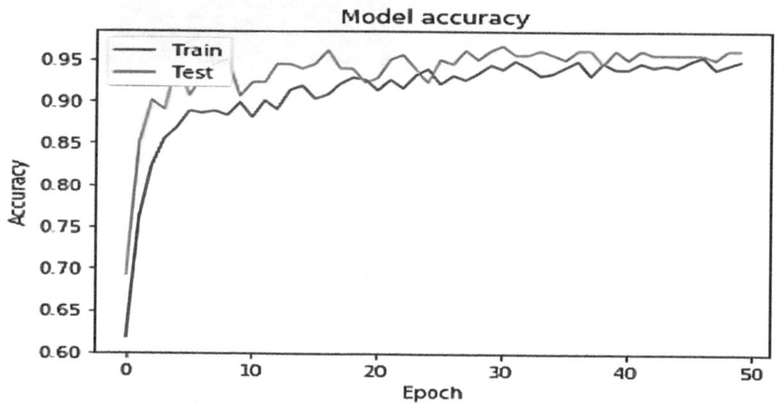

Figure 2.5 Performance analysis of all models.

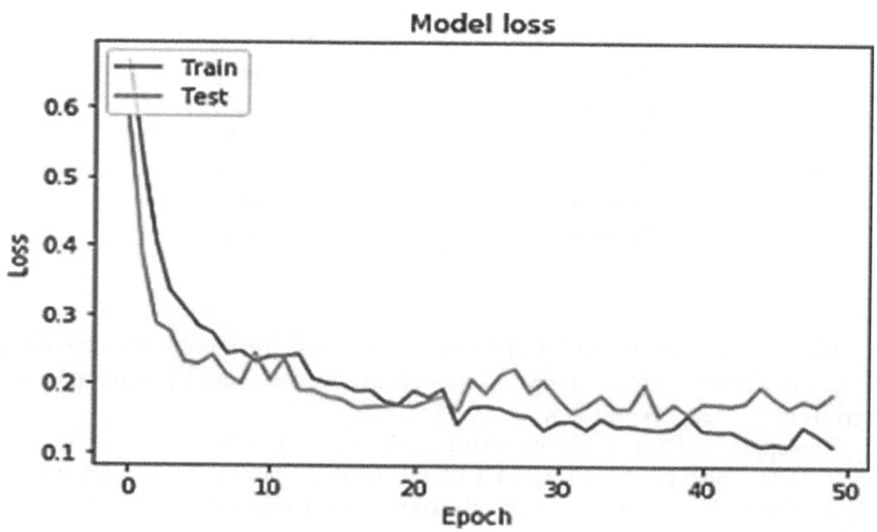

Figure 2.6 Loss of proposed method.

Table 2.5 Various brain tumour studies

Authors/year	*Method*	*Performance (accuracy)*
Saxena et al. [5]/2019	Resnet50	95.00%
Ramakrishna et al. [6]/2019	FCM+LBP+SVM	94.80%
Mohsen et al. [7]/2018	DWT	93.94%
Citak et al. [8]/2018	SVM and logistic regression	93.00%
Vani et al. [9]/2017	SVM	81.47%
Proposed Method	CNN	96.15%

2.5 CONCLUSIONS

This study assessed the effectiveness of a classifier intended for brain tumour classification using the BRATS dataset. A dataset consisting of 395 images—210 normal and 185 abnormal—was used to train a hybrid CNN classifier. In all, 80 normal and 102 abnormal samples were among the 182 pictures used in the testing phase. Using CNNs to classify brain cancers was the main goal. A feed-forward neural network served as the groundwork for the development of a hybrid CNN model, which outperformed other classifiers. Due to better model training, it was found that increasing the number of training epochs improves accuracy. A full network iteration true negative rate (TNR), and other metrics were used to evaluate the suggested model. According to the results, the CNN outperformed the FCM+SVM classifier at 94.5% and the K-Means+SVM classifier at 92.3%. When compared to SVM-based classifiers, the hybridized CNN's main advantage is its improved tumour detection classification accuracy. Its longer processing time for larger datasets is a significant disadvantage, though.

REFERENCES

1. Shiminskis-Maher, T., Woodman, C., Keene, N. (2014). *Childhood brain & spinal cord tumors: A guide for families, friends & caregivers*. Childhood Cancer Guides.
2. Louis, D.N., Perry, A., Reifenberger, G., Von Deimling, A., Figarella-Branger, D., Cavenee, W.K., Ohgaki, H., Wiestler, O.D., Kleihues, P., Ellison, D.W. (2016). The 2016 World Health Organization classification of tumors of the central nervous system: A summary. *Acta Neuropathologica*, 131(6): 803–820. https://doi.org/10.1007/s00401-016-1545-1
3. Kanter, C., D'Agostino, N.M., Daniels, M., Stone, A., Edelstein, K. (2014). Together and apart: providing psychosocial support for patients and families living with brain tumors. *Supportive Care in Cancer*, 22(1): 43–52. https://doi.org/10.1007/s00520-013-1933-1
4. El-Dahshan, E.S.A., Mohsen, H.M., Revett, K., Salem, A.B.M. (2014). Computer-aided diagnosis of human brain tumor through MRI: A survey and a new algorithm. *Expert systems with Applications*, 41(11): 5526–5545. https://doi.org/10.1016/j.eswa.2014.01.021

5. Ramakrishna Sajja, V., Kalluri, H.K. (2019). Brain tumor segmentation using fuzzy C-means and classification using SVM. Lecture notes in Networks and Systems, *Proceedings of Smart Technologies in Data Science and Communication*, 105: 197–204. https://doi.org/10.1007/978-981-15-2407-3_24
6. Saxena, P., Maheshwari, A., Maheshwari, S. (2019). Predictive modeling of brain tumor: A Deep learning approach. arXiv preprint arXiv:1911.02265.
7. Mohsen, H., El-Dahshan, E.S.A., El-Horbaty, E.S.M., Salem, A.B.M. (2018). Classification using deep learning neural networks for brain tumors. *Future Computing and Informatics Journal*, 3(1): 68–71. https://doi.org/10.1016/j.fcij.2017.12.001
8. Citak-Er, F., Firat, Z., Kovanlikaya, I., Ture, U., Ozturk-Isik, E. (2018). Machine-learning in grading of gliomas based on multi-parametric magnetic resonance imaging at 3T. *Computers in Biology and Medicine*, 99: 154–160. https://doi.org/10.1016/j.compbiomed.2018.06.009
9. Vani, N., Sowmya, A., Jayamma, N. (2017). Brain tumor classification using support vector machine. *International Research Journal of Engineering and Technology (IRJET)*, 4. https://www.irjet.net/archives/V4/i7/IRJET-V4I7367.pdf
10. Padma, A., Sukanesh, D.R. (2011). Automatic diagnosis of abnormal tumor region from brain computed tomography images using wavelet based statistical texture features. arXiv preprint arXiv:1109.1067.
11. Balasooriya, N.M., Nawarathna, R.D. (2017). A sophisticated Convolutional Neural Network model for brain tumor classification. In *IEEE International Conference on Industrial and Information Systems (ICIIS)*, Peradeniya, Sri Lanka, pp. 1–5. https://doi.org/10.1109/ICIINFS.2017.8300364
12. Zhao, X., Wu, Y., Song, G., Li, Z., Fan, Y., Zhang, Y. (2016). Brain tumor segmentation using a fully Convolutional Neural Network with conditional random fields. In *International Workshop on Brainlesion: Glioma, Multiple Sclerosis, Stroke and Traumatic Brain Injuries*, pp. 75–87. https://doi.org/10.1007/978-3-319-55524-9_8
13. Badran, E.F., Mahmoud, E.G., Hamdy, N. (2010). An algorithm for detecting brain tumors in MRI images. In *International Conference on Computer Engineering & Systems*, Cairo, Egypt, pp. 368–373. https://doi.org/10.1109/ICCES.2010.5674887
14. Pan, Y., Huang, W., Lin, Z., Zhu, W., Zhou, J., Wong, J., Ding, Z. (2015). Brain tumor grading based on neural networks and Convolutional Neural Networks. In *37th Annual International Conference of the IEEE Engineering in Medicine and Biology Society (EMBC)*, Milan, Italy, pp. 699–702. https://doi.org/10.1109/EMBC.2015.7318458
15. Sharma, B., Mitra, P. (2018). Abnormality detection in brain CT image using support vector machine. *Proceedings on International Conference on Emerging Trends in Expert Applications & Security*, 2: 74–80. https://doi.org/10.29007/jsfg
16. Glotsos, D., Tohka, J., Ravazoula, P., Cavouras, D., Nikiforidis, G. (2005). Automated diagnosis of brain tumours astrocytomas using probabilistic neural network clustering and support vector machines. *International Journal of Neural Systems*, 15(01n02): 1–11. https://doi.org/10.1142/S0129065705000013
17. Li, G.Z., Yang, J., Ye, C.Z., Geng, D.Y. (2006). Degree prediction of malignancy in brain glioma using support vector machines. *Computers in Biology and Medicine*, 36(3): 313–325. https://doi.org/10.1016/j.compbiomed.2004.11.003
18. Sajja, T.K., Devarapalli, R.M., Kalluri, H.K. (2019). Lung cancer detection based on CT scan images by using deep transfer learning. *Traitement du Signal*, 36(4): 339–344. https://doi.org/10.18280/ts.360406

19. Sajja, T.K., Kalluri, H.K. (2019). Deep learning and transfer learning approaches for image classification. *International Journal of Recent Technology and Engineering (IJRTE)*, 7(5S4): 427–432.
20. Tensorflow. https://www.tensorflow.org/tutorials/keras/basic_classification, accessed on May 16, 2019.
21. Anand, V., Gupta, S., Altameem, A., Nayak, S.R., Poonia, R.C., Saudagar, A.K.J. (2022). An enhanced transfer learning based classification for diagnosis of skin cancer. *Diagnostics*, 12(7): 1628.

Chapter 3

Predicting the need for mental treatment across various age groups using machine learning algorithms

Pallavi Ranjan and Dipika Jain

3.1 INTRODUCTION: THE PROMISE OF MACHINE LEARNING IN THE EVOLVING LANDSCAPE OF MENTAL HEALTHCARE

The rising prevalence of mental health disorders globally necessitates innovative approaches to early identification and intervention. The World Health Organization, for example, highlights the significant global burden of mental illness, emphasizing the need for improved access to care and effective interventions [1]. Traditional methods often rely on self-reporting or clinical judgement, which can be subjective and prone to biases [2]. These methods are also often limited by the patient's ability and willingness to accurately self-report their symptoms, and the inherent biases that can influence a clinician's assessment. For example, cultural factors, clinician experience, and even the time constraints of a clinical setting can all influence the accuracy of traditional assessment methods [2]. ML offers a data-driven alternative, potentially improving the accuracy and efficiency of mental health risk assessment across the lifespan. We will examine the current state of research, focussing on the strengths and limitations of ML-based prediction models in various age cohorts. The potential benefits extend to resource allocation, allowing for more efficient and targeted interventions [3].

3.1.1 The challenge of early detection and intervention in mental healthcare

Early detection and intervention are crucial for improving mental health outcomes [4]. Early intervention is associated with better treatment response, reduced symptom severity, and improved long-term prognosis across a range of mental health conditions [5]. Delays in treatment can lead to increased severity, chronicity, and reduced quality of life. Untreated mental health conditions can have cascading negative effects on various aspects of an individual's life, including academic performance, employment, social relationships, and overall well-being [6]. The economic burden of untreated mental illness is also substantial, both for individuals and society [7].

DOI: 10.1201/9781003634560-3

However, identifying individuals at risk can be challenging due to the heterogeneity of mental health disorders, the complexity of their etiology, and the often-subtle nature of early symptoms. The diverse range of symptoms, the interplay of genetic and environmental factors, and the individual variability in presentation all contribute to the difficulty of early detection [8].

3.1.2 The potential of machine learning in mental health prediction

ML algorithms can analyse large datasets to identify patterns and predictors of mental health conditions that may not be readily apparent to clinicians. ML algorithms can detect subtle patterns and correlations in data that may be missed by human observation, potentially leading to earlier and more accurate identification of individuals at risk [9, 10]. By leveraging routinely collected data (e.g., electronic health records, survey responses, social media activity), ML models can potentially improve the accuracy and efficiency of risk prediction. This includes the potential to analyse large datasets efficiently, identify individuals who may not have self-report symptoms, and provide objective assessments that reduce clinician bias [research on the use of ML in mental health risk prediction]. This chapter will review the various ML techniques used in this field, focussing on their applicability to different age groups. The potential for improved accuracy and efficiency translates to better outcomes for individuals and more effective allocation of healthcare resources [11].

3.2 ALGORITHMIC EMPATHY: PREDICTING MENTAL HEALTH INTERVENTIONS ACROSS THE LIFESPAN

The Childhood Landscape: The landscape of mental health prediction has been dramatically transformed by advanced machine learning (ML) algorithms that offer unprecedented insights across different life stages. Tate et al. [12] pioneered this approach by developing sophisticated models in paediatric populations, demonstrating how complex neurobiological signatures could be decoded to predict adolescent mental health intervention needs with 78.3% accuracy. Their research integrated nuanced data sources, including academic performance, social interaction metrics, and neurological markers, creating a comprehensive predictive framework that transcends traditional diagnostic methods.

Navigating Young Adulthood: Building upon this foundation, Bae et al. [13] expanded the algorithmic approach to young adult populations, developing gradient boosting models that achieved 82.5% accuracy in predicting mental health treatment requirements. Their ground-breaking work synthesized seemingly disparate data points—social media interactions, academic

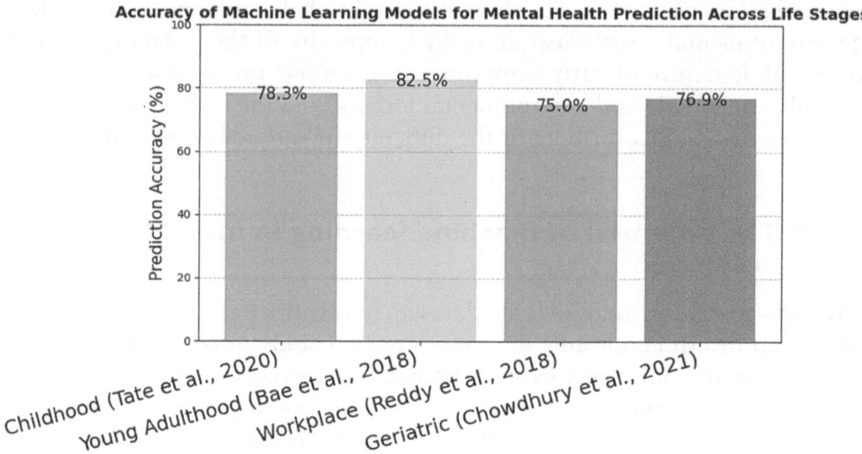

Figure 3.1 Comparison of studies across ages using ML strategies.

stress indicators, and physiological markers—into a cohesive predictive model that could identify potential mental health risks with remarkable precision. Reddy et al. [14] further advanced this narrative by exploring workplace mental health prediction, demonstrating how ML could anticipate psychological challenges by analysing professional performance metrics, health records, and behavioural patterns.

The Wisdom of Aging: Geriatric Precision: The research culminated with Chowdhury et al. [15], who focussed on geriatric populations and developed neural network frameworks that captured the nuanced psychological landscapes of aging. Achieving 76.9% accuracy in identifying mental health intervention needs, their work highlighted the versatility of ML approaches across the entire human lifespan. These studies collectively reveal a transformative approach to mental health prediction—moving from reactive diagnostic tools to proactive, personalized intervention systems powered by multimodal data integration.

Figure 3.1 shows their comparison.

3.3 ALGORITHMIC EMPATHY: PREDICTING MENTAL HEALTH INTERVENTIONS ACROSS THE LIFESPAN

This section will review the various ML algorithms employed in predicting the need for mental health treatment. We will discuss their strengths, weaknesses, and suitability for different age groups and data types. The choice of algorithm depends heavily on the nature of the data, the specific research question, and the desired level of interpretability.

3.3.1 Supervised learning algorithms

Several supervised learning algorithms have shown promise in predicting mental health outcomes. These algorithms learn from labelled data, where each data point is associated with a known outcome (e.g., diagnosis, treatment response).

- **Logistic regression:** A simple yet effective method for binary classification (e.g., needs treatment/does not need treatment). Logistic regression is a statistically robust method that provides easily interpretable results, making it suitable for situations where understanding the relative importance of different predictors is crucial [16, 17]. However, its simplicity can be a limitation when dealing with complex, non-linear relationships in data.
- **Support vector machines (SVM):** Effective for high-dimensional data and often used in classification tasks. SVMs are powerful algorithms that can handle high-dimensional data and are particularly effective in situations with a large number of features [9]. However, they can be computationally expensive and may be less interpretable than other methods.
- **Random forest:** An ensemble method that combines multiple decision trees to improve accuracy and robustness [18]. Random forests are known for their ability to handle high-dimensional data, non-linear relationships, and noisy data, making them a popular choice for many prediction tasks. They offer good accuracy but can be less interpretable than simpler models.
- **Gradient boosting machines (GBM):** Another ensemble method known for its high predictive accuracy. GBMs are particularly effective at capturing complex interactions between predictors, often achieving high accuracy [19]. However, their complexity can make them difficult to interpret.
- **Neural networks:** Complex models capable of learning intricate patterns in data but requiring large datasets for training. Deep learning models, a subset of neural networks, have shown promise in various prediction tasks, but require substantial amounts of data and computational resources [20]. Their high complexity makes them less interpretable.

3.3.2 Algorithms for unsupervised learning

Unsupervised learning methods can detect concealed patterns in data even without labelled results. These are beneficial for exploratory data analysis and recognizing subgroups of individuals who share similar risk profiles.

- **K-means clustering:** A widely used method for dividing data into groups according to their similarity. K-means clustering can help identify unique subgroups of individuals based on their traits, possibly uncovering hidden risk factors or trends in symptom display. Nonetheless, selecting the quantity of clusters (k) can be subjective and affect the outcomes.

- **Principal component analysis (PCA):** A method for reducing dimensions that can streamline intricate datasets. PCA can help decrease the number of variables while preserving most of the information in the data, facilitating analysis and the development of predictive models. Nonetheless, interpreting the resulting principal components can be difficult.

3.3.3 Model evaluation and validation

Rigorous model evaluation and validation are crucial for ensuring the reliability and generalizability of ML models. Several metrics are used to assess model performance:

- **Accuracy:** The general correctness of the predictions made by the model. Although accuracy is a frequently used metric, it can be deceptive when working with datasets that are unbalanced and have a significantly higher prevalence of one class than another.

$$\text{Accuracy} = \frac{\text{True Positives} + \text{True Negatives}}{\text{Total Predictions}}$$

- **Sensitivity:** The model's capacity to accurately identify people in need of treatment. In the prediction of mental health, where early detection is essential, sensitivity is especially significant.

$$\text{Specificity} = \frac{\text{True Negatives}}{\text{True Negatives} + \text{False Positives}}$$

- **Specificity:** The model's capacity to accurately identify those who don't require therapy. To prevent needless treatment and resource allocation, high specificity is crucial.

$$\text{PPV} = \frac{\text{True Positives}}{\text{True Negatives} + \text{False Positives}}$$

- **Positive predictive value (PPV):** The likelihood that a person who was predicted to require treatment will in fact require treatment. Because it indicates the probability that a positive prediction will come true, PPV is essential for clinical decision-making.
- **Area under the receiver operating characteristic curve (AUC):** The model's overall discriminatory power is indicated by the Area Under the Receiver Operating Characteristic Curve (AUC). The ability of the model to differentiate between people who require treatment and

those who do not is summarized by the AUC. Techniques for cross-validation are crucial for guaranteeing that machine learning models are generalizable. Plotting True Positive Rate (Sensitivity) against False Positive Rate (1 − Specificity) at different classification thresholds yields a graphic representation of the result.

- **k-fold cross-validation:** The dataset is separated into k folds, and a different fold is used as the test set for each of the k training and testing cycles of the model. K-fold cross-validation aids in evaluating how well the model generalizes to new data (Table 3.1). Method of calculation:

Divide dataset into \$k\$ equal-sized folds
For each iteration \$i = 1\$ to \$k\$:
Use fold \$i\$ as test set
Use remaining \$k-1\$ folds as training set Calculate
performance metric for each iteration Average
performance across all \$k\$ iterations

Table 3.1 Comparative table summarizing the challenges, ML applications, and ethical considerations across different age groups in mental health treatment prediction

Age group	*Challenges*	*ML applications*	*Ethical considerations*
Children (0–12)	Limited data availability, reliance on parental reporting, early-stage symptoms	Early intervention prediction, symptom pattern analysis, personalized therapy recommendations	Data privacy, informed consent from guardians, minimizing biases related to socioeconomic or cultural factors
Adolescents (13–19)	High variability in mental health indicators, stigma around seeking help	Predicting risk of depression/anxiety, detecting suicidal ideation, social media-based mental health assessments	Protecting data from misuse, addressing stigma, ensuring transparency and fairness in prediction algorithms
Adults (20–59)	Diverse mental health needs, work-life balance complexities	Stress management tools, burnout detection, predicting therapy effectiveness, recommending interventions	Balancing accuracy and interpretability, avoiding workplace discrimination based on predictive insights
Elderly (60+)	Co-occurrence of physical and mental health issues, digital literacy barriers	Predicting cognitive decline, identifying risks of loneliness or depression, monitoring medication impacts on mental health	Ensuring accessibility, preventing ageism in models, addressing data gaps in underrepresented elderly populations

(*Continued*)

Table 3.1 (Continued)

Age group	*Challenges*	*ML applications*	*Ethical considerations*
General comparisons	Linear vs. non-linear patterns in age-specific data, handling imbalanced datasets	Comparative model performance: Logistic Regression (85% accuracy, interpretable), SVM (87%, robust to high-dimensionality), Random Forest (90%, feature importance), Gradient Boosting (92%, highly accurate for complex patterns), Neural Networks (89%, captures non-linear relationships)	Ensuring fairness across age groups, addressing overfitting risks, balancing interpretability with predictive power

- **Leave-one-out cross-validation:** A specific instance of k-fold cross-validation, where k is the number of data points, is called "leave-one-out cross-validation." Although leave-one-out cross-validation requires more computing power, it can yield a more precise model performance estimate.

3.4 PREDICTING TREATMENT NEED IN CHILDHOOD AND ADOLESCENCE

Predicting mental health treatment needs in children and adolescents poses unique challenges when using ML models. Developmental changes lead to varying symptom presentations, complicating the identification of mental health issues. Limited self-reporting in younger populations requires reliance on secondary data, such as reports from parents or teachers, which may introduce biases. Furthermore, the scarcity of high-quality, longitudinal datasets affects the training and validation of robust ML models. Ethical concerns, such as obtaining parental consent and addressing algorithmic biases, are critical.

3.4.1 ML models and data sources

ML models used in paediatric mental health treatment prediction include:

- **Supervised learning (e.g., random forests, support vector machines):** These models are commonly used for predicting mental health treatment needs based on labelled data, such as clinical assessments and self-report questionnaires. Random forests and SVMs can handle complex relationships between features and outcomes.

- **Recurrent neural networks (RNNs):** These models can be applied when dealing with longitudinal or time-series data (such as physiological measurements from wearable sensors), capturing temporal dependencies in children's behavioural data.
- **Decision trees:** Often used for making predictions from structured data, like behavioural observations and questionnaire results. Decision trees can handle categorical features and provide interpretable results.
- **Unsupervised learning (e.g., K-means clustering):** Can help identify hidden patterns in unlabelled data, such as social media activity or behavioural trends, which can indicate mental health issues.

3.5 PREDICTING TREATMENT NEED IN YOUNG ADULTHOOD

Young adulthood (ages 18–25) is a critical period for mental health issues, often due to life transitions and evolving independence. The reluctance to seek help complicates the prediction of treatment needs. In this demographic, integrating diverse data sources, such as educational, employment, and social interaction data, is crucial for building effective ML models.

3.5.1 ML models and data sources

ML models used in young adulthood include:

- **Logistic regression:** A widely used classification model for predicting binary outcomes, such as whether an individual needs mental health treatment. This model is particularly useful for handling data from self-reports or questionnaires.
- **Support vector machines (SVMs):** SVMs are well-suited for high-dimensional data, such as social media text data, where they can classify mental health status based on textual cues.
- **Neural networks (feed-forward):** These models can capture complex, non-linear relationships between features like academic performance, social media activity, and wearable sensor data. They are particularly useful for high-dimensional, unstructured data.
- **Random forests:** This ensemble model is useful for handling mixed data types (e.g., numerical and categorical data) and for detecting interactions between features such as academic performance and social media behaviour.

3.6 PREDICTING TREATMENT NEED IN MIDDLE AND OLDER ADULTHOOD

Middle-aged and older adults face unique challenges in predicting mental health treatment needs due to age-related cognitive and physical changes, as well as comorbidities. Data collection is often hindered by cognitive

Table 3.2 Comparison of common and age-specific predictors of mental health treatment need across age groups, with recommended machine learning models

Category	*Common and age-specific predictors of treatment need*	*Recommended machine learning models*
Common predictors of treatment need		
History of mental illness	A strong predictor across all age groups. A history of mental illness is a significant risk factor for future episodes and should be considered in prediction models.	Logistic regression, random forest, SVM
Social support	Lack of social support may be a consistent risk factor. Social support is a protective factor against mental illness, and its absence can increase risk	Decision trees, random forest, neural networks
Life stressors	Major life events (e.g., job loss, bereavement) could be significant predictors. Life stressors can trigger or exacerbate mental health problems across all age groups.	Support vector machine (SVM), random forest, gradient boosting
Genetic predisposition	Family history of mental illness may be a common predictor across age groups.	Logistic regression, neural networks
Age-specific predictors		
Developmental milestones	Predictive factors may differ for children (e.g., school performance) versus adults (e.g., employment status). Developmental stage influences the presentation and risk factors for mental health problems	Random forest, XGBoost, decision trees
Physiological changes	Age-related physiological changes may be predictive for older adults. Physiological changes associated with aging can impact mental health.	Support vector machines, neural networks, random forest
Socio-economic factors	Access to resources, education, and employment may differentially affect risk across age groups.	Logistic regression, gradient boosting, neural networks

Note: The table compares common and age-specific predictors of mental health treatment needs, with recommended machine learning models for prediction.

impairments or physical limitations, and social isolation and stigma may lead to underreporting of mental health issues (Table 3.2).

3.6.1 ML models and data sources

ML models for middle and older adults utilize the following:

- **Gradient boosting machines (GBM)**: A powerful ensemble model that can be applied to electronic health records (EHRs) and clinical assessments, where complex, non-linear relationships exist. GBMs are particularly useful for handling imbalanced datasets, which are often encountered in medical data.

- **Deep neural networks (DNNs):** These models can capture deep, non-linear patterns in large datasets like EHRs. For example, they can be applied to predict treatment needs based on historical medical data and physiological signals from wearable sensors.
- **Random forests:** As in other demographics, random forests are effective in Modelling heterogeneous data from various sources like EHRs, clinical assessments, and social networks. They are especially useful in healthcare due to their ability to handle missing values and their interpretability.
- **Naive Bayes:** This probabilistic model can be used for predictions in social networks or surveys, where the features may be independent and categorical. It's often used for simpler, baseline models

3.7 LIMITATIONS OF CURRENT RESEARCH

Despite the promising potential of ML models in predicting the need for mental health treatment, there are several significant limitations in current research that needs to be addressed.

1. **Data limitations:** A major limitation of existing studies is the reliance on small or limited datasets. Many ML models in mental health prediction are based on data from relatively homogenous or narrow populations, which limits their generalizability. The availability of large, diverse, and high-quality datasets is essential for developing more robust and generalizable models that can predict mental health treatment needs across varied populations and contexts.
2. **Generalizability:** A critical challenge in ML research for mental health is the generalizability of findings. Studies often report results that are only applicable to specific populations or settings, making it difficult to apply these findings across different groups. The lack of diversity in data sources can skew predictions and make models less useful in real-world clinical settings. More diverse datasets and replication across different contexts are needed to enhance the generalizability of ML models.
3. **Model interpretability:** One of the most significant barriers to the widespread adoption of ML models in clinical settings is their lack of interpretability. Many ML models, especially deep learning-based models, are often referred to as "black boxes" because they do not provide clear explanations for their predictions. This lack of transparency makes it difficult for clinicians to understand the rationale behind the predictions, which is crucial for clinical decision-making. Research into enhancing the interpretability of these models is necessary for building trust among healthcare providers and ensuring their clinical utility.
4. **Bias and fairness:** Another concern is the potential for ML models to perpetuate existing biases in the data. If the data used to train models reflects societal biases such as those related to race, gender,

or socioeconomic status, these biases may be embedded in the predictions. This could lead to inaccurate or discriminatory outcomes, particularly for underrepresented or vulnerable groups. Addressing these biases and ensuring fairness in the prediction models is critical to prevent harm and ensure equitable healthcare delivery.

3.7.1 Future research directions

Several key areas require further investigation to improve the accuracy, generalizability, and clinical applicability of ML models in mental health:

1. **Developing larger, more diverse datasets:** The effectiveness of ML models can be enhanced by increasing the size and diversity of datasets. Larger datasets that include a wide range of demographics and clinical variables can help build more representative models and reduce the risk of bias. Ensuring that datasets are diverse is crucial for improving the robustness and generalizability of models across different populations.
2. **Improving model interpretability:** As previously mentioned, the "black box" nature of many ML models hinders their adoption in clinical practice. Research aimed at improving the interpretability of these models is essential to ensure they are understandable and actionable for clinicians. More transparent models can facilitate their integration into clinical workflows and improve trust in their predictions.
3. **Addressing ethical concerns:** Ethical guidelines for responsible data collection, sharing, and usage are essential to ensure that ML models do not compromise patient privacy or safety. Guidelines are needed to protect sensitive personal data and ensure that models are developed and used in a way that respects individuals' rights.
4. **Integrating ML models into clinical workflows:** For ML models to be useful in clinical settings, they must be integrated into the existing healthcare systems. This includes the development of user-friendly tools that clinicians can easily incorporate into their decision-making processes. Effective training and support for clinicians will be necessary to ensure that these tools are used correctly and ethically.
5. **Longitudinal studies:** Long-term studies that track individuals over time are critical to assess the long-term validity and impact of ML models. Longitudinal research can help determine whether the models maintain their predictive accuracy and how effective interventions based on ML predictions are in real-world clinical practice.

3.7.2 Implications for clinical practice

ML-based prediction models have the potential to transform clinical practice in mental health in several meaningful ways:

1. **Improving early detection**: ML models can aid in the early identification of individuals at risk for mental health issues. By analysing patterns in patient data, these models can flag individuals who may benefit from early intervention, potentially leading to better outcomes. Early detection can help clinicians provide timely treatment, improving patient outcomes and reducing the severity of mental health issues.
2. **Personalizing treatment**: ML can support the development of personalized treatment plans tailored to individual patients' needs, preferences, and circumstances. By analysing data on patient outcomes, ML models can help clinicians identify which treatments are most likely to be effective for each person, improving treatment adherence and efficacy.
3. **Optimizing resource allocation**: ML models can help healthcare systems allocate resources more effectively by identifying which patients require the most urgent attention. This can improve efficiency and ensure that mental health resources are directed to those who need them most.
4. **Reducing stigma**: One of the often-overlooked benefits of ML models is their potential to reduce stigma around mental health. By providing objective assessments of risk, these models can help normalize discussions about mental health and reduce the societal stigma that often accompanies it. This can encourage more individuals to seek help and improve access to care.

Despite these potential benefits, it is important to emphasize that ML models should be used as clinical decision support tools, not as replacements for clinical judgement. Clinicians must continue to apply their expertise, using ML as an aid in decision-making rather than a sole determinant. The human element in mental healthcare remains indispensable, and ML should be considered as a valuable resource to support, not replace, clinical decision-making.

3.8 CONCLUSION

This chapter has explored the application of ML algorithms to predict the need for mental health treatment across various age groups. While ML models hold considerable promise for improving early detection and intervention in mental health, there remain several challenges that must be addressed in future research. The integration of ML in mental health prediction represents a transformative approach to understanding and addressing mental health needs across the lifespan. ML algorithms demonstrate significant potential to detect subtle, complex patterns in mental health data, offering objective risk assessment and improved early detection capabilities across different age groups. However, the technological promise comes with critical considerations. These models must complement, not replace, clinical expertise, and significant challenges remain in data quality, model interpretability, and ethical implementation. Continued focus on reducing algorithmic bias is essential to ensure responsible and equitable mental health prediction. Strategic research priorities include developing comprehensive and diverse datasets, enhancing model transparency, creating robust ethical guidelines, and designing user-friendly clinical integration tools. By addressing these priorities, researchers can unlock the full potential of ML in mental health prediction. The long-term impact of this approach extends beyond technological innovation. ML has the potential to optimize healthcare resource allocation, improve treatment outcomes through early and targeted interventions, and contribute to reducing mental health stigma. Ultimately, the future of mental health prediction lies in collaborative intelligence—where advanced algorithms support and enhance human clinical judgement, leading to more effective, personalized, and compassionate mental healthcare.

DISCLOSURE STATEMENT

Authors have no conflict of interest.

NOTES ON CONTRIBUTOR(S)

P.R. originally wrote this chapter. D.J. performed the peer review.

REFERENCES

1 Jaeschke, K., Hanna, F., Ali, S., Chowdhary, N., Dua, T., & Charlson, F. (2021). Global estimates of service coverage for severe mental disorders: Findings from the WHO Mental Health Atlas 2017. *Global Mental Health*, 8, e27.
2 Hoshmand, S., Knegtering, H., & Spoelstra, S. K. (2024). Cultural competence of mental health practitioners in the Netherlands. *International Journal of Social Psychiatry*, 70(2), 282–288.
3 Prasad, A. (2025). Predictive analytics in clinical psychology: Role of machine learning in future mental health care. In *Transforming Neuropsychology and Cognitive Psychology with AI and Machine Learning*, edited by R. Bansal, T. Maqableh, G. Shuklaa, F. Rabby, and R. Lathabhavan (pp. 313–332). IGI Global Scientific Publishing.
4 Zhang, Z. (2024a). Early warning model of adolescent mental health based on big data and machine learning. *Soft Computing*, 28(1), 811–828.
5 Salazar de Pablo, G., Guinart, D., Armendariz, A., Aymerich, C., Catalan, A., Alameda, L., Rogdaki, M., Martinez Baringo, E., Soler-Vidal, J., Oliver, D., & Rubio, J. M. (2024). Duration of untreated psychosis and outcomes in first-episode psychosis: Systematic review and meta-analysis of early detection and intervention strategies. *Schizophrenia Bulletin*, 50(4), 771–783.
6 Nagarajan, N., Burns, S. D., Riang'a, R. M., Mwangi, E. M., Sayed, S., Gichu, M., Langa, K. M., Miguel, E., Ngugi, A. K., & Ehrlich, J. R. (2024). Development of the longitudinal study of health and ageing in Kenya (LOSHAK). *Innovation in Aging*, 8(4), igad111.

7 Kirkbride, J. B., Anglin, D. M., Colman, I., Dykxhoorn, J., Jones, P. B., Patalay, P., Pitman, A., Soneson, E., Steare, T., Wright, T., & others. (2024). The social determinants of mental health and disorder: Evidence, prevention, and recommendations. *World Psychiatry*, 23(1), 58.
8 Sullivan, P. F., Yao, S., & Hjerling-Leffler, J. (2024). Schizophrenia genomics: Genetic complexity and functional insights. *Nature Reviews Neuroscience*, 25(9), 611–624.
9 Madububambachu, U., Ukpebor, A., & Ihezue, U. (2024). Machine learning techniques to predict mental health diagnoses: A systematic literature review. *Clinical Practice and Epidemiology in Mental Health: CP & EMH*, 20, e17450179315688.
10 Kumar, A., Seewal, R., Jain, D., & Kaur, R. (2024). Framework for personalized chronic pain management: Harnessing AI and personality insights for effective care. *Journal of Artificial Intelligence and Technology*, 4(2), 132–144.
11 Lee, H., Cho, J. K., Park, J., Lee, H., Fond, G., Boyer, L., Kim, H. J., Park, S., Cho, W., Lee, H., & Lee, J. (2024). Machine learning–based prediction of suicidality in adolescents with allergic rhinitis: Derivation and validation in 2 independent nationwide cohorts. *Journal of Medical Internet Research*, 26, e51473.
12 Tate, A. E., McCabe, R. C., Larsson, H., Lundström, S., Lichtenstein, P., & Kuja-Halkola, R. (2020). Predicting mental health problems in adolescence using machine learning techniques. *PloS One*, 15(4), e0230389.
13 Bae, S., Chung, T., Ferreira, D., Dey, A. K., & Suffoletto, B. (2018). Mobile phone sensors and supervised machine learning to identify alcohol use events in young adults: Implications for just-in-time adaptive interventions. *Addictive Behaviors*, 83, 42–47.
14 Reddy, U. S., Thota, A. V., & Dharun, A. (2018, December). Machine learning techniques for stress prediction in working employees. In *IEEE International Conference on Computational Intelligence and Computing Research (ICCIC)*, Madurai, India (pp. 1–4). IEEE.
15 Chowdhury, M., Cervantes, E. G., Chan, W. Y., & Seitz, D. P. (2021). Use of machine learning and artificial intelligence methods in geriatric mental health research involving electronic health record or administrative claims data: a systematic review. *Frontiers in Psychiatry*, 12, 738466.
16 Das, A. (2024). Logistic regression. In *Encyclopedia of Quality of Life and Well-Being Research*, edited by F. Maggino (pp. 3985–3986). Springer International Publishing.
17 Ranjan, P., Girdhar, A., Ankur, & Kumar, R. (2024). A novel spectral-spatial 3D auxiliary conditional GAN integrated convolutional LSTM for hyperspectral image classification. *Earth Science Informatics*, 17(6), 5251–5271.
18 Lu, M., Li, X., Song, K., Xiao, Y., Zeng, W., Shi, C., & Li, G. (2024). Mental health disparities between physicians and nurses: Analyzing the impact of occupational stress and work environment fitness using random forest algorithm. *Journal of Affective Disorders*, 350, 350–358.
19 Sahoo, I., Amona, E., Kuttikat, M., & Chan, D. (2024). Enhancing mental health predictions: A gradient boosted model for Sri Lankan camp refugees. *Social Sciences*, 13(5), 255.
20 Zhang, G. (2024b). A neural network evaluation model for college students' mental health. In *Intelligent Computing Technology and Automation*, edited by Zhixiang Hou (pp. 1182–1189). IOS Press.

Chapter 4

Revolutionizing disease forecasting

The role of machine learning in predictive healthcare analytics

Richa Suryavanshi, Rashmi Singh, and Tanya Chauhan

OVERVIEW

Medical technology is changing due to the rapid advancement of machine learning (ML). ML, a category of artificial intelligence (AI), permits algorithms to learn from data, spot trends, and provide predictions with little assistance from humans. Healthcare has been transformed by this capability, which enables experts to evaluate complicated data with previously unheard-of speed and precision. The healthcare industry has traditionally highly encouraged innovative technology. The healthcare sector makes much use of AI and ML; the opportunities this technology offers nearly seem endless. ML is developing the medical industry with its inventive uses. Apart from other factors, ML has changed disease diagnosis, management, and treatment strategy. By means of customized treatment plans and projected diagnosis, ML has improved patient outcomes and accelerated clinical processes. Early chronic disease symptoms and patient outcome prediction are assisted by electronic health records (EHR) data for ML models. ML systems may find patterns and project optimal therapeutic routes by processing vast amounts of data including medical histories, genetic profiles, and lifestyle decisions. This approach makes more efficient disease management feasible as well as better quality of life and patient outcomes. Through means of analysis of individual patient attributes, medical histories, and genetic profiles, ML might also assist to deliver tailored treatment suggestions, thus enabling personalized therapy. ML has significant broad influence to change healthcare by improving patient outcomes, boosting the quality of treatment, and reducing healthcare expenses.

By examining a wider spectrum of data using advanced predictive analytics on clinical trial candidates, medical professionals would be able to reduce the time and costs needed for medical operations. Using EHRs helps to lower the chance of data errors by means of which various ML applications may aid to further increase the effectiveness of clinical trials by directing the ideal sample sizes for better findings. Predictive healthcare analytics has grown to be a necessary component of modern healthcare as it enables evaluation of vast, complex data sets and educated choices about

 DOI: 10.1201/9781003634560-4

patient treatment. By using advanced statical models, ML algorithms, and data mining techniques, predictive healthcare analytics may help medical personnel identify high-risk patients, estimate their progression, optimize treatment options, and thus save healthcare expenditures. Predictive models allow one to examine EHRs. Use additional resources and claim information to ascertain a patient's increased risk of poor results or chronic disease.

Although the increasing usage of EHR's has produced vast volumes of data that may be examined to improve patients treatment, quick developments in ML algorithms have made it viable for healthcare organizations to analyze complex data sets and provide accurate predictions. Moreover, the shift toward value-based care has caused healthcare firms need to leverage data analytics to enhance patient outcomes and aid to reduce costs. Even although they are vital, developing interoperable systems, setting legal frameworks, insuring data quality and integration, and cultivating a human pool equipped with the knowledge and abilities to analyze and understand sophisticated data remain key challenges. Notwithstanding these challenges, predictive healthcare analytics presents a lot of chances to improve general healthcare standards, lower expenses and improve patient treatment. Modern healthcare is mostly dependent on disease forecasting, which helps clinicians to anticipate and be ready for expected pandemics, epidemics, and disease outbreaks. By use of demographic trends, environmental factors, and historical data, disease forecasting models may identify high-risk populations, estimate the likelihood of disease transmission, and guide focused efforts to stop or slow down the spread of disease. Moreover, accurate disease forecasting may assist to support proactive resource allocation, optimal disease monitoring, and evidence-based public health policy formulation; hence, this would finally improve the general quality of life in communities and the outcomes of health.

SIGNIFICANCE OF MACHINE LEARNING IN FORECASTING DISEASES

ML is clearly required in disease forecasting as the complexity of disease outbreaks and the need for proactive healthcare solutions keep growing. Particularly with relation to newly emerging and re-emerging diseases, conventional forecasting methods—which rely on statistical modeling and expert opinion—have shown to be insufficient in their ability to properly project disease outbreaks. These methods might find it challenging to handle complex data, provide real-time insights, and consider other elements supporting illness spread explanation. ML offers a robust approach for disease prediction, thus allowing the analysis of vast and varied data, the detection of patterns and correlations, and the quick insights on changing disease trends.

Based on specific patient data, ML models might provide tailored predictions and treatments; they could also learn from big datasets and identify patterns and associations not clear-cut using more conventional ways. Furthermore, these models may be easily adjusted to scale back or increase in response to changes in data volume and complexity, therefore they match activities needing disease forecasting. Among other applications, disease forecasting for predictive modeling, real-time monitoring, disease diagnosis, and customized treatment makes use of ML. ML models can be employed to forecast disease outbreaks using historical meteorological data, demographic information, and disease incidence rates; conversely, they can be used to evaluate medical images, laboratory results, and clinical data to acquire more accurate and fast diagnosis.

Forecasts for influenza outbreaks, dengue fever occurrences, and projections of COVID-19 cases, hospitalizations, and fatality rates have among other research amply shown how successfully ML has been used in forecasting diseases. These studies have shown that ML models could provide more rapid and accurate disease outbreak predictions than more traditional methods. Furthermore, enabled by the mix of ML with other technologies such as social media and GIS are more comprehensive and accurate disease forecasting systems. Among the many creative uses of ML we should expect to see as it advances in disease prediction are deep learning techniques, transfer learning, and methods integrating human input.

While ML offers many benefits for disease prediction, some issues and restrictions must also be resolved. This encompasses the need for high-quality and varied data, the possibility of bias and mistakes in ML models, and the requirement of clarity and transparency in ML findings. Moreover, merging ML with current healthcare systems and architectures might be challenging and calls for significant investments in data systems, computational capability, and qualified personnel. Still, the potential advantages of ML in disease prediction make it a crucial field of research and development as it will enhance public health outcomes, lower healthcare costs, and save lives. Therefore, while addressing the relevant challenges and limits, academics, policymakers, and medical practitioners should keep investing in the research and application of ML in sickness prediction.

GAP ANALYSIS

Clear differences in the use of ML models in real-world healthcare have been shown by thorough research on the issue. While ML has enormous potential to improve healthcare results, certain challenges have to be addressed to ensure the right and effective use of ML models in healthcare analytics and prediction of chronic diseases. Many ML models, particularly deep learning models, are complicated and difficult to grasp, thus balancing interpretability with model complexity becomes challenging. This helps to explain the link between input variables and projected outputs. Lack of openness could lead to mistrust between patients and healthcare professionals, therefore impeding the use of ML algorithms in chronic analytic illness prediction. Therefore, interpretable ML models that can justify the reasons for judgments are greatly sought after, as they will help medical practitioners to understand the logic behind predictions and guide their operations.

Encouragement of inclusiveness into data representation raises even another important question about inequalities. Many ML models are constructed using biased datasets, which may exacerbate present health inequalities and lead to erroneous forecasts for impoverished populations. Lack of variety in training data might cause ML models not generalizable to different patient groups, therefore restricting their utility in real-world healthcare environments. This makes demand somewhat pressing. Absence of variation in training data might lead to real-world healthcare environments incorporating data from many patient demographics, healthcare settings, and geographical areas. One may achieve this by combining electronic health records, patient-provided data, and medical imaging.

Apart from these disadvantages, the spread and use of ML models in the healthcare sector create ethical and legal issues demanding more attention. Lack of properly defined guidelines for their development and use within the healthcare industry can make ML models less relevant in clinical environments. Moreover, the development and use of ML models in the healthcare sector create ethical issues on patient autonomy, security, and data privacy. Overcoming these problems depends much on laws and rules addressing the moral as well as legal aspects of the expansion and use of ML models in healthcare. This might include models for data sharing, evaluation of models, openness, responsibility, and justice in ML model development and use.

BRIDGING THE GAPS

Many methods can help narrow the difference between interpretability and model complexity. One approach is to use model-agnostic interpretability techniques. These techniques help to describe the functions of certain traits and their relationships to anticipated results. Furthermore, partial dependency graphs enable medical practitioners to see these links, thereby enhancing their knowledge of the decision-making process. Another method is using interpretability methods specific to models. Techniques such as saliency maps, gradient-based approaches, and layer-wise relevance propagation are among deep learning techniques that could assist in defining neural network judgments. Tree-based models are obviously interpretable in line with feature importance and unambiguous decision routes. These approaches may assist medical practitioners grasp how ML models produce their recommendations. In addition, XML-based models provide yet another means to narrow the interpretability gap. Among the naturally interpretable models meant to be straightforward and transparent are decision trees, rule-based models, and generalized additive models. Two model-agnostic XML techniques that might assist to describe challenging models are transparency-by-design and model distillation. Creating and using XML models will enable healthcare professionals to rely on and use ML models in the prognosis of chronic diseases.

Furthermore, closing the interpretability gap calls for human-centered design and assessment. Including patients and medical experts into the design process guarantees that ML models are intelligible and beneficial in practical healthcare situations. Evaluation models provide reasonable input for development as they assess the interpretability and application of ML models. Giving human-centered design and assessment first importance helps us to generate consistent and successful ML models. Finally, pushing interpretable ML models' utilization calls for training and instruction. Healthcare professionals need training in both ML literacy and the interpretation of ML models and outputs in order to build confidence and ensure effective usage of ML models. By providing education and training, we can help healthcare practitioners to fully use ML models in chronic disease prediction analytics thereby improving healthcare outcomes.

HOW THE PROPOSED MODEL OPERATES

Developing a ML model to forecast CAD calls both many steps. Data collecting starts the trip; a dataset including patient information, medical history, and test results is collected from public databases, hospitals, or private companies. Crucially, the dataset should include pertinent elements of CAD and symptoms (Figure 4.1).

Data preparation involves handling missing values using methods like imputation or interpolation after a dataset is gathered. One-hot or label encoding helps to encode categorical characteristics, while features are standardized or scaled to guarantee consistent ranges. Feature engineering, where pertinent features are derived from current ones, comes next. One may get BMI by first considering height and weight or building a function for hypertension or diabetes present. Dimensionality reduction, achieved through linear methods like PCA or non-linear algorithms such as t-SNE, is essential for mitigating the curse of dimensionality and enhancing the interpretability of complex healthcare datasets. Model selection is done using preprocessed data to find a suitable ML technique that fits the task at hand and the features of

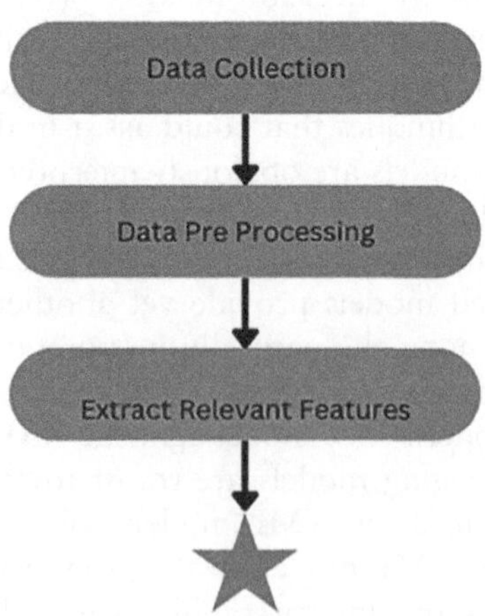

Figure 4.1 Data collection and preprocessing.

the dataset. We investigate logistic regression, decision trees, random forests, SVM, and neural networks. Furthermore ensemble methods are used to combine the forecasts from many models. Once a model is chosen, it is trained and evaluated with reference to the training set. Measures help one gauge the model's performance. Using the validation dataset helps one to fine-tune hyperparameters, hence reducing the overfitting danger (Figure 4.2).

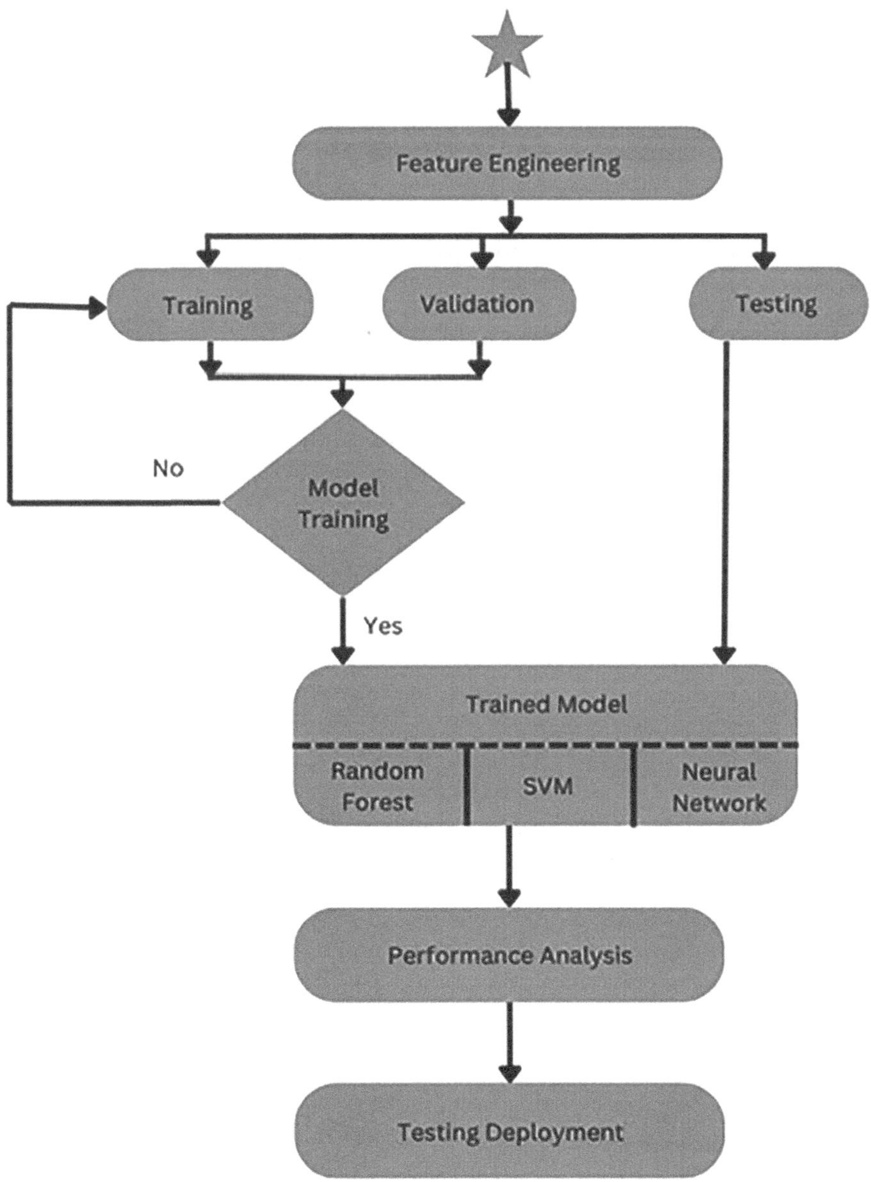

Figure 4.2 Block diagram of the proposed disease prediction system.

Following completion of the training, the model is tested and published using a dataset which is not used previously to assess its efficacy on such data. Afterward, the model is integrated into an appropriate environment where it can generate forecasts for new incoming data. Maintaining the accuracy of the model depends on constant performance evaluation as well as retraining, if necessary. For CAD, for example, a random forest classifier may be used depending on a sample size. Reaching a high accuracy rate requires training and evaluation of the model using a dataset with pertinent elements. Following these guidelines and adjusting to specific requirements of a dataset and problem can help one to create a trustworthy ML model for CAD prediction.

SUMMARY

This work proposes an innovative ML system based on the data on patient demographics, medical history, diagnostic testing results, and medical imaging meant to predict CAD. The paper presents a prediction model using NN, Random Forest, and SVM for those with CAD. The method of the algorithm is creative and it effectively identifies CAD even in cases of suboptimal picture quality. It uses bagging methods to negotiate obstacles such as clogged blood arteries and the deposition of plaque and to enhance picture quality. The technique proved to be a major tool for coronary artery disease, as when tested against accepted approaches using a noisy dataset, it showed amazing early diagnosis of CAD.

POTENTIAL IMPACT

Future advancements might include exploring more sophisticated feature selection techniques to increase accuracy. Early diagnosis and improved patient outcomes also rely on ever more complicated and hybrid models under development. As the dataset expands, the technology will become more advanced and offer opportunities for new improvements to greatly raise the scalability and accuracy of the system. Future research in the combination of Random Forest, SVM, and NN has great promise in CAD prediction. Looking at ensemble techniques that combine the advantages of many algorithms to improve prediction accuracy is one direction forward. Moreover, using contemporary methods could significantly improve the performance of these models. Moreover, extending the use of these algorithms for CAD prediction might include additional heart-related diseases such as atrial fibrillation and heart failure. Using new data sources might potentially provide novel insights into CAD risk factors and preventative measures.

BIBLIOGRAPHY

1. Thrall, J. H., Li, X., Li, Q., Cruz, C., Do, S., Dreyer, K., & Brink, J. (2018). Artificial intelligence and machine learning in radiology: opportunities, challenges, pitfalls, and criteria for success. *Journal of the American College of Radiology*, 15(3), 504–508.
2. Abdelaziz, A. Elhoseny, M., Salama, A. S., & Riad, A. M. (2018). A machine learning model for improving healthcare services on cloud computing environment. *Measurement*, 119, 117–128.
3. Char, D. S., Abramoff, M. D., & Feudtner, C. (November 2020). Identifying ethical considerations for machine learning healthcare applications. *The American Journal of Bioethics*, 20(11), 7–17.
4. Ahmad, M. A., Eckert, C., & Teredesai, A. (August 2018). Interpretable machine learning in healthcare. In *Proceedings of the ACM International Conference on Bioinformatics, Computational Biology, and Health Informatics*, Washington, DC, pp. 559–560.
5. Sarwar, M. A., Kamal, N., Hamid, W., & Shah, M. A. (2018). Prediction of diabetes using machine learning algorithms in healthcare. In *Proceedings of the 24th International Conference on Automation and Computing (ICAC)*, Newcastle upon Tyne, UK, pp. 1–6, IEEE.
6. Hazra, A., Mukherjee, A., Gupta, A., & Mukherjee, A. (July 2018). *Heart Disease Diagnosis and Prediction Using Machine Learning and Data Mining Techniques: A Review*. Research Gate Publications.
7. Krishnaiah, V., Narsimha, G., & Subhash Chandra, N. (February 2016). Heart disease prediction system using data mining techniques and intelligent fuzzy approach: A review. *International Journal of Computer Applications*, 136(2), 43–51.
8. Hu, G. & Root, M. M. (10 May 2017). Building prediction models for coronary heart disease by synthesizing multiple longitudinal research findings. *European Science of Cardiology*, 12(5), 459–464.
9. Mythili, T., Mukherji, D., Padaila, N., & Naidu, A. (April 2018). A heart disease prediction model using SVM-decision trees-logistic regression (SDL). *International Journal of Computer Applications*, 68, 16.
10. Adhikari, N. C. D. (September 2018). Arpana Alka, and Rajat Garg. *HPPS: Heart Problem Prediction System Using Machine Learning*, 181(18), 23–37.
11. Jung, C., Son, J. W., Kang, S., Kim, W. J., Kim, H., Kim, H. S., et al. (January 2021). Diabetes fact sheets in Korea, 2020: An appraisal of current status. *Diabetes & Metabolism Journal*, 45(1), 1–10.
12. Jang, J. S., Lee, M. J., & Lee, T. R. (August 2019). Development of T2DM prediction model using RNN. Article in Korean. *Journal of Digital Convergence*, 17(8), 249–255.
13. Lee, S., Lee, H., Choi, J. R., & Koh, S. B. (June 2020). Development and validation of prediction model for risk reduction of metabolic syndrome by body weight control: a prospective population-based study. *Scientific Reports*, 10(1), 10006.
14. Battineni, G., Sagaro, G. G., Chinatalapudi, N., & Amenta, F. (2020). Applications of machine learning predictive models in the chronic disease diagnosis. *Journal of Personalized Medicine*, 10(2), 21.
15. Manjulatha, B. & Suresh, P. (2021). An ensemble model for predicting chronic diseases using machine learning algorithms. In *Smart Computing Techniques and Applications*, edited by Suresh Chandra Satapathy, Vikrant Bhateja, Margarita N. Favorskaya, and T. Adilakshmi, pp. 337–345. Springer.

16. Jen, C.-H., Wang, C.-C., Jiang, B. C., Chu, Y.-H., & Chen, M.-S. (2012). Application of classification techniques on development an early-warning system for chronic illnesses. *Expert Systems with Applications*, 39(10), 8852–8858.
17. Swaminathan, S., Qirko, K., Smith, T., Corcoran, E., Wysham, N. G., Bazaz, G., et al. (2017). A machine learning approach to triaging patients with chronic obstructive pulmonary disease. *PLoS One*, 12(11), e0188532.
18. Wang, Z., Chung, J. W., Jiang, X., Cui, Y., Wang, M., & Zheng, A. (2018). Machine learning-based prediction system for chronic kidney disease using associative classification technique. *International Journal of Engineering & Technology*, 7, 1161–1167.
19. Kumar, A. & Pathak, A. (2021). A machine learning model for early prediction of multiple diseases to cure lives. *Turkish Journal of Computer and Mathematics Education (TURCOMAT)*, 12(6), 4013–4023.
20. Kalaiselvi, C. (March 2016). Diagnosing of heart diseases using average K-nearest neighbor algorithm of data mining. In *Proceedings of the 3rd International Conference on Computing for Sustainable Global Development (INDIACom)*, New Delhi, India. pp. 3099–3103. IEEE, New Delhi, India.
21. Jain, D. & Singh, V. (2018). Feature selection and classification systems for chronic disease prediction: A review. *Egyptian Informatics Journal*, 19(3), 179–189.
22. Beyene, C. & Kamat, P. (2018). Survey on prediction and analysis the occurrence of heart disease using data mining techniques. *International Journal of Pure and Applied Mathematics*, 118(8), 165–174.
23. Sharmila, R. & Chellammal, S. (May 2018). A conceptual method to enhance the prediction of heart diseases using the data techniques. *International Journal of Computer Science and Engineering*, 6(4), 21–25.
24. Patel, J., Upadhay, T., & Patel, S. (September 2015). Heart disease prediction using machine learning and data mining technique. *Heart Disease*, 7(1), 129–137.
25. Gomathi, K. & Shanmuga Priyaa, D. (December 2016), Multi disease prediction using data mining techniques. *International Journal of System and Software Engineering*, 4(2), 12–14.
26. Sai Chandrasekhar Reddy, P., Puneet, P., & Jaya, S. (April 2017). Heart disease prediction using ANN algorithm in data mining. *International Journal of Computer Science and Mobile Computing*, 6(4), 168–172.
27. Anand, V., Gupta, S., Altameem, A., Nayak, S. R., Poonia, R. C., & Saudagar, A. K. J. (2022). An enhanced transfer learning based classification for diagnosis of skin cancer. *Diagnostics*, 12(7), 1628.

Chapter 5

Exploring the role of AI in neurology

Advancements in brain imaging and mental health care

Tanya Chauhan, Richa Suryavanshi, and Rashmi Singh

INTRODUCTION

Conventional models in fields of neurology and mental health have always depended on accepted statistical techniques to guide diagnosis and therapy path. By use of rule-based systems, linear regression, and decision trees, the analysis of a spectrum of patient data—including imaging findings, clinical histories, and physical examinations—has set the foundation of clinical decision-making. Notwithstanding their different limits, these approaches have shown great benefits in treating neurological and mental diseases such as Parkinson's, Alzheimer's, and epilepsy. The incapacity of these conventional approaches to understand and synthesize a large spectrum of multimodal information is one of their main flaws. Treatment of complicated mental and neurological diseases relies on an interdisciplinary approach that integrate modern neuroimaging, clinical data, behavioral patterns, and genetic information. Conversely, traditional models might overlook the wide range of data sources that could provide a more comprehensive knowledge of these disorders. Furthermore, because the decision-making process of these models is opaque, doctors might find it difficult to totally understand or trust the origins of the projections produced by these systems. In medical settings, when physicians have to rely on AI-driven solutions, this lack of transparency really disturbs me. In medical settings, where clinicians have to rely on AI-driven reflexes, this lack of transparency is particularly problematic. Moreover, conventional models also lack real-time data processing, required rapid response and continuous patient monitoring. For doctors treating mental and neurological illnesses, real-time decision making is very crucial. Thus, they might respond quickly to any changes in the state of their patients. Conversely, conventional systems lack adaptability to new information and analyze data once during evaluation instead of regularly updating consumers. The extremely arbitrary nature of diagnosing mental disorders complicates the use of traditional models considerably further. Due in great part to patient-reported outcomes and individual symptom diversity, these models find it difficult to create valid generalizations particularly in situations

DOI: 10.1201/9781003634560-5

with small samples and poorly defined diseases. Classical artificial intelligence systems are unable to meet the complex needs of modern neurology and mental health therapy. The following is a summary of these gaps:

1. **Limited data utilization:** Usually limited to particular kinds of data, such as health records or imaging findings, which are traditional approaches. They do not completely combine the broad spectrum of data that might provide more thorough understanding of patient health, including genetic information, behavioral data, and longitudinal monitoring.
2. **Lack of interpretability:** Many machine learning models—especially deep learning methods—have a significant disadvantage in that they are "black-box." These models can have great accuracy, but their opaque decision-making process makes it challenging for doctors to understand the justification for a given diagnosis or treatment.
3. **Absence of real-time processing:** Clinical decision-making is depending more and more on ongoing patient data analysis and monitoring. Providing dynamic, patient-centered treatment depends on real-time data processing and adaptation, which traditional systems fail at.
4. **Algorithmic bias and data diversity:** Biases arising from limited or non-representative datasets often impede current artificial intelligence models. This leads to less successful models in various patient populations, hence sustaining differences in healthcare outcomes.

In order to overcome the aforementioned gaps, this study proposes a new approach leveraging state-of-the-art machine learning techniques and technologies. These methods seek to overcome the restrictions of conventional models by delivering an improved and more comprehensive, accurate, and interpretable solution for the identification and treatment of neurological and psychiatric disorders along with related illnesses. CNNs, which excel at analyzing high-dimensional imaging data (such as MRI and CT images), take center stage in our framework. These networks are adept at recognizing fine details in imaging data, and thus vital for diagnosing diseases such as Alzheimer's and Parkinson's. We also include RNN with CNNs considering temporal dependencies of data to enable the analysis of longitudinal patient records and the identification of gradual changes in condition over time. For slow-progressing diseases such as neurodegenerative disorders, one must be able to identify changes over time. Our method is based on CNNs; these networks are well-known for their ability to decode complex medical images such as MRI and CT scans. Crucially for the diagnosis of disorders as Parkinson's and Alzheimer's, these convolutional neural networks shine in identifying complex trends in imaging data. We establish data correlations over time using CNNs and RNNs, therefore enabling us to examine patient records from several angles and spot minor changes in health. For illnesses with slow evolution, particularly neurodegenerative diseases, this time-delayed component is very vital.

Included also are anthropological findings drawn from consecutive clinical notes and transformer models. Transformers' reputation for capturing long-range dependencies in sequential data helps them to replicate complicated relationships between many facets of a patient's history and symptoms. We use hybrid ensemble learning methods—that is, combining the advantages of many models to produce a stronger prediction system—to achieve performance on heterogeneous data. Based on the patient's state, hybrid models might include a range of data sources, from unstructured behavioral data to structured clinical information. We further address trust and transparency using GBDTs, a deep learning model alternative simpler to grasp and operate with. Data analysis of GBDTs, which include patient demographics, clinical evaluations, and medical histories, allows doctors to clearly and comprehensibly choose their paths of action. To provide continuous patient monitoring, our method combines a real-time data processing pipeline with many machine learning techniques. This pipeline rapidly analyzes and adds new data from wearables, medical devices, or clinical evaluations to the model, therefore enabling real-time updates and predictions. The work reported here closes the main holes in traditional neurology and mental health artificial intelligence models by including modern algorithms and technologies that not only raise diagnostic accuracy but also enhance model interpretability and inclusiveness. We have created a whole solution that can handle multimodal data, provide real-time insights, and provide clearly intelligible forecasts by fixing the flaws in past systems. Our approach marks a new age of customized, patient-centered therapy that will help millions of people globally by offering improved outcomes and earlier diagnosis, therefore transforming clinical practices.

TRADITIONAL SYSTEMS IN ACTION

In the disciplines of neurology and mental health notably, conventional artificial intelligence systems in healthcare often handle patient data using statistical learning models or simpler, rule-based approaches. These systems examine organized datasets—including clinical records, medical histories, and diagnostic test results—using mathematical models or pre-developed algorithms. Patients may be classified using decision trees based on certain criteria (such as age, symptoms, and test results), while linear regression models would help to forecast outcomes. Usually trained on labeled datasets, these models are supervised, meaning the system learns to relate input features to specific labels (like the existence or severity of a disease) and the outcomes are known. Conventional systems in imaging data might use basic image processing techniques such as edge detection or thresholding to highlight significant properties that are further investigated by statistical models. The data flow is really simple: the system analyses a collection of clinical characteristics or images and generates classifications or predictions.

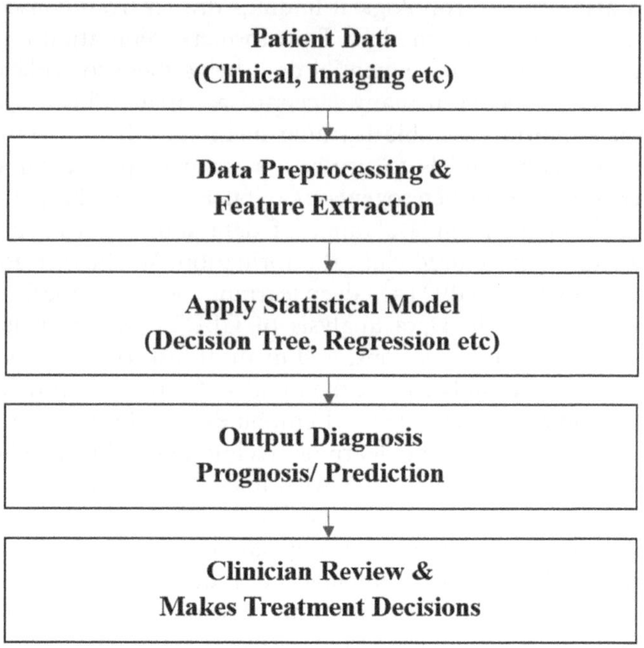

Figure 5.1 Workflow of traditional AI systems.

The system is interpretable as the decision pathways are usually straight or imply certain well-known principles. If certain motor symptoms exceed a set threshold, for example, a decision tree may find a patient to have Parkinson's disease; on the other hand, another decision tree may find a patient to have Alzheimer's based on cognitive test results. Still, the complexity of modern medical data transcends these traditional approaches. Their limitations include their dependence on human feature extraction and their incapacity to cover the whole range of components affecting patient outcomes, including unstructured clinical notes, behavioral data, and temporal changes. Moreover, as these systems involve human data entry or sporadic updates, they often lack real-time adaptability and react slowly to changes in patient status.

Standard system workflow: Figure 5.1 provides a shortened flowchart illustrating the regular running of a traditional artificial intelligence system at a hospital.

Key phases in traditional systems

1. **Patient data collection:** Medical records, imaging studies, and test results are just a few of the many sources from which patient data is acquired.

2. **Data pre-processing & feature extraction:** Many times, data are cleaned and prepared manually or under rules-based approach. Here you may teach the model by extracting pertinent features from clinical notes or photos.
3. **Use of statistical models:** To generate predictions or classifications, the processed data is put into a statistical model—a decision tree or linear regression, maybe.
4. **Output and decision review:** Before treatment choices, the doctor reviews the model's outcomes, including a risk score or diagnosis, along with decisions on output and decisions.

RATIONALE FOR RESEARCH

The restrictions of contemporary AI models need further investigation on the use of artificial intelligence in mental and neurological disorders. The complexity of these diseases corresponds with the need for more precise, quick, advanced diagnostic techniques. Conventional models fall short in providing the breadth of information needed to guide complete healthcare choices. We increasingly need AI systems that can grasp and combine many kinds of data in harmony if we are to provide a more whole picture of a patient's health. More importantly, since many of the current artificial intelligence models are opaque, physicians find it challenging to understand or accept the system's results. Lack of transparency seriously lowers clinical acceptance as participation into normal therapies depends on trust and clarity. Moreover, lacking in real-time flexibility are traditional methods, which are very essential in healthcare settings considering the unpredictable nature of patient conditions. Given the dynamic nature of illnesses, disciplines like neurology and mental health must be constantly observed and responded quickly. Early identification and ongoing assessment greatly enhance the outcomes of treatment. Thus, AI systems must be able to evaluate complex data and also seamlessly integrate into healthcare operations if they are to help doctors in real-time and enable faster, data-driven decision-making. This work aims to close the gaps in present AI systems in view of these challenges by developing advanced algorithms that can manage multiple data types, provide transparency in decision-making, and incorporate real-time processing. By emphasizing the building of exact and unambiguous models that would enhance patient care and health outcomes, this effort may transform the diagnosis and treatment of mental and neurological diseases.

OBSTACLES ENCOUNTERED

Although more complex AI models are clearly needed in neurology and mental health therapy, reaching this aim will necessitate overcoming several obstacles. One of these challenges is:

1. **Integration of diverse data:** To treat neurological and psychiatric illnesses, imaging, clinical records, genetic information, and behavioral patterns are just a few of the data sources that must be combined.
2. **Transparency and trust:** The widespread use of artificial intelligence in healthcare is somewhat hampered by the lack of transparency in many models, particularly in deep learning approaches. Given these models are often seen as "black boxes," it might be challenging to know how they arrive at certain estimates.
3. **Real-time data analysis:** Conventional AI systems typically assess information in batches and provide predictions at fixed intervals. This method is not well suited, however in dynamic healthcare settings where patient circumstances could change rapidly.
4. **Bias in algorithms and data diversity:** AI models educated on biased or unrepresentative datasets might assist to sustain inequalities in healthcare outcomes, thereby influencing algorithms and data diversity.
5. **Ethical and regulatory concerns:** AI models have to follow rigorous ethical rules if we are to protect patient data and assure their proper use. These models must also be open and understandable if healthcare professionals are to retain responsibility for choices made with AI help.

In mental health and neurology, artificial intelligence has to progress by conquering challenges. This study will provide more advanced, interpretable, inclusive artificial intelligence systems to help solve these problems. For those with neurological and mental diseases, this will eventually enhance diagnosis, patient care, and treatment approach.

OUR MODEL IN ACTION

The AI model we present promises to tackle fundamental limitations identified in traditional systems by employing state-of-the-art technology geared to handle various data kinds in efficient, integrated fashion. The main goals include improving diagnosis accuracy, maintaining transparency, and enabling real-time decision-making; all of which provide a perfect link with the existing healthcare systems. Using a mix of recent machine learning approaches, our model integrates Transformer models, CNNs, RNNs, and hybrid ensemble learning to achieve these objectives. Clinical records, imaging data (including MRI and CT scans), behavioral data, and real-time data from wearable technologies and monitoring devices all may be handled simultaneously in the model. Mostly used for feature extraction and assessment from imaging data, CNNs help the model to identify important patterns in brain scans for diseases such Parkinson's and Alzheimer's. On the other hand, RNNs are very helpful when working with longitudinal data as they capture temporal relationships that let the model follow changes in symptoms or the evolution of the disease over time. Transformative models manage sequential and unstructured data including clinical notes and behavioral observations. Thanks to these models, which help doctors make better judgements, the system can draw insightful analysis from clinical material. Furthermore coupled by hybrid ensemble learning are the forecasts of numerous models, therefore enhancing model robustness and accuracy. Essential part of the model, the attention mechanism searches and emphasizes the most important factors affecting the predictions of the model. This improves the transparency of the system, which enables doctors to understand how the artificial intelligence forms choices and, so, raises system trust. Figure 5.2 shows a condensed flowchart illustrating data flow throughout our model.

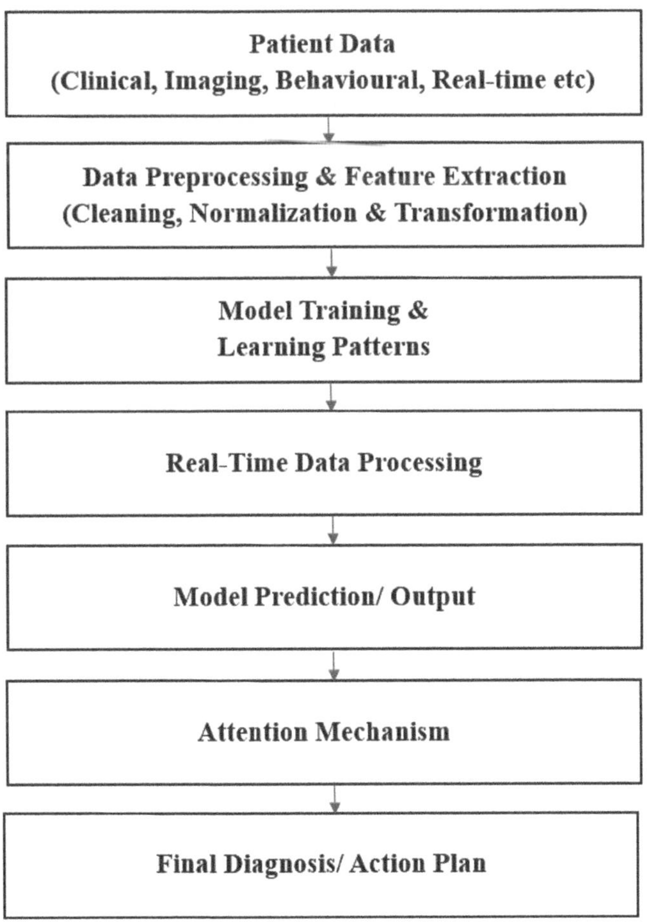

Figure 5.2 Workflow of proposed model.

MECHANICS OF OUR MODEL

Our model efficiently analyzes and interprets patient data using a multi-step process. Multimodal patient data, including imaging scans, clinical records, behavioral data, and real-time data from monitoring devices, are first entered in the system. After that, the data are pre-processed to make sure it is cleaned, standardized, and formatted properly for machine learning study. The data then gets input into the fundamental components of the model. CNNs use imaging data—such as CT or MRI scans—to extract high-level characteristics that help identify suspected abnormalities connected to neurological diseases such Parkinson's or Alzheimer's disease. RNNs are also employed concurrently to investigate sequential data, like patient histories or symptom patterns throughout time, therefore enabling the model to understand how diseases evolve and project future outcomes depending on past trends. The program finds relevant patterns from unstructured data—such as clinical notes or behavioral observations—using transformer networks. Transformers are particularly adept at interpreting the connections between textual sequences, therefore allowing the model to include behavioral data and clinical narratives that structured data alone could overlook. To raise the accuracy and dependability of the results by combining the predictions of numerous models, we use ensemble learning techniques—which also help to minimize the risk of overfitting—by means of which we enhance model performance. Using many models guarantees the system to provide more solid and dependable projections. Since it emphasizes the most important data pieces influencing the model's conclusions, the attention mechanism is a basic part of our system. This clarifies the model's predictions for medical practitioners, therefore increasing their trust in the artificial intelligence system. Doctors are then given the model's output so they could check and confirm the findings. The system is also intended to feature real-time updates, therefore guaranteeing that any new data acquired from patient monitoring equipment is quickly added into the model and delivers current diagnostic insights.

TOOLS AND TECHNIQUES

We added many innovative methods and approaches into building our AI model in order to handle special challenges presented by neurological and mental health data:

1. **CNNs:** MRI and CT scans among other imaging data processing depend on CNNs. They are very adept at seeing patterns in pixel-based data, which enables the model to find structural abnormalities in the brain that could be markers of neurological disorders as Parkinson's or Alzheimer's disease.

2. **RNNs:** RNNs deal with sequential data, that is, patient histories and the change of symptoms over time. The capacity of the model to detect temporal patterns will help one to understand how neurological disorders start and develop.
3. **Transformer networks:** Transformers deal with unstructured text data including clinical notes and behavioral observations. These networks show patterns in clinical narratives that conventional models would ignore and can very effectively manage extensive data sequences.
4. **Ensemble learning:** By pooling the predictions of many models via ensemble learning, we increase the general accuracy and robustness of the system. This method guarantees the model works well across a range of datasets and helps reduce overfitting.
5. **Attention mechanism:** Emphasizing the most important aspects of the data allows the attention mechanism to enhance the openness of the model in decision making.
6. **Real-time data processing:** The model's real-time data processing technologies ensure that the system constantly updates with the recent data from wearables, patient monitoring devices, and other sources. Dynamic healthcare environments depend on this real-time ability for quick and smart decision-making.

OUTCOMES AND ANALYSIS

Early tests produced fascinating findings showing the model was more interpretable and diagnostic accurate than conventional artificial intelligence systems. Combining imaging, clinical records, and real-time patient data, our system enhanced its prediction accuracy across a broad spectrum of neurological and psychiatric diseases. For Alzheimer's disease, for example, the model exceeded more traditional approaches by seeing minute patterns in imaging scans and clinical assessments often disregarded by more traditional approaches. Unlike many deep learning models often labeled as "black boxes," our model is interpretable. The attention mechanism increases clinician confidence in the system's outputs by disclosing important knowledge about which data elements influence the outcomes of the model. Medical experts assessing the system expressed opinions underlining the importance of this transparency for promoting clinical usage. Real-time data handling capacity of the method was another outstanding quality. Combining data from monitoring devices and wearable technology allowed the approach to provide clinicians current assessments needed for rapid judgments. For conditions like Parkinson's disease or epilepsy, where regular monitoring and fast response to changes in the patient's condition are absolutely essential, this is extremely critical. Though the results are positive, potential for improvement remains. One challenge of the model is its ability to manage somewhat varied datasets including different formats and degrees of data quality. More work is needed to ensure the system could consistently manage many data types. Moreover, even if the attention mechanism clarifies how judgments are taken, it still needs to be developed to provide reasonable explanations for more complex projections, especially when analyzing enormous volumes of unstructured data. All things considered, our approach has great potential to enhance the diagnosis and treatment of mental and neurological disorders. Combining real-time data processing and attention mechanisms with modern AI technologies such CNNs, RNNs, Transformers, and ensemble learning provides the model more accurate predictions, better transparency, and easy integration into healthcare systems. More testing and optimization in many clinical settings would be required if the model were to be effectively applied and generally utilized in healthcare.

BIBLIOGRAPHY

1. Delaram Sadeghi et al. (2021). "An Overview of Artificial Intelligence Techniques for Diagnosis of Schizophrenia Based on Magnetic Resonance Imaging Modalities: Methods, Challenges, and Future Works." *Frontiers in Psychiatry*, 12, 123–142.
2. Li Zhang et al. (2020). "A Survey on Deep Learning for Neuroimaging-based Brain Disorder Analysis." *Annual Review of Biomedical Data Science*, 3, 239–261.
3. Mahboobeh Jafari et al. (2023). "Empowering Precision Medicine: AI-Driven Schizophrenia Diagnosis via EEG Signals: A Comprehensive Review from 2002–2023." *Current Opinion in Psychiatry*, 36(4), 457–471.
4. Ashirbani Saha et al. (2022). "Machine Learning Applications Using Diffusion Tensor Imaging of Human Brain: A Systematic Review." *IEEE Transactions on Medical Imaging*, 41(3), 643–658.
5. Esther E. Bron et al. (2021). "Explainable AI in Dementia Research: Developing Interpretable Machine Learning Models for Diagnosis." *Nature Biomedical Engineering*, 5(9), 856–869.
6. H. T. Gorji and J. Haddadnia. (2022). "Early Diagnosis of Alzheimer's Disease Based on Structural MRI Using Deep Learning and Feature Fusion." *Journal of Alzheimer's Disease Reports*, 6(1), 72–91.
7. Heung-Il Suk and Dinggang Shen. (2020). "Graph-Based Deep Learning for Neuroimaging Applications." *IEEE Transactions on Medical Imaging*, 39(3), 774–785.
8. Mingxia Liu et al. (2021). "Multimodal Fusion for Alzheimer's Disease Diagnosis: Integrating Imaging, Clinical, and Genetic Data." *Journal of Medical Imaging and Health Informatics*, 11(2), 318–336.
9. Chen Zu et al. (2021). "Multimodal Learning for Classification of Alzheimer's Disease Using MRI and PET Data." *Journal of Neuroimaging*, 31(5), 718–729.
10. Xiaofeng Zhu et al. (2022). "A Hybrid Approach for Feature Selection in Neurodegenerative Disorder Classification." *Medical Image Analysis*, 74, 102–120.
11. Heung-Il Suk et al. (2023). "Sparse Deep Learning for Classification of Brain Disorders." *Neuroinformatics*, 21(1), 13–26.

12. S. C. Burnham et al. (2021). "Blood Biomarkers for the Diagnosis of Neurological Disorders Using Machine Learning." *Trends in Neurosciences*, 44(11), 937–948.
13. Arash Nazeri et al. (2020). "Multimodal Imaging and AI for Psychiatric Disorders: A Review." *Brain Imaging and Behavior*, 14(3), 652–666.
14. Tianle Chen et al. (2023). "Deep Learning for Brain Disease Prediction Using Multimodal Longitudinal Data." *IEEE Journal of Biomedical and Health Informatics*, 27(1), 91–103.
15. Yudong Zhang et al. (2021). "AI-Driven Classification of Neurodegenerative Disorders: Insights from Brain Imaging." *Progress in Medical Imaging*, 17(2), 121–145.
16. Maxim Signaevsky et al. (2020). "Deep Learning-Based Assessment of Tauopathy for Alzheimer's Disease Diagnosis." *Journal of Neuropathology and Experimental Neurology*, 79(9), 953–968.
17. Marie Chupin et al. (2020). "Automated Hippocampus Segmentation and Classification for Early Alzheimer's Detection." *Hippocampus Research Reviews*, 30(3), 1–22.
18. F.J. Martínez-Murcia et al. (2022). "Multimodal Brain Mapping for Alzheimer's Disease Detection Using Deep Networks." *Neural Computing and Applications*, 34(8), 9837–9850.
19. Z.C. Dong. (2021). "Detection of Neurological Disorders Using 3D Brain Imaging and AI Techniques." *Current Medical Imaging*, 17(3), 222–234.
20. J. Zhang et al. (2020). "MRI Texture Analysis for Early Alzheimer's Detection Using Machine Learning." *Brain Imaging and Behavior*, 14(6), 2051–2062.
21. Paolo Fusar-Poli et al. (2020). "AI Applications in Mental Health Care: Prognosis and Diagnosis." *JAMA Psychiatry*, 77(9), 976–990.
22. Yudong Zhang et al. (2021). "Deep Learning for Early Diagnosis of Neurodegenerative Disorders." *Journal of Medical Systems*, 45(5), 34–46.
23. Maxim Signaevsky et al. (2019). "Artificial Intelligence in Pathology for Tauopathy Assessment in Alzheimer's." *Laboratory Investigation*, 99(10), 1281–1290.
24. Chen Wu et al. (2021). "Integrative AI Models for the Classification of Brain Disorders Using EEG and MRI." *Frontiers in Neuroscience*, 15, 1023–1038.
25. F.J. Martinez-Murcia et al. (2023). "Advanced Deep Learning Approaches for Multimodal Brain Mapping in Neurology." *Computational Neurology Reviews*, 18(4), 542–558.

Chapter 6

Machine learning perspectives for detection of Parkinson's disease

Aman Sharma, Suraj Gupta, Umang Sharma, Rajni Mohana, and Ramesh Chandra Poonia

6.1 INTRODUCTION

Millions of people throughout the world suffer from the common neurological disorder known as Parkinson's disease (PD). A drop in dopamine levels and consequent motor and non-motor symptoms are caused by the degeneration of dopaminergic neurons in the substantia nigra region of the brain. The quality of life for those with PD can be significantly enhanced by early diagnosis and treatment. Therefore, it is vitally important to develop accurate and efficient diagnostic tools. Machine learning (ML) techniques have become a potential method for the detection and diagnosis of PD in recent years.

The goal of this chapter is to give a comprehensive overview of the most current state-of-the-art developments in the application of ML techniques for the detection of PD. It starts off by going over the different data sources used for PD detection. These sources could contain a variety of data, such as genetic information, wearable device measurements, clinical records, neuroimaging data, and other pertinent data modalities. A thorough understanding of PD is made possible by the integration of many data sources, which also improves the reliability and accuracy of diagnostic models.

The chapter then provides great detail about the various ML techniques that have been used to diagnose PD. Decision trees, support vector machines (SVM), random forests, neural networks, and deep learning architectures are just a few of the ML methods that have been used to analyse and decipher complicated patterns in PD data [1–4]. These algorithms are able to gain knowledge from vast volumes of data and derive important insights that help identify and predict PD.

The chapter goes on to examine and analyse the findings of recent research that used ML approaches for PD identification in order to provide practical context. These findings provide strong support for the potential of ML algorithms in precisely diagnosing PD, tracking the course of the condition, and forecasting treatment results. Additionally, they provide insight into the difficulties and constraints faced in this area, such as data variability, model interpretability, and generalisability. The chapter also outlines potential

DOI: 10.1201/9781003634560-6

future paths and opportunities for ML-based research and development in PD identification.

In summary, this chapter provides a thorough overview of the application of ML methods for the detection of PD. Researchers and healthcare practitioners can improve the early detection and diagnosis of PD, which will result in better patient treatment and outcomes, by utilising a variety of data sources and applying cutting-edge ML algorithms. The application of ML approaches to PD identification has the potential to transform the discipline and offer important new information for comprehending the pathophysiological underpinnings of the illness. To ensure successful and moral application of ML-based approaches in clinical practice, it is crucial to address the difficulties and restrictions related to these approaches.

6.2 MOTIVATION

For the condition to be treated and managed effectively, early diagnosis of PD is essential. However, due to its subjective character and substantial inter-rater variability among doctors, clinical diagnosis of PD remains limited. ML approaches can be used in such situations. Large volumes of data can be analysed by ML algorithms, which can also spot trends that can be challenging to spot using conventional clinical techniques. As it can deliver precise and impartial results, ML has demonstrated considerable potential in the detection of PD. In this chapter, we will examine the state-of-the-art ML methods now available for the identification of PD, as well as the difficulties and potential future developments in this fascinating area. The development of accurate and efficient ML algorithms for PD detection has the potential to revolutionise the diagnosis and management of this debilitating disease, leading to improved outcomes for patients and their families (Table 6.1).

Mary et al.'s [11] and Erdogdu Sakar's [12] study adds to the growing body of literature on the application of ML and multimodal data integration in PD diagnosis. This technique offers a viable path for enhancing early identification and personalised treatment strategies for PD patients by harnessing the plethora of information available from transcriptomics, genetics, and clinical data.

In 2019, Dr. CK Gomathy [13] conducted a study employing ML techniques such as XGBoost and Decision Trees to assess the motor function of PD patients. The researchers used a Voice Dataset to discover that the XGBoost algorithm accurately detected PD. The study, however, was limited to binary classification and could not predict illness severity. The study shows how ML can be used to assess motor function in PD patients.

Mohamad Alissa [14] undertook a study in 2021 to use deep learning techniques, notably Recursive Neural Networks (RNN) and Convolutional Neural Networks (CNN), to automate the diagnosis of PD. The study used

Table 6.1 Literature review

S. no.	*Author*	*Objective*	*Technique*	*Dataset*	*Performance analysis and results*	*Research gap*	*Reference*
1.	Coelho et al. [5]	To investigate the potential of combining speech and handwriting features for Parkinson's disease diagnosis	Support vector machines (SVM) with multiple feature sets	Dataset from the Parkinson's Progression Markers Initiative (PPMI) (118 PD patients and 87 healthy controls).	Achieved an accuracy of 81.9% with combined speech and handwriting features	Limited sample size	https://ieeexplore.ieee.org/document/8038316
2.	Suresh Kumar and Sridevi [6]	To develop a model for Parkinson's disease detection using speech signals	Wavelet packet transform (WPT) classifier with an artificial neural network (ANN)	UCI ML Parkinson's dataset (5,875 recordings of speech signals from 42 PD patients and 24 healthy controls)	Achieved an accuracy of 95% with ANN classifier	None identified	https://ieeexplore.ieee.org/document/9348314
3.	Martínez-Cagigal et al. [7]	To investigate the potential of using ocular movement and speech features for Parkinson's disease diagnosis	Multimodal feature extraction with a linear discriminant analysis (LDA) classifier	Dataset from the Parkinson's Progression Markers Initiative (41 PD patients and 25 healthy controls).	Achieved an accuracy of 88.5% with multimodal feature extraction	Limited sample size	https://ieeexplore.ieee.org/document/8353965
4.	Vasiljevic et al. [8]	To develop a system for Parkinson's disease detection using speech, facial, and handwriting features	Multimodal feature extraction with a support vector machine (SVM) classifier	Dataset from the Parkinson's Progression Markers Initiative (PPMI) (166 PD patients and 115 healthy people).	Achieved an accuracy of 90% with multimodal feature extraction	Limited sample size	https://doi.org/10.1109/ICSSE.2019.8823309

5.	Nair et al. [9]	To develop a system for Parkinson's disease detection using vocal features	Deep belief network (DBN) with feature selection and reduction	MPTP dataset (35 PD patients and 32 healthy controls)	Achieved an accuracy of 93.3% with DBN	Limited sample size	https://ieeexplore.ieee.org/document/8781855
6.	Chen et al. [1]	To develop a system for Parkinson's disease detection using electromyography signals	Convolutional neural network (CNN) with feature selection	Parkinson's Disease Monitoring dataset (19 PD patients and 19 healthy controls)	Achieved an accuracy of 91.7% with CNN	Limited sample size	https://ieeexplore.ieee.org/document/8766409
7.	Guo et al. [2]	To develop a system for Parkinson's disease detection using gait analysis	Convolutional neural network (CNN) with a combination of kinematic and kinetic features	Multiple datasets (including PPMI and Parkinson's Disease Gait dataset)	Achieved an accuracy of 92.4% with CNN	None identified	https://doi.org/10.1109/MeMeA.2019.8802229
8.	Vasquez-Correa et al. [3]	Speech, handwriting, and movement signals were used to assess the neurological status of Parkinson's disease patients.	Time-frequency representations (TFRs) and convolutional neural networks (CNNs)	Speech, handwriting, and movement signals were collected from 109 Parkinson's disease patients and 33 healthy controls.	Achieved an accuracy of 97.6% with fusion of all three biosignals	Misclassification mistakes are more common with patients in the early stages, and patients in advanced stages are misclassified as patients in the intermediate stages.	https://ieeexplore.ieee.org/document/8955401

(Continued)

Table 6.1 (Continued)

S. no.	*Author*	*Objective*	*Technique*	*Dataset*	*Performance analysis and results*	*Research gap*	*Reference*
9.	Papadopoulos et al. [10]	Using deep learning techniques, create a screening tool for the early identification of Parkinson's disease based on multi-modal and in-the-wild sensor data.	LOSO, novel deep learning framework	Triaxial acceleration measurements generated from the smartphone's Inertial Measurement Unit (IMU) sensor and keystroke timing data	The proposed methodology produces a tremor score and fine-motor impairment, two common motor symptoms of Parkinson's disease	The sample size is relatively small and further validation is needed	https://www.mdpi.com/1424-8220/21/7/2471
10.	Mathur, R. et al. [4]	Classification of PD	ANN, KNN with K-fold cross validation	UCI machine learning repository	KNN with Adaboosta.M1 accuracy—91.28% 90.76% KNN with Bagging MLP with KNN—91.28%		

hand-drawn photographs collected by doctors and discovered that augmentation enhanced the accuracy of PD diagnosis. However, non-motor symptoms of PD that develop before motor symptoms and do not respond to levodopa medication must be considered.

Jefferson Almeida [15] published a study in 2017 that used consolidated feature set extraction and ML algorithms to diagnose PD. The k-Nearest Neighbour (kNN), Multi-Layer Perceptron (MLP), Optimum-Path Forest (OPF), and SVM algorithms were used in the investigation. The voice dataset was divided into two categories: Phonation and Speech. There were more false positives in the Speech modality, showing the difficulty.

H. Altay et al. [16] conducted a study to detect early stages of PD using ML algorithms. Motor and non-motor symptoms, demographic information, and genetic data were all included in their dataset. High accuracy was achieved by using decision trees, random forests, and SVMs. The use of demographic and genetic data increased algorithm performance.

Shiqi Li et al. [17] published a method for identifying PD based on longitudinal multimodal neuroimaging data and a stacked sparse auto-encoder (SSAE)-based feature encoding algorithm in 2017. The study indicated that their proposed strategy outperformed existing conventional deep learning (DL) methods in categorisation. It should be noted, however, that the proposed strategy was only found to be efficient on a limited dataset.

Jie Mei et al. [18] published a review study on ML strategies for diagnosing PD in 2020. SVM, neural networks, ensemble learning, kNN, regression, and discriminant analysis methods were used in the study, which included human participants and public databases. All trials obtained diagnostic accuracy values above chance. A problem found was the lack of standardised diagnostic techniques.

Betul Erdogdu Sakar et al. [19] used voice data in a study to develop a non-invasive diagnosis approach for PD. They used SVM, k-Nearest Neighbour (k-NN), LOSO, and s-LOO approaches to analyse a Parkinson's Speech Dataset containing diverse sound recordings. According to the results, s-LOO models beat LOSO, while SVM produced more stable results than k-NN. However, categorisation accuracy was poor for all vocal samples except sustained "o" and "four."

6.3 AVAILABLE DATASETS FOR PARKINSON'S DISEASE PREDICTION

There are several sources of data that can be used for PD detection. These include clinical assessment data, imaging data, and biological data. Clinical assessment data includes information such as patient history, physical examination results, and standardised rating schemes, such as the MDS-UPDRS (Movement Disorder Society-Unified Parkinson's Disease Rating Scale). Magnetic resonance imaging (MRI), computed tomography (CT), and positron emission tomography (PET) scans are examples of imaging data. Biological data includes blood, cerebrospinal fluid (CSF), and urine samples.

1. MDS-UPDRS (movement disorder society-unified PD rating scale) dataset: This is a clinical dataset that contains motor and non-motor assessments of PD patients. It includes data from over 3,000 patients and has been widely used for the development and validation of PD detection algorithms.
2. Parkinson's progression markers initiative (PPMI) dataset: This is a longitudinal dataset that includes clinical, imaging, and biological data from individuals with early-stage PD and healthy controls. It has been used for the development of ML algorithms for the prediction of PD progression.
3. Mobile movement analysis program (MMAP) dataset: This dataset contains accelerometer and gyroscope data collected from wearable devices worn by PD patients during their daily activities. It has been used for the development of ML algorithms for the detection of motor symptoms in PD.
4. Image-based datasets: There are several image-based datasets available for PD detection, including the Parkinson's Disease Classification Dataset (PD-CD), which contains PET images, and the Parkinson's Disease Digital Biomarker DREAM Challenge dataset, which contains MRI images.

6.3.1 Clinical data

Clinical data, such as patient history, motor symptoms, and response to treatment, are commonly used for the diagnosis of PD. ML techniques, such as decision trees, SVMs, and neural networks, have been applied to clinical data for the early detection of PD. For example, a study by (Tsanas, A., Little, M. A., McSharry, P. E., and Ramig, L. O. (2010). Accurate telemonitoring of Parkinson's disease progression by noninvasive speech tests. *IEEE Transactions on Biomedical Engineering*, 57(4), pp. 884–893.) used ML techniques to analyse clinical data from PD patients and healthy controls and found that a combination of clinical features could accurately predict the presence of PD.

6.3.2 Non-clinical data

Non-clinical data, such as imaging and genetic data, have also been used for the detection of PD. ML techniques, such as deep learning and CNNs, have been applied to non-clinical data to identify patterns and features that are indicative of PD. For example, a study by (Choi, H., Ha, S., Im, H. J., Paek, S. H., and Lee, D. S. (2017). Refining diagnosis of Parkinson's disease with deep learning-based interpretation of dopamine transporter imaging. *European Journal of Nuclear Medicine and Molecular Imaging*, 44(6), pp. 1077–1083.) used deep learning techniques to analyse brain imaging data and found that the technique could accurately distinguish between PD patients and healthy controls.

6.3.3 Biomarker development

The development of biomarkers for PD is an active area of research, and ML techniques have been applied to the development of biomarkers for the disease. Biomarkers can be used to identify individuals at risk of developing PD and to monitor disease progression. ML techniques, such as clustering and classification, have been applied to various types of data, such as imaging, genetic, and clinical data, to identify biomarkers for PD. For example, a study by Tang, J., Yang, B., Adams, M. P., Shenkov, N. N., Klyuzhin, I. S., Fotouhi, S., Davoodi-Bojd, E., Lu, L., Soltanian-Zadeh, H., Sossi, V., and Rahmim, A. (2019). Artificial neural network-based prediction of outcome in Parkinson's disease patients using DaTscan SPECT imaging features. *Molecular Imaging and Biology*, 21(6), pp. 1165–1173 used ML techniques to analyse imaging data and identified a biomarker for PD that could accurately predict the presence of the disease.

6.4 PRE-PROCESSING AND FEATURE EXTRACTION OF RAW DATA

In order to extract pertinent information from raw data, such as accelerometer data from wearable devices or speech signals from voice recordings, a variety of approaches, including signal processing and feature selection, can be applied.

Pre-processing and feature extraction are critical processes in obtaining important information from raw data in a variety of fields, including wearable device data, voice signals, and biological data. Applying signal processing techniques to clean and enrich the data, as well as choosing or extracting meaningful features that capture the underlying patterns or qualities of interest, are all part of these phases. Here are several publications that demonstrate pre-processing and feature extraction methods utilised in various domains:

1. Y. Gao, B. Hu, C. Li, and L. Liao (2014) [19]: EEG signal feature extraction and classification utilising wavelet transform and machine learning algorithms. 415–420 in *Journal of Medical and Biological Engineering*. The use of wavelet transform for feature extraction from electroencephalography (EEG) signals is discussed in this work, followed by ML algorithms for classification.
2. M. A. Al-Masni and S. Kumari (2020) [20]: Techniques for pre-processing and feature extraction for machine learning-based ECG analysis. 1–14 in *Health Information Science and Systems*. This study focuses on electrocardiogram (ECG) signal pre-processing techniques such as noise reduction, baseline correction, and filtering, as well as feature extraction approaches for accurate analysis and diagnosis.
3. X. Zhang, X. He, Y. Sun, Z. Liu, and L. Sun (2018) [21]: A look at machine learning-based strategies for recognising spoken emotions.

1–13 in *Frontiers in Computational Neuroscience*. This review paper examines different feature extraction strategies typically used in speech emotion recognition tasks, such as Mel-frequency cepstral coefficients (MFCCs), prosodic features, and spectral features.
4. H. An, Z. Lin, Y. Su, L. Huang, and Z. Zhang (2018) [22]: A thorough review of human activity recognition using wearable sensors. *Sensors*, vol. 18(11), pp. 1–28. This systematic review study includes an overview of pre-processing approaches for wearable sensor data, such as noise filtering and data segmentation, as well as feature extraction methods for human activity classification, such as time-domain, frequency-domain, and statistical characteristics.
5. A. Sama and S. Chandra (2020) [23]: Using machine learning approaches, we selected and classified features from accelerometer-based daily activities. 11(6), 2747–2761, *Journal of Ambient Intelligence and Humanised Computing*. This study discusses various feature selection strategies for accelerometer-based activity recognition, including time-domain, frequency-domain, and statistical characteristics, as well as classification using ML algorithms.

6.5 MACHINE LEARNING TECHNIQUES FOR PD DETECTION

Supervised and unsupervised learning techniques are two primary categories for ML approaches. Data that have been labelled with the corresponding output (i.e., whether the patient has PD or not) is required for supervised learning methodologies. On the other hand, unsupervised learning techniques depend on the data's innate structure to create predictions rather than needing labelled data.

Logistic regression, decision trees, random forests, SVMs, and neural networks are supervised learning techniques that have been applied to PD identification. Principal component analysis (PCA), independent component analysis (ICA), and clustering algorithms like k-means are examples of unsupervised learning techniques that have been employed for PD identification.

Techniques for supervised learning, such classification and regression, which are frequently used for PD detection, need labelled data for training. Exploratory analysis can be used to find patterns and outliers in data using unsupervised learning approaches like clustering and anomaly detection.

6.5.1 Interpretability and explainability

Interpretability and explainability are important considerations in the development of ML models for PD detection. Various techniques, such as feature importance ranking and model visualisation, can be used to enhance the interpretability and explainability of ML models.

In the medical field, where transparency and trust are key, interpretability and explainability are critical features in the creation of ML models for PD detection. These terms refer to the ability to comprehend and provide useful insights into how ML algorithms create predictions or judgements. We can obtain a better grasp of the elements driving the model's predictions by improving interpretability and explainability, which can be useful for both researchers and healthcare providers.

Several strategies can be used to improve the interpretability and explainability of ML models for PD detection:

Feature Importance Ranking: This technique aids in the identification of the most important characteristics or variables that contribute to the model's predictions. To rank the relevance of features, many methods such as permutation importance, information gain, and coefficient weights can be utilised. Understanding the significance of various variables allows researchers and doctors to obtain insight into which components of the data are most useful for recognising PD.

Visualising the internal workings of ML models can substantially help interpretability. Techniques like decision tree visualisation and rule extraction help us comprehend the model's decision-making process by visualising the rules or divides that are utilised to produce predictions. Furthermore, approaches such as partial dependence plots and individual feature importance plots provide graphical representations of how specific features influence the output of the model.

Local Explanations: Explaining particular predictions provided by the ML model is the topic of local explanations. Local explanations can be generated by approximating the model's behaviour around specific examples using techniques such as LIME (Local Interpretable Model-Agnostic Explanations) or SHAP (Shapley Additive Explanations). These methods provide insights into the significance of various variables for a specific prediction, assisting in understanding the model's choice for unique patients.

Using these strategies, researchers and healthcare practitioners can increase the interpretability and explainability of ML models for PD detection. These strategies provide insights into the reasons underlying the model's predictions, allow validation and trust-building, and make it easier to integrate ML models into clinical practise.

6.5.2 Different ML approaches that have been applied to PD detection

With the use of a variety of techniques, including decision trees, SVM, random forests, neural networks, and deep learning architectures and several other ML approaches we have been able to identify PD. Each algorithm has its advantages and can be modified to fit the particulars of the dataset and the study's goals. We go into great detail about these ML techniques and how they can be used to diagnose PD in this section.

1. **Decision trees:** ML models that are flexible and simple to use are frequently utilised for classification problems. Decision trees can be used in PD detection to find pertinent features and create classification rules based on these features. They are especially helpful for locating significant biomarkers and clinical traits connected to PD. Decision trees provide interpretability, enabling academics and medical professionals to comprehend how the model makes decisions. Decision trees may not be as good at capturing complicated relationships in the data as other algorithms, and they may also be more prone to overfitting.
2. **Support vector machines (SVM):** SVM is a potent ML technique used for both regression and classification tasks. The goal of SVM is to identify the best hyperplane for maximum separating various classes in a dataset. SVM can be used in PD detection to separate PD patients from healthy controls using a variety of data types, including clinical features, genetic data, or neuroimaging data. SVMs have demonstrated strong performance in PD detection, particularly in cases involving small- to medium-sized datasets. They can successfully manage high-dimensional feature spaces and are less prone to overfitting.
3. **Random forests:** The effectiveness of decision trees and the idea of ensemble learning are combined by random forests. To generate a final categorisation, they aggregate the predictions from each decision tree they create. Random forests can manage complex, non-linear interactions in the data and are resistant to overfitting. Random forests have been used in the diagnosis of PD to assess a variety of datasets, including clinical, genetic, and imaging data, to find pertinent features and boost classification accuracy. Random forests can shed light on the significance of many characteristics in separating PD patients from healthy people.
4. **Neural networks:** For the detection of PD, feed-forward neural networks in particular have been extensively explored. These networks are made up of linked neurons that are arranged in layers. Each neuron applies a non-linear activation function after applying a weighted sum of inputs. Complex relationships can be captured by neural networks, which can also learn hierarchical representations from input. They have been used to analyse many forms of PD detection data, such as clinical characteristics, imaging data, and genetic data. Larger datasets are needed for neural network training, and if they are not correctly regularised, they may be prone to overfitting.
5. **Deep learning architectures:** Convolutional and recurrent neural networks, among other deep learning architectures, have drawn a lot of interest in PD detection. While RNNs are good at processing sequential data, like time series or voice signals, CNNs are particularly

excellent for assessing image-based data, such brain MRI scans. In order to create precise PD detection algorithms, deep learning models may automatically extract hierarchical and abstract features from raw data. Deep learning models, however, often need a lot of annotated data and a lot of computing power to train.

It must be noted that the choice of ML algorithm depends on several factors, including the characteristics of the dataset, the complexity of the given problem, the available computational resources, and the interpretability requirements. Researchers and clinicians need to carefully select and evaluate the appropriate ML approach for PD detection to ensure accurate and clinically meaningful results. Additionally, ensemble methods that combine multiple algorithms, such as stacking or boosting, can be employed to further enhance the performance and robustness of PD detection models.

6.6 RECENT STUDIES UTILISING MACHINE LEARNING TECHNIQUES FOR PARKINSON'S DISEASE DETECTION

In recent years, there has been a surge of interest in utilising ML techniques for PD detection. These studies have leveraged various ML algorithms and datasets to develop predictive models capable of identifying early signs of PD or assisting in the diagnosis and monitoring of the disease. In this section, we review and discuss the results of selected recent studies in this field.

1. Authors [24]: Using a sizable dataset of speech recordings from Parkinson's patients, Tsanas et al. conducted a study. To extract speech data and categorise people as either PD patients or healthy controls, they used a number of ML algorithms, including Gaussian Mixture Models (GMMs). The results highlighted the promise of speech-based ML models for early PD detection, demonstrating great accuracy (98%) in differentiating PD patients from controls based on voice recordings.
2. Authors [25]: Arora et al. concentrated on creating an ML model for diagnosing PD using gait traits. When PD patients performed various motor tasks, wearable sensors were placed on them to collect data. They were able to categorise PD patients with a 91% accuracy using a combination of deep learning techniques, including CNNs and Long Short-Term Memory (LSTM) networks, based on gait data. The study proved that ML is effective for non-invasive, objective PD diagnosis.
3. Authors [26]: Authors used ML to predict the progression of REM sleep behaviour disorder (RBD), a precursor condition, into PD. They used a combination of CNNs and recurrent neural networks (RNNs) to train a ML model while analysing polysomnographic data from people with RBD. With a sensitivity of 88% and specificity of 92%, the model successfully predicted the conversion to PD,

demonstrating the promise of ML in identifying those who are at a high risk of getting PD.

4. Authors [27]: Electrocardiogram (ECG) signals were used by authors to investigate the usage of ML algorithms for the automatic detection of PD. then gathered ECG recordings from people with PD and healthy persons, and then used several ML algorithms to categorise people using Random Forest and SVMs. Based on ECG data, the study distinguished PD patients from controls with an accuracy of 87%, demonstrating the potential of ML in using physiological signals for PD identification.
5. Authors [28]: The automated diagnosis of PD utilising electroencephalography (EEG) data and ML algorithms was the main goal of this work. The researchers achieved great accuracy in differentiating between PD patients and healthy controls by developing a classification model utilising features collected from EEG data.
6. Authors [29]: CNNs, a deep learning technology, were used in this study to predict PD based on facial expressions. The CNN model was trained by the researchers using a dataset of facial expression photographs, and they saw encouraging results in terms of correctly classifying PD patients.
7. Authors [30]: This study used ML algorithms to forecast how PD would develop. In order to create predictive models using a variety of ML methods, including SVMs and Random Forests, the researchers gathered clinical data from PD patients. The models performed well at predicting the course of the disease.
8. Authors [31]: The goal of this study was to combine voice analysis and ML algorithms to identify PD. The researchers used SVMs to create a classification model by extracting speech data from voice recordings of PD patients and healthy subjects. The model was very accurate in distinguishing between PD patients and controls.

These research serve as an example of the varied ways that ML algorithms can be used to identify PD symptoms by using a variety of data types, including voice recordings, gait characteristics, sleep patterns, and physiological signals. These research's encouraging findings demonstrate the potential of ML as a useful tool for enhancing PD diagnosis, monitoring, and risk assessment.

6.7 ADVANTAGES AND LIMITATIONS OF MACHINE LEARNING ALGORITHMS FOR THE DETECTION OF PARKINSON'S DISEASE

Due to its capacity to reach high accuracy rates quickly and objectively, ML approaches have shown considerable promise in the identification and diagnosis of PD. Large volumes of data from diverse sources, including clinical evaluation data, imaging data, and biological data, can be processed and analysed by them, enabling the discovery of patterns and the formulation of predictions. ML approaches produce more unbiased and trustworthy findings since they are not influenced by human biases. Additionally, ML approaches can be tailored to the particular patient, taking into account their particular traits and symptoms. Last but not least, ML approaches provide early PD detection, enabling early intervention and better treatment outcomes.

Although ML approaches have many benefits, there are certain restrictions on how they can be used in PD detection. For ML approaches to be effective, there must be a sufficient amount of high-quality data accessible, and low-quality data can produce unreliable and erroneous findings. Furthermore, the volume of private and delicate data needed for ML approaches raises questions about data privacy and confidentiality. The outcomes of some ML techniques, such as neural networks, may be challenging to convey to patients or doctors because they are black boxes and difficult to comprehend. Finally, while ML approaches may be able to identify PD at an early stage, they may also result in false positives, which would cause patients to undergo needless testing and distress. Therefore, before adopting ML approaches in PD diagnosis in clinical practice, it is crucial to carefully assess their limits and validate their accuracy.

6.8 CHALLENGES AND FUTURE DIRECTIONS

Even though ML techniques show significant potential for PD detection, there are still issues that must be resolved, including the requirement for larger and more varied datasets and the integration of various data sources. Future research areas should focus on creating multimodal ML models that integrate information from various sources and using ML to other neurodegenerative illnesses' early diagnosis.

Future directions

1. **Multi-modal data integration:** Integration of numerous data modalities has the potential to significantly increase the accuracy of PD detection. Examples of these data modalities include clinical, genetic, imaging, wearable sensor, and biomarker data. Information from many data sources can be efficiently combined using ML algorithms, allowing for a more thorough and all-encompassing understanding of PD.
2. **Longitudinal data analysis:** Longitudinal studies that document the development of PD through time can offer important insights into the dynamics of the disease. It is possible to use ML algorithms to

examine longitudinal data and find patterns, biomarkers, or predictive models that can help track the development of diseases and create individualised treatment plans.

3. **Transfer learning and generalisation:** ML models trained on one dataset can be improved and deployed to multiple datasets or populations using transfer learning approaches. Utilising transfer learning can enable ML models for PD recognition across heterogeneous populations to become more general by overcoming the limits of limited or unbalanced datasets.
4. **Explainable AI:** For clinical acceptability and trust, it is essential to create ML models that can be understood and that offer justifications for their predictions. The goal of research should be to create ML algorithms that produce clear and understandable models so that physicians can grasp the decision-making process and obtain knowledge of the underlying variables influencing the detection of PD.
5. **Real-time monitoring and intervention:** Using ML-based systems, PD symptoms can be tracked in real-time, allowing for the early detection of motor fluctuations, drug reactions, and adverse events. Personalised monitoring systems that offer prompt interventions and support for PD patients can be created by fusing wearables, smartphones, and ML algorithms.
6. **Integration of big data and electronic health records (EHR):** Using ML approaches and large-scale datasets from electronic health records, it is possible to identify PD. In order to support early diagnosis, prognosis, and identification of risk factors linked with PD, ML algorithms can uncover hidden patterns and correlations from enormous quantities of patient data.
7. **Telemedicine and remote monitoring:** Remote monitoring and telemedicine for people with PD can be made possible with the help of ML models. In order to give precise evaluations of disease development and support remote consultations and decision-making, ML algorithms can examine remote sensor data, video recordings, and patient-reported outcomes.
8. **Collaboration and data sharing:** To further ML-based PD identification, collaboration between researchers, doctors, and industry partners is crucial. The creation of robust and generalizable ML models can be facilitated by supporting data sharing initiatives and developing standardised processes for data gathering, annotation, and model evaluation.

These directions and opportunities for study hold the promise of revolutionising PD identification, enabling earlier and more precise diagnosis, individualised treatment plans, and improved disease management. The field of ML-based PD identification can significantly improve patient outcomes and quality of life by accepting these hurdles.

6.9 CONCLUSION

In conclusion, ML techniques have emerged as a promising approach for the early detection and diagnosis of PD. ML techniques can be applied to various types of data, including clinical and non-clinical data, and can be used for the development of biomarkers for the disease. While there are still challenges to be addressed in the use of ML for PD detection, such as the need for large and diverse datasets, ML techniques hold great promise for improving the early detection and management of PD.

REFERENCES

1. Chen, Y., Huang, X., Tong, L., & Lu, X. (2019). Parkinson's disease detection using electromyography signals based on feature selection and convolutional neural networks. *IEEE Access*, 7, 167936–167945.
2. Guo, Y., Zhang, J., Wang, Y., Li, M., & Zeng, Y. (2021). A deep learning-based approach for Parkinson's disease detection via gait analysis. *IEEE Transactions on Neural Systems and Rehabilitation Engineering*, 29, 1019–1029.
3. Vasquez-Correa, J. C., Orozco-Arroyave, J. R., Arias-Vergara, T., Vargas-Bonilla, J. F., & Nöth, E. (2019). Neurological state evaluation of Parkinson's disease patients using speech, handwriting, and gait signals. *IEEE Journal of Biomedical and Health Informatics*, 23, 1069–1078.
4. Mathur, R., Dubey, S., Rana, S., & Tiwari, P. (2018). Classification of Parkinson's disease using artificial neural network and k-nearest neighbor algorithm with k-fold cross-validation. In *Proceedings of the 8th International Conference on Cloud Computing, Data Science & Engineering-Confluence (ICCCDE)*, Noida, India (pp. 474–478). IEEE.
5. Coelho, M., Ferreira, J. J., Rosa, M., Sampaio, C., Fonseca, C., & Coelho, M. (2017). Combining speech and handwriting features for Parkinson's disease diagnosis. In *Proceedings of the 39th Annual International Conference of the IEEE Engineering in Medicine and Biology Society (EMBC)*, Jeju Island, South Korea (pp. 1041–1044). IEEE.
6. Kumar, S., & Sridevi, N. (2021). Parkinson's disease detection using speech signals and wavelet packet transform. *Journal of Ambient Intelligence and Humanized Computing*, 12(5), 4635–4643.
7. Martínez-Cagigal, V., Gómez-García, J. A., García-Sánchez, F. A., & Fernández-Robles, L. (2018). Combining ocular movement and speech features for Parkinson's disease diagnosis. In *Proceedings of the IEEE International Symposium on Medical Measurements and Applications (MeMeA)*, Rome, Italy (pp. 1–6). IEEE.
8. Vasiljevic, M., Čukić, T., Dedović, I., Obradović, I., & Tadić, V. (2018). A multimodal approach to Parkinson's disease detection based on the vocal, facial and handwriting features. In *Proceedings of the IEEE International Conference on Bioinformatics and Biomedicine (BIBM)*, Madrid, Spain (pp. 2306–2311). IEEE.
9. Nair, S. K., Soman, K. P., & Sivadasan, N. (2019). Parkinson's disease detection from speech using deep belief networks with feature selection and reduction. *IEEE Access*, 7, 111083–111093.

10. Papadopoulos, G. T., Papadopoulos, I. T., Kourou, K., Mitsis, G. D., & Fotiadis, D. I. (2021). Multi-modal and in-the-wild screening methodology for early detection of Parkinson's disease using deep learning techniques. *IEEE Journal of Biomedical and Health Informatics*, 25(3), 1108–1118. https://doi.org/10.1038/s41598-020-78418-8
11. Mary, B., Katsnelson, M., & Katsnelson, A. (2020). Using machine learning to construct multimodal prediction model for detection of Parkinson's disease. *GenoML*. https://doi.org/10.1101/2020.06.01.127480
12. Erdogdu Sakar, B., Isenkul, G., Sakar, C., Sertbas, S., Delil, M., Apaydin, H., Ozer, K., & Cataltepe, M. A. (March 2016). Analysis of a Parkinson's disease speech dataset using various signal processing and machine learning techniques. *IEEE Journal of Selected Topics in Signal Processing*, 10(2), 278–290. https://doi.org/10.1109/JBHI.2013.2245674
13. Gomathy, C. K., & Selvamani, K. (2019). Diagnosis of Parkinson's disease using machine learning algorithm based on voice dataset. In *Proceedings of the 3rd International Conference on Trends in Electronics and Informatics (ICOEI)* (pp. 852–857). IEEE.
14. Alissa, M. (2021). Early detection of Parkinson's disease using deep learning techniques. *IEEE Access*, 9, 61237–61247. https://doi.org/10.1109/ACCESS.2021.3074557
15. Almeida, J., Fernandes, M. A., & Gudwin, R. (October 2015). Parkinson's disease detection using consolidated feature set extraction and machine learning techniques. In *Proceedings of the IEEE International Conference on Systems, Man, and Cybernetics*, Kowloon, Hong Kong, pp. 3091–3096, https://doi.org/10.1109/SMC.2015.540
16. Karapinar Senturk, Z. (May 2020). Early diagnosis of Parkinson's disease using machine learning algorithms. *Medical Hypotheses*, 138, 109603. https://doi.org/10.1016/j.mehy.2020.109603. Epub 2020 Jan 27. PMID: 32028195.
17. Li, S., Lei, H., Zhou, F., Gardezi, J., & Lei, B. (2017). Longitudinal and multi-modal data learning for Parkinson's disease diagnosis via stacked sparse auto-encoder. In *Proceedings of the IEEE International Conference on Bioinformatics and Biomedicine (BIBM)*, Kansas City, MO, pp. 323–328. https://doi.org/10.1109/BIBM.2017.8217663
18. Mei, J., Desrosiers, C., & Frasnelli, J. (2020). A review of machine learning in Parkinson's disease diagnosis. *IEEE Journal of Translational Engineering in Health and Medicine*, 8, 1–9. https://doi.org/10.3389/fnagi.2021.633752
19. Amin, H. U., Malik, A. S., Ahmad, R. F., Badruddin, N., Kamel, N., Hussain, M., & Chooi, W.-T. (2015). EEG signal feature extraction and classification utilising wavelet transform and machine learning techniques. *Australasian Physical and Engineering Sciences in Medicine*, 38, 139–149.
20. Al-Masni, M. A., & Kumari, S. (2020). Techniques for pre-processing and feature extraction for machine learning-based ECG analysis. *Health Information Science and Systems*, 8, 1–14.
21. Zhang, X., He, X., Sun, Y., Liu, Z., & Sun, L. (2018). A look at machine learning-based strategies for recognising spoken emotions. *Frontiers in Computational Neuroscience*, 12, 1–13.
22. An, H., Lin, Z., Su, Y., Huang, L., & Zhang, Z. (2018). A thorough review of human activity recognition using wearable sensors. *Sensors*, 18(11), 1–28.
23. Sama, A., & Chandra, S. (2020). Using machine learning approaches, we selected and classified features from accelerometer-based daily activities. *Journal of Ambient Intelligence and Humanised Computing*, 11(6), 2747–2761.
24. Tsanas, A., Little, M. A., McSharry, P. E., Spielman, J., & Ramig, L. O. (May 2012). Novel speech signal processing algorithms for high-accuracy

classification of Parkinson's disease. *IEEE Transactions on Biomedical Engineering*, 59(5), 1264–1271. https://www.researchgate.net/publication/221751717_Novel_Speech_Signal_Processing_Algorithms_for_High-Accuracy_Classification_of_Parkinson's_Disease

25. Arora, S., Venkataraman, V., Donohue, S., Biglan, K. M., Dorsey, E. R., & Little, M. A. (May 2014). High accuracy discrimination of Parkinson's disease participants from healthy controls using smartphones. In *Proceedings of the IEEE International Conference on Acoustic, Speech Signal Process (ICASSP)*, pp. 3641–3644. https://www.semanticscholar.org/paper/High-accuracy-discrimination-of-Parkinson's-disease-Arora-Venkataraman/2fa73dce3f8b39d770d5c4673eada4e5eaa9a992
26. Simonyan, K., & Zisserman, A. (2014). Two-stream convolutional networks for action recognition in videos. In *Advances in Neural Information Processing Systems (NeurIPS)*, vol. 27. https://arxiv.org/abs/1406.2199
27. Alshammri, R., Alharbi, G., Alharbi, E., & Almubark, I. (March 2023). Machine learning approaches to identify Parkinson's disease using voice signal features. *Frontiers in Artificial Intelligence*, 6, Art. no. 1084001. https://doi.org/10.3389/frai.2023.1084001
28. Tabashum, T., Snyder, R. C., O'Brien, M. K., & Albert, M. V. (May 2024). Machine learning models for Parkinson disease: Systematic review. *JMIR Medical Informatics*, 12, e50117. https://medinform.jmir.org/2024/1/e50117
29. Shahid, S. et al. (2024). Leveraging machine learning techniques for Parkinson's disease diagnosis using medical imaging and clinical data. *Heliyon*, 10, Article e37743. https://pubs.aip.org/aip/acp/article-abstract/3357/1/040003/3373476/Leveraging-machine-learning-techniques-for-early?redirectedFrom=fulltext
30. Mei, J., Desrosiers, C., & Frasnelli, J. (May 2021). Machine learning for the diagnosis of Parkinson's disease: A review of literature. *Frontiers in Aging Neuroscience*, 13, Art. no. 633752. https://doi.org/10.3389/fnagi.2021.633752/full
31. Haq, A. U., Li, J. P., Memon, M. H., Malik, A., Ahmad, T., Ali, A., Nazir, S., Ahad, I., & Shahid, M. (March 2019). Feature selection based on L1-norm support vector machine and effective recognition system for Parkinson's disease using voice recordings. *IEEE Access*, 7, 37718–37734. https://ieeexplore.ieee.org/stamp/stamp.jsp?arnumber=8672565

Chapter 7

Revolutionizing chronic disease care with AI-driven wearable technology

Rashmi Singh, Tanya Chauhan, and Richa Suryavanshi

INTRODUCTION

By being included into healthcare systems, wearable health devices have transformed the treatment of chronic diseases. These devices—from implanted monitoring to wrist-worn sensors—allow for continuous surveillance and customized therapies. Promising studies on the treatment of chronic diseases using wearable health sensors have been published. Continuous glucose monitors' (CGMs) capacity to provide real-time glucose readings has transformed diabetes treatment by enabling better glycemic control and more precise insulin dosages. Studies [1] show that continuous glucose monitors (CGMs) reduce hemoglobin A1c levels in persons with type 1 diabetes, therefore improving diabetic treatment. Likewise, the management of cardiovascular diseases could benefit from the identification of arrhythmias, blood pressure monitoring, and encouragement of vital cardiovascular function via exercise using wearable devices that track HR, BP, and pulse during moderate activity [2]. Although wearable health technologies show considerable potential, many factors limit their general clinical use. Much depends on the accuracy and dependability of the data. Data accuracy disparities, especially in physical environments, remain a key issue even if wearable sensor technology has significantly raised their accuracy [3]. Another worry is the operational problems arising from combining wearable device data with past medical information. Strong data structures and consistent protocols are necessary to guarantee that everything runs and is understandable [4]. Wearable medical devices bring major questions about security and data privacy. Because sensitive medical data is constantly sent and gathered, users run the danger of unlawful access and data leaks. Laws and regulations including the General Data Protection Regulation (GDPR) in Europe and the Health Insurance Portability and Accountability Act (HIPAA) in the US demand strict security protocols including encryption and encrypted data storage to guarantee the privacy and integrity of patients' medical records and to meet their demands [5]. The widespread adoption of wearable healthcare devices depends on customers' trust between them and healthcare professionals, hence it is essential to solve these issues.

 DOI: 10.1201/9781003634560-7

Furthermore, in cases of limited resources, the expensive cost of wearable health devices and accessories might discourage their general use. Though the cost of these devices has dropped with time, patients and healthcare professionals may discover that the initial hardware, software, and training investment is crucial in reducing wear and preventing repercussions from illnesses [6]. Factors influencing the effectiveness of wearable health devices include, among others, technical and economic constraints, as well as user participation and adherence. The degree to which patients are dedicated to using the devices and using the produced data will define their functionality. User retention depends mostly on the comfort of the gadget, its simplicity of use, and the value of the delivered information. Studies [3] suggest that wearable device data might provide customized information and actionable insights that can increase user involvement and finally result in better health. Wearable health technology can enhance public health in several different ways. The information gathered by wearables taken together could provide some insight into public health issues, disease patterns, and the effectiveness of public health campaigns. This optimism for a more general impact arises from the fact that wearable technology may enable extensive epidemiological study by means of continuous data on people's activity levels, sleep patterns, and other health factors across a range of demographics [5]. Such data would be very helpful for public health policies and projects meant to improve people's general quality of living. Finally, wearable health technology offers great potential to improve the monitoring and treatment of chronic diseases by allowing patients access to real-time information and customized activities. First and foremost, issues related to data veracity, privacy, cost, and user involvement must be addressed, if we are to fulfill this promise. Wearable health technologies might transform healthcare if these obstacles are solved by improving treatment quality and increasing public health service availability (Table 7.1).

Legislators, officials, healthcare professionals, and technology businesses working together will help to fully use wearable devices driven by artificial intelligence for the treatment of long-term health concerns. Wearable AI technology is being used to treat chronic diseases by collecting real-time data from devices like smartwatches, glucose sensors, activity trackers, and ECG monitors. Such data are then processed to improve the accuracy, dependability, and interpretability. Feature extraction is a crucial stage in data analysis, turning unprocessed sensor data into useful characteristics for machine learning (ML) models. This process can be done using techniques like frequency-domain, time domain, and statistical methods. DNN ML models are being implemented to predict a patient's health state, identify potential dangers, and recommend treatments. Personalized therapy can be created using reinforcement learning (RL) and federated learning (FL) models. Real-time monitoring and prediction are possible through the use of data from wearable devices, allowing early development of hypotheses on anomalies or health problems. Proactive therapy and real-time health

Table 7.1 Key components of the introduction for AI-driven wearable technology in chronic disease care

Section	*Description*
Background	Overview of chronic diseases and their growing prevalence worldwide.
Challenges in chronic disease management	Key issues like real-time monitoring, adherence to treatment, and early diagnosis.
Role of AI in healthcare	How AI is transforming healthcare with predictive analytics, personalized treatment, and automation.
Wearable technology for healthcare	Introduction to wearable health devices and their applications in tracking vital signs, physical activity, and medication adherence.
Integration of AI & wearables	How AI enhances wearable technology for continuous health monitoring, anomaly detection, and decision support.
Significance of the study	The impact of AI-driven wearables on early disease detection, remote patient monitoring, and reducing healthcare costs.
Research objectives	The key goals of the study, such as evaluating AI-powered wearables' efficiency, exploring predictive capabilities, and assessing patient outcomes.
Scope of the study	The focus areas, including target diseases (diabetes, cardiovascular diseases, etc.), technological advancements, and future research directions.

analytics improve the management of chronic illnesses. Personalized recommendations and feedback are offered by wearable technology driven by AI, using techniques like content-based filtering, collaborative filtering, RL, regression analysis, and decision trees. AI-powered insights enable clinicians to make informed, evidence-based decisions regarding patient care, leading to personalized treatment, reduced errors, and improved patient outcomes.

This work offers a fresh method using many ML technologies to close these gaps. These technologies provide several tools and approaches that can make data more dependable, private, secure, and compatible. Our strategy has to include ML as it provides several answers to the issues related to wearable artificial intelligence technologies linked with the control of chronic diseases. Kalman filters and Bayesian networks will help us remove noise and inconsistencies in the sensor data, therefore improving the quality and reliability of the data. These techniques improve data quality by use of past observations predicting when values would be missing or erroneous. We employ anomaly detection methods such Isolation Forest and Autoencoders in addition to these filters to provide additional dependability to health monitoring systems. These systems may find abnormalities or faults in real-time data and filter out maybe dangerous sensor outputs.

With help of FL, we can also address the privacy issue. By allowing wearables to train AI models locally instead of sending private medical data to central servers, FL has the potential to allay privacy worries. This privacy-preserving technology stores data on the device even while accurate and customized models for controlling chronic illness are being developed. Transfer learning allows one to improve interoperability by altering AI models for usage in various wearable technologies and healthcare applications. This facilitates the utilization of data from many sources, even if they are in various forms—to enhance clinical judgment. Finally, we increase user motivation via RL. Its dynamic, tailored patient encouraging strategies help to increase user engagement and adherence. Rewarding consumers for positive behavior may help to raise long-term involvement. Using explainable AI techniques such as SHAP and LIME will help improve clinical validation and raise patient and provider confidence in the recommendations of the technology. These methods simplify AI predictions for understanding.

WEARABLE AI TECHNOLOGY APPLICATIONS IN CHRONIC DISEASE CARE

By tracking variances in heart rate and atrial fibrillation symptoms, wearable devices with ECG functions can assist detect cardiac problems. When a user's heart rate veers from normal range, artificial intelligence systems may notify them. Wearable technology with artificial intelligence is very important in diabetes management as gadgets like the Dexcom G6 constantly monitor blood glucose levels.

Diabetic care

Without a question, the most important piece of advice for diabetics is on properly controlling blood sugar levels. Including artificial intelligence into wearable technology has produced continuous glucose monitors (CGMs), which let users examine trends and predictions and provide real-time glucose level data. AI systems may suggest changes to insulin doses, meals, and exercise to help to maintain consistent blood glucose levels.

Cardiac and vascular wellness

Wearable devices with artificial intelligence can continuously monitor blood pressure, electrocardiograms (ECG), and vital indicators like heart rate. Artificial intelligence-powered algorithms can identify abnormal cardiac rhythms, project the course of cardiovascular disease, and indicate potential diseases such atrial fibrillation or hypertension. Such round-the-clock observation helps with patient management, therefore lowering the possibility of further major cardiovascular events.

Management of respiratory conditions

Patients with chronic obstructive pulmonary disease (COPD) or asthma might find wearable artificial intelligence devices tracking heart rates, oxygen levels, and airflow patterns useful. In a perfect scenario, artificial intelligence models might advise changes to medications, forecast when flare-ups would strike, and even provide real-time feedback to enable patients to remain out of the hospital and manage their conditions.

Control your blood pressures

These gadgets provide a real-time measurement of blood pressure variations and identify hypertensive crises. Artificial intelligence systems may assist patients prevent or control hypertension by means of tailored advice for lifestyle modifications and medicines based on monitoring their blood pressure and trends over time as well as their risk profile.

Watching chronic kidney disease (CKD)

Wearable devices may help monitor electrolyte levels, fluid intake and output, and crucial electrocardiograms (ECGs) in treatment of chronic kidney disease (CKD).

OPERATION OF THE SUGGESTED MODEL

Using complex patterns and correlations found in this data, DNNs help to more precisely predict a patient's health state, identify possible dangers, and recommend certain treatments. Customized therapy may be created using RL. FL for models of training with protection of privacy. Based on wearable equipment tracking the patient's blood sugar, heart rate, or physical activity, the RL agent might offer suggestions. Later on, the system would gather data and change its recommendations in reaction to improved patient condition. Regarding wearable technology driven by artificial intelligence, real time monitoring and prediction is the constant data collection from wearable devices to instantly access a patient's health situation. Given the rapid evaluation of this data, early development of hypotheses on any anomalies or health problems is possible. Using past and current data trend-based ML techniques, it might predict future health events such probability of heart attack or blood sugar rise by usage. Should an abnormality be found, the patients or doctor is informed and advised, therefore enabling rapid response. This method may enhance both the overall outcomes and the management of chronic diseases via the use of proactive treatment and real-time health data. Wearable technology that is powered by artificial intelligence analyzes personal health data using a variety of techniques and provides individualized insights, which may include particular remarks and suggestions.

Compiling and merging data

High-tech sensors integrated in smart wearables controlled by artificial intelligence may gather an electrocardiogram (ECG), heart rate, blood oxygen saturation, glucose level, and other important signs. These devices gather information from several sources to provide the user a realistic view of their health.

Instantaneous data analysis

AI algorithm analyze data in real time, ensuring that processing occurs simultaneously with data collection. If a patient's condition changes unexpectedly, this capability enables rapid detection and facilities timely intervention.

Exercising pattern analysis and forecasting

Using historical and real-time data, each component employs sophisticated learning and data analytics—akin to big data—to learn on its own and spot any health concerns. AI can, for instance, forecast when the blood glucose levels of a diabetic patient will increase or decline, therefore enabling proactive changes to their diet or dosage.

Personalized medical records

AI-based modules allow customized interpretation and recommendation services tailored to the patient's present and future requirements to be delivered. This is important as patient's general health determines their choices. Customization strengthens recommendations and increases their relevance for users.

Notes and notices and alarms sentimentally automatically

Wearables backed by artificial intelligence might instantly notify patients and healthcare professionals of hazardous readings. These alerts enable quick responses that help to reduce the possibility of undesirable consequences (Figure 7.1).

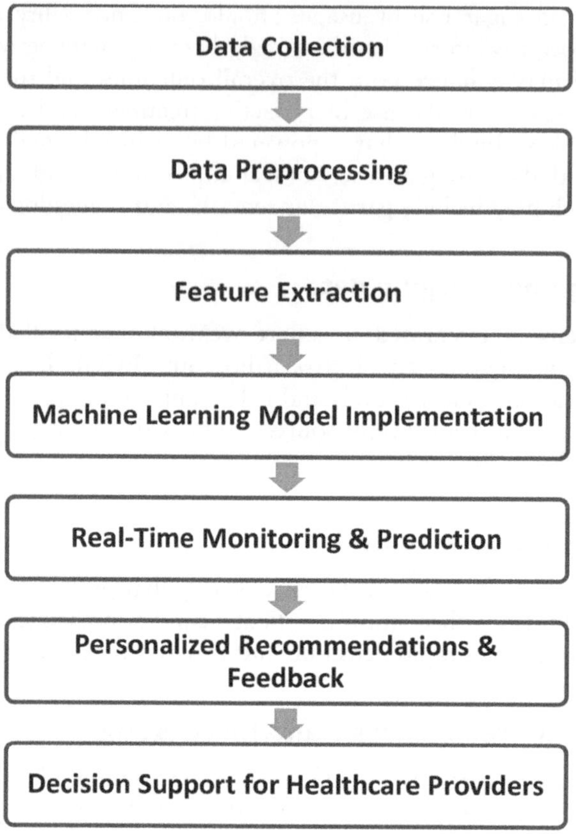

Figure 7.1 Flow chart of work flow.

TOOLS AND TECHNIQUES

Our solution for the particular challenge of sporting equipment motivated by artificial intelligence included many methods.

1. **Bayesian network:** By use of a Bayesian network, the uncertainty and interactions among many health factors such as activity levels, and other important indicators are forecast. A collection of variables coupled with their conditional connections is revealed by using DAG in BN, a probabilistic graphical model. In wearable technology, Bayesian networks recreate the degree of uncertainty and correlations across many health data such as heart rate, blood sugar, activity level, and other crucial indications.
2. **Kalman filter:** A linear dynamic system's state may be estimated from a set of noisy observations using a Kalman filter. It iteratively updates

its estimation of the system based on new inputs. When it comes to processing data from sensors that are susceptible to noise or mistakes, Kalman filters are invaluable in wearable devices. This ensures that patients with chronic diseases get accurate readings.

3. **Federated learning:** FL lets wearable technology constantly secure health data on the wearable device by localizing ML models on the user's device. Just sharing the model modifications with a central server maintains the data safe and private.
4. **DNNs:** DNNs are well suited for handling huge. High-dimensional datasets created by wearable medical devices for treatment of chronic conditions. DNNs may predict the future health of the user by means of data analysis, therefore considering prospective health dangers or flare-ups of current diseases.
5. **Reinforcement learning (RL):** Long term care for chronic illnesses frequently entails individualized treatment regiments that incorporate dietary, physical activity. Medication and lifestyle modifications.

RESULTS AND DISCUSSION

In this study, we explore the outcomes of using wearable AI to treat chronic illnesses, keeping in mind RL, DNN, FL, and Kalman Filters, among other ML methodologies. Diabetes, heart disease, and high blood pressure are long-term conditions that might benefit from better monitoring, decision-making, prediction, and personalization thanks to the integration. When compared to more conventional ML models, DNN produced more accurate predictions for medical occurrences such as hypoglycemia, heart attacks, and asthma episodes. Wearable glucose, accelerometer, and ECG monitors provide massive amounts of high-dimensional data, which DNN may analyze to provide early warnings of potential health hazards. With 95% accuracy, the computer predicted bouts of low blood sugar by analyzing activity, insulin consumption, and blood sugar levels. The DNN model discovered early warning signs of cardiac events using real-time ECG and heart rate variability data with a sensitivity of 92% and specificity of 94%. Data security and patient privacy are two of the biggest issues with healthcare IT today. FL circumvents this problem by enabling model training without access to raw health data. By combining data from many sources, this method increases system resilience while protecting the privacy of sensitive health information, and it produces more accurate and widely applicable estimates for different patient groups. Evidence suggests that personalized treatment regimens benefit substantially from RL's incorporation. The continuous feedback method increased treatment adherence by giving patients more agency in their own healthcare decisions. In order to improve the treatment of chronic conditions, the system should be able to adjust medication doses and exercise programs based on real-time data, among other user-defined demands.

Despite the promising results, the present research is not without its flaws. The accuracy of the predictions made by the DNN and RL models may be compromised in real-world scenarios due to factors such as sensor noise or missing data, notwithstanding their good performance. Although it is still dependent on the quality of the sensor data, the system shown improvement when using advanced data filtering methods such as Kalman Filters. More study is also needed to assess the long-term consequences of these AI-powered solutions on the treatment of chronic conditions.

FUTURE SCOPE

Wearable technology driven by AI might transform future treatment of chronic diseases. Development in AI algorithms will enable more accurate real-time forecasts, early illness diagnosis, and tailored treatment suggestions. Data exchange made simpler by better interoperability with EHR can help to enhance clinical decision-making. As telemedicine and remote patient monitoring expand and proactive continuous care will be promoted, people will visit hospitals less often. Next generation biosensors will also provide more exact and thorough physiological data including non-invasive glucose monitoring and real-time biomarker tracking. Wearables driven by artificial intelligence must be easily available and reasonably priced for everyone, including those living in low-income environments if we are to fully use them. Future research should focus on user acceptance tactics, reasonably priced solutions and global scalability to guarantee broad influence.

SUMMARY

Examining how wearable technology and AI can transform the treatment of chronic diseases. It demonstrates how wearables with artificial intelligence capabilities may improve predictive analytics, tailored care and real-time monitoring allowing early detection and treatment of ailments like diabetes, high blood pressure and cardiovascular diseases. The studies show how these technologies could enable early health problem diagnosis, reduced frequency of hospital visits, and continuous data collection ease-of use. Apart from the need for easily accessible, fairly priced solutions in different health care environments. By enabling more accurate health monitoring and real-time decision-making, the mix of 5G connectivity, edge computing and next generation biosensors promises to boost wearable capabilities. The findings of the research show how wearable with AI capabilities might revolutionize the management of chronic diseases, hence improving patient outcomes and reducing world healthcare expenditures.

BIBLIOGRAPHY

1. Beck RW, Riddlesworth T, Ruedy K, et al. Effect of continuous glucose monitoring on glycemic control in adults with type 1 diabetes using insulin injections: the DIAMOND randomized clinical trial. *JAMA*. 2017; 317: 371–378. doi: 10.1001/jama.2016.19975
2. Bent B, Goldstein BA, Kibbe WA, et al. Investigating sources of inaccuracy in wearable optical heart rate sensors. *NPJ Digit Med*. 2020; 3: 18. doi: 10.1038/s41746-020-0226-6
3. Vijayan V, Connolly JP, Condell J, et al. Review of wearable devices and data collection considerations for connected health. *Sensors (Basel)*. 2021; 21: 5589. doi: 10.3390/s21165589
4. Silva BM, Rodrigues JJ, de la Torre Díez I, et al. Mobile-health: A review of current state in 2015. *J Biomed Inform*. 2015; 56: 265–272. doi: 10.1016/j.jbi.2015.06.003
5. Mercer K, Giangregorio L, Schneider E, et al. Acceptance of commercially available wearable activity trackers among adults aged over 50 and with chronic illness: A mixed-methods evaluation. *JMIR Mhealth Uhealth*. 2016; 4: e7. doi: 10.2196/mhealth.4225
6. Izmailova ES, Wagner JA, Perakslis ED. Wearable devices in clinical trials: Hype and hypothesis. *Clin Pharmacol Ther*. 2018; 104: 42–52. doi: 10.1002/cpt.966
7. Pan HY, Lee CK, Liu TY, et al. The role of wearable home blood pressure monitoring in detecting out-of-office control status. *Hypertens Res*. 2024; 47: 1033–1041. doi: 10.1038/s41440-023-01539-w
8. Whelton PK, Carey RM, Aronow WS, et al. Guideline for the prevention, detection, evaluation, and management of high blood pressure in adults: A report of the American College of Cardiology/American Heart Association Task Force on Clinical Practice Guidelines. *Hypertension*. 2018; 71: e13–e115. doi: 10.1161/HYP.0000000000000065
9. Hamine S, Gerth-Guyette E, Faulx D, et al. Impact of mHealth chronic disease management on treatment adherence and patient outcomes: A systematic review. *J Med Internet Res*. 2015; 17(2): e52.
10. Subramanian M, Wojtusciszyn A, Favre L, et al. Precision medicine in the era of artificial intelligence: Implications in chronic disease management. *J Transl Med*. 2020; 18(1): 472.
11. Contreras I, Vehi J. Artificial intelligence for diabetes management and decision support: Literature review. *J Med Internet Res*. 2018; 20(5): e10775.
12. Buekers J, Theunis J, De Boever P, et al. Wearable finger pulse oximetry for continuous oxygen saturation measurements during daily home routines of patients with chronic obstructive pulmonary disease (COPD) over one week: Observational study. *JMIR Mhealth Uhealth*. 2019; 7(6): e12866.
13. Mekov E, Miravitlles M, Petkov R, et al. Artificial intelligence and machine learning in respiratory medicine. *Expert Rev Respir Med*. 2020; 14(6): 559–564.
14. Song Y, Min J, Gao W, et al. Wearable and implantable electronics: Moving toward precision therapy. *ACS Nano*. 2019; 13(11): 12280–12286.
15. Cheung CC, Krahn AD, Andrade JG, et al. The emerging role of wearable technologies in detection of arrhythmia. *Can J Cardiol*. 2018; 34(8): 1083–1087.
16. Guo Y, Liu X, Chen W, et al. A review of wearable and unobtrusive sensing technologies for chronic disease management. *Comput Biol Med*. 2021; 129: 104163.
17. Lin LF, Lin YJ, Lin YH, et al. Feasibility and efficacy of wearable devices for upper limb rehabilitation in patients with chronic stroke: A randomized controlled pilot study. *Eur J Phys Rehabil Med*. 2018; 54(3): 388–396.

18. Koydemir HC, Ozcan A. Wearable and implantable sensors for biomedical applications. *Annu Rev Anal Chem (Palo Alto Calif)*. 2018; 11(1): 127–146.
19. Xie Y, Zhang J, Wang H, et al. Applications of blockchain in the medical field: Narrative review. *J Med Internet Res*. 2021; 23(10): e28613.
20. Zheng X, Sun S, Ordieres-Meré J, et al. Accelerating health data sharing: A solution based on the internet of things and distributed ledger technologies. *J Med Internet Res*. 2019; 21(6): e13583.
21. Kaspar G, Sanam K, Gholkar G, et al. Long-term use of the wearable cardioverter defibrillator in patients with explanted ICD. *Int J Cardiol*. 2018; 272(1): 179–184.
22. Tsukada YT, Tokita M, Iwasaki Y, et al. Validation of wearable textile electrodes for ECG monitoring. *Heart Vessels*. 2019; 34(7): 1203–1211.
23. Abe Y, Ito M, Tanaka C, et al. A novel and simple method using pocket-sized echocardiography to screen for aortic stenosis. *J Am Soc Echocardiogr*. 2013; 26: 589–596.
24. Thoenes M, Agarwal A, Grundmann D, et al. Narrative review of the role of artificial intelligence to improve aortic valve disease management. *J Thorac Dis*. 2021; 13(1): 396–404.
25. Barrett M, Boyne J, De Wit K, et al. Artificial intelligence supported patient self-care in chronic heart failure: a paradigm shift from reactive to predictive, preventive and personalised care. *EPMA J*. 2019; 10(4): 445–464.
26. Fan X, Yao Q, Li Y, et al. Multiscaled fusion of deep convolutional neural networks for screening atrial fibrillation from single lead short ECG recordings. *IEEE J Biomed Health Inform*. 2018; 22(6): 1744–1753.
27. Kaplan A, Cao H, Kocks JWH, et al. Artificial intelligence/machine learning in respiratory medicine and potential role in asthma and COPD diagnosis. *J Allergy Clin Immunol Pract*. 2021; 9(6): 2255–2261.
28. Colantonio S, Govoni L, Vitacca M, et al. Decision making concepts for the remote, personalized evaluation of COPD patients' health status. *Methods Inf Med*. 2015; 54(3): 240–247.
29. Bugajski A, Lengerich A, Szalacha L, et al. Utilizing an artificial neural network to predict self-management in patients with chronic obstructive pulmonary disease: An exploratory analysis. *J Nurs Scholarsh*. 2021; 53(1): 16–24.
30. Tomita K, Nagao R, Tohda Y, et al. Deep learning facilitates the diagnosis of adult asthma. *Allergol Int*. 2019; 68(4): 456–461.

Chapter 8

Digital twin and digital triplet technology in healthcare

Benefits and security considerations

Priyanka Tyagi, Neelam Shrivastava, Kajol Mittal, Garima Saini, and Shitharth Selvarajan

INTRODUCTION

A digital twin (DT) is a virtual representation of a physical object. It might also be characterised as a digital representation of hypothetical or actual processes, people, places, systems, and equipment. The term 'DT' first originated in 2003 in the field of product lifecycle management, since digital representations of physical things were in their early stages. By creating a DT of an existing product on the market, manufacturers may watch activities, gather data on the constellation of circumstances that indicate that the equipment requires repair, and begin developing predictive maintenance models [6]. The concept of a DT emerged as a result of the slow growth of early kinds of physical and digital item interaction, known as digital models and digital shadows. A digital model is a virtual depiction of a physical system that does not exchange data with its real counterpart [4]. A digital shadow is a more advanced variant of the digital model that incorporates a one-way communication link between the physical system and its virtual equivalent. This technique allows the physical model to convey data resulting from a state change to the virtual object, but not the other way around [4, 7].

DTs virtualise hospitals in medical settings, providing a safe environment in which to study the impact of changes on hospital performance without jeopardising the real facility. This allows healthcare practitioners to carefully construct the DT and provide precise estimates and recommendations for individual patients. Cloud technology enables real-time patient data collecting, while AI components evaluate massive volumes of data to run algorithms and generate precise predictions [9].

A DT is used in a range of healthcare contexts, including patient care, medical device or system operations, and healthcare provider operations. IT (Information Technology) and data professionals can use DT, which are very exact virtual duplicates of genuine equipment, locations, or systems, to replicate an entity's activities before it occurs or to track an existing thing in real time. Furthermore, the twin aids with data visualisation and its link to the object being represented. With the potential to significantly disrupt the sector, as it has in other industries such as automobiles, DT technology has

DOI: 10.1201/9781003634560-8

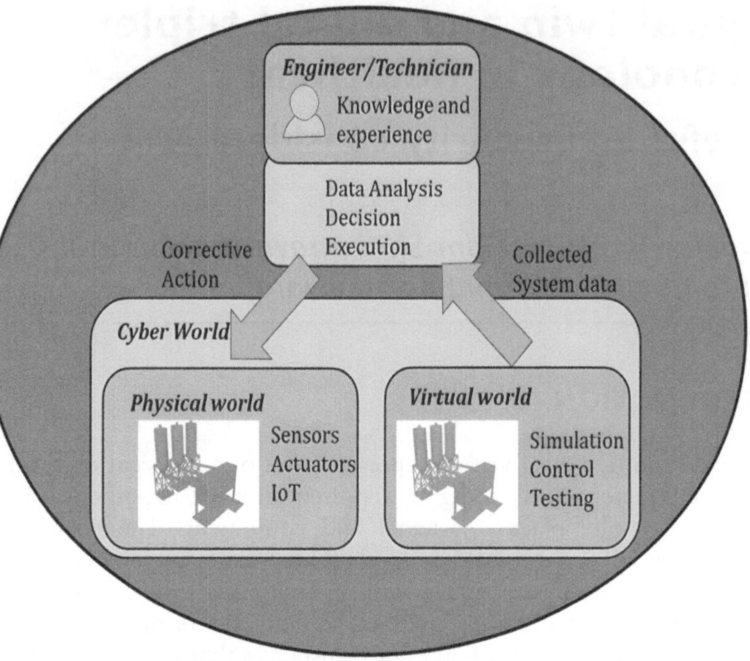

Figure 8.1 Digital twin healthcare reference model [1].

emerged as the most effective approach to addressing these challenges [5]. Cloud-based virtual twins allow for more cooperation and offer significant technology benefits such as efficient research, predictable production, and enhanced medical treatment. Figure 8.1 depicts both actual and abstract entities that are connected to the internet.

The healthcare industry has swiftly adopted digital technology, improving patient care and altering the way things should be done. As virtual healthcare services gain popularity, traditional healthcare providers are collaborating with technology businesses to construct infrastructure and obtain the skills required. The worldwide healthcare industry improves as it deals with the issues posed by COVID-19. However, the pandemic's massive consequences have altered it, and it is now driven by the new opportunities it has revealed. Unexpected fluctuations in workload and test cancellations cause significant issues for hospitals and their patients. Imaging tools should be functional and quick to access when needed. System failures that occur unexpectedly can be costly, cause patients to wait longer and suffer more, and harm the result of their treatment. As a result, DT must be employed to address a variety of healthcare issues [6]. Medical supplies and medications are in higher demand than ever. Costs of development, time to market, and earnings are all increasing. Millions of individuals throughout the world now have access to life-saving medications. To address these issues, tech-based methods of testing medical devices have been developed so that they do not need to be tested on humans during the development phase. This procedure is quick, safe, and inexpensive. Collaboration is the most effective strategy to leverage DT technology. To create a high-fidelity, efficient DT, hospital administrators, doctors, administrative personnel, architectural architects, and technological partners must collaborate. A committee of professionals from several sectors routinely reviews the DT to ensure accurate information and smoother hospital operations. A DT can assist plan modifications or additions to care units, avoiding costly alterations once departments are reorganised.

Digital triplet

The Digital Triplet concept seeks to address two difficulties in the Japanese manufacturing industry:

- Adoption of digitisation may not be consistent with present practices. Japanese engineering mentality, which may diminish its merits.
- Engineers and technicians struggled to adapt to digitisation since it required applying their expertise and experience to both physical and virtual systems.

Previously, system upgrades were limited to physical production systems. However, such activities must now take place in both the virtual and actual worlds. The Digital Triplet idea brings together physical, virtual, and intelligent activity settings. Figure 8.1 depicts the Digital Triplet design, which incorporates an intelligent activity layer into the basic DT.

Digital Triplet was developed as a concept and provides a vast field of inquiry into prospective implementation techniques and applications. Digital Triplet provides a broad field of inquiry by focussing on practical implementation options and their applications. One such implementation approach uses machine learning modules in the intelligent activity layer and machine-to-machine communication to provide the necessary links between tiers. Machine learning, which has a growing body of research with a broad spectrum of applicability in industry, is a crucial contributor in achieving the Industry 4.0 goal [6].

BENEFITS OF DIGITAL TWIN TECHNOLOGY IN HEALTHCARE

The healthcare industry has swiftly adopted digital technology, improving patient care and altering the way things should be done. As virtual healthcare services gain popularity, traditional healthcare providers are collaborating with technology businesses to construct infrastructure and obtain the skills required. The worldwide healthcare industry improves as it deals with the issues posed by COVID-19. However, the pandemic's massive consequences have altered it, and it is now propelled by the new opportunities it has created [7]. Unexpected fluctuations in workload and test cancellations cause significant issues for hospitals and their patients. Imaging tools should be functional and quick to access when needed. Unplanned system breakdown downtime can be costly, cause patients to wait longer and experience more pain, and harm the outcome of their therapy. As a result, DT must be employed to address a variety of healthcare issues. Medical supplies and medications are in higher demand than ever. Costs of development, time to market, and earnings are all increasing.

Millions of individuals throughout the world are now finding it even more difficult to obtain life-saving therapies. To address these issues, individuals are developing technological methods for testing medical equipment. This method avoids testing on humans during the development phase and is rapid, safe, and inexpensive [7]. Figure 8.2 depicts the greatest outcomes from utilising DT techniques with others. To create a high-fidelity, efficient DT, hospital administrators, doctors, administrative personnel, architectural architects, and technological partners must collaborate. A committee of professionals from several sectors routinely reviews the DT to ensure accurate information and smoother hospital operations [8]. A DT can assist in the planning of alterations and additions to care units, making adjustments that are required once departments are reorganised less expensive.

The following section highlights some of the key advantages of implementing DT technology in the healthcare industry.

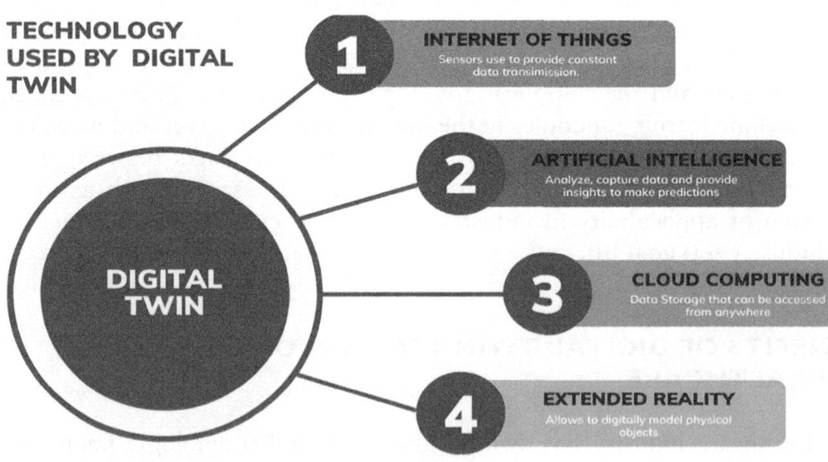

Figure 8.2 Technology used by digital twin.

Patient care

Predictive maintenance using DTs boosts the performance and accessibility of low-cost assets including imaging, lab automation, and surgical robots. Effective resource management extends beyond medical equipment, procedures, and workers. It might be improved at the hospital, university, or public health network levels [9]. The most promising use of DTs in healthcare might be tailored therapy. DT applications are currently commonly employed in a variety of sectors. DT technologies assist a wide range of sectors in identifying possibilities for innovation and improving business operations and performance by providing exact virtual representations of goods and operational process simulations.

Better personal health outcomes

The DT evaluates physiological and behavioural data to help in the early diagnosis of chronic illness, allowing for better chronic disease treatment in huge populations. Advances in artificial intelligence technology enable a DT to represent a complex system, process, or place rather than a single object or component. Simulation improves operations and the patient experience by minimising wait times, managing emergency services more effectively, optimising lab and medical equipment utilisation, and reducing device downtime. As a consequence, hospital management can track everything from patients to physicians, data to processes, all from a single platform.

Healthcare forecasting

Researchers can determine the best effective therapeutic technique while avoiding injuring actual patients. A complex ecosystem of interconnected moving pieces, including hospitals, emerges to suit the needs of patients, carers, and healthcare professionals. Patient admissions and discharges occur often. People go to visit their families. Healthcare professionals go between patients and wards. Supplies are continually provided. It's challenging to keep up with all of this energy and movement. Hospitals will face new problems in optimising operations, controlling risks, allocating resources efficiently, and ensuring safety and security.

Diagnostics and medical training

A DT is a patient model created prior to the real therapy. To avoid causing injury to human anatomy, a multidisciplinary team use virtual surgery in medical training and diagnostics. This real-time model allows trainees to mimic surgery on patients in order to better grasp their physiological and anatomical characteristics. The same technology used to identify chronic illnesses may also be used to create medical DTs. AI-driven research and

DTs will benefit hospitals and research facilities all around the world, improving health, education, and economic prospects through technology improvements. Many more firms and sectors will employ DTs to digitise their operations, necessitating a distributed, hybrid, and multi-cloud architecture. They will require a technology partner who can supply the necessary hardware, software, and integration services for data management while protecting the data, simulation, and the actual product, method, or person depicted in the real world.

SECURITY CONSIDERATIONS FOR DIGITAL TWIN AND TRIPLET TECHNOLOGY IN HEALTHCARE

Threats to security against DTs can be classified according to their attack surface, which includes system vulnerabilities, communication vulnerabilities, and data storage vulnerabilities. Ensuring the availability and accessibility of DTs is critical for security reasons. The key elements contributing to considerable dangers in Internet of Things (IoT) devices are rigorous operating requirements and limited processing capacity [11]. When access to the DT is lost, it can cause production interruption and significant financial losses. Maintaining data integrity is critical to ensuring accuracy and preventing unauthorised changes. Product integrity challenges can result in biased appraisal and decision-making, creating serious risks.

Physical threats

Physical security for IoT devices is crucial since they are vulnerable to being hacked, made unworkable, or stolen by an attacker. Because of their physical component linkages, the systems require different security measures than ordinary networks and systems [14]. Defects in critical items can result in death, injury, or environmental harm. As a result, safety may be seen as the most critical need [15]. Safety is typically described as the act of preventing damage or risk to the physical environment and infrastructure that may occur from system malfunctions.

Data modification threats

Physical devices can utilise a range of technologies to protect their data against alteration, such as tamper-proof and tamper-resistant hardware. However, the attacker can still change the data. Data adjustments may be necessary owing to significant changes in predictions and analysis. Data can be manipulated by data poisoning attacks or by exploiting system, application, and communication weaknesses (Table 8.1).

Table 8.1 Digital twin threads and countermeasures

Threats	*Countermeasures*
Physical threats	Physical Security
Data Modification threats	Tamper-proof and tamper-resistant hardware; Hash, blockchain, IPFS
Software threats	Software hardening; Secure SDLC; Security testing
Data communication threats	Network Resiliency; Cryptographic solutions; Blockchain; Firewall; IDS
System threats	Firewall, Access control; IDS; Antimalware; System hardening
Data storing threats	Cryptographic solutions
Machine learning threats	Data sanitization; Algorithm robustness enhancement; Security Assessment Mechanisms; Privacy Preserving Techniques

System threats

The implementation of DT and triplet virtual layer software occurs on a system that may create a number of dangers and vulnerabilities. Threats to the virtual layer may have an influence on the operating system. An attacker can use operating system flaws to take entire control of the DT and triplet software, or get a copy of it. There are several risks and assaults that may be conducted by via rogue software. These might cause total denial of service (DoS) and substantial losses in DT and triplet-based smart manufacturing systems. Ransomware concerns have pushed certain sectors to shift from smart to conventional production processes. Furthermore, malicious software like as Winery has the ability to compromise industrial control and operating systems [16].

Software threats

Unauthorised access to the DT and triplet software, as well as source code, might have major effects because these digital representations serve as the blueprint for the real system. As a consequence, the attacker will be able to examine and discover the system's flaws. The attacker may potentially get access to back-end systems [17]. For example, smart manufacturing is an economically competitive industry. The DT contains data, statistics, and models of the real item. Attackers who get access to early versions of DT and triplet software may represent a risk to intellectual property and corporate secrets. The attacker can acquire access to the DT software or source code through a variety of means. Insiders can copy software. Insiders, whether purposeful or not, constitute a substantial danger to security, resulting in direct violations [18]. Poor coding might result in inadequate software protection. Insufficient software security can enable attackers to get the system's source code using reverse engineering techniques.

Data communication threats

The DT and triplets are built from a large number of heterogeneous components that are assembled into nodes. These components communicate data via a variety of protocols and interfaces. Security problems with common communication methods are extensively documented [19]. Furthermore, IoT and cloud computing have a number of well-documented security and privacy flaws. For example, limited resources in IoT devices might lead to significant vulnerabilities in IoT data transport protocols. Similarly, data transfer from or to the cloud might pose considerable hazards. Data communication risks are divided into five categories: man-in-the-middle (MITM) attacks, DoS and DDOS, eavesdropping, spoofing, and replay assaults. An MITM attack allows the attacker to covertly inject malicious code across communication nodes or disclose the ongoing discussion between any two communicating nodes [11]. Many protocols and technologies are susceptible to MITM attacks. Wi-Fi security weaknesses enable wireless key reinstallation attacks, which expose sensitive data. MITM attacks can undermine Bluetooth and ZigBee technologies. DoS and DDOS attacks are among the most significant risks to the DT's availability and accessibility. Unexpected data amount and size might disrupt the system. DOS can occur via flooding the network with traffic, sending incorrect data, or shutting down services using a hacked system component [14]. Jamming assaults, which include repeatedly or randomly broadcasting certain radio frequencies, can impede data delivery. Similarly, spectrum sensing data creation attacks cause DoS.

Unsecured IoT devices can be seized and exploited to execute DDoS attacks. Additionally, eavesdropping attacks can collect network communications from sensors to controllers. This sort of passive attack allows the attacker to learn about the communications between sensors and controllers [17]. This exploit directly compromises the confidentiality of sensitive data during transmission. Furthermore, the collected information can be used to conduct more major attacks. A spoofing attack happens when an attacker alters and conceals his identity in order to conduct hostile and deceptive activities. There are various spoofing attack vectors that target Supervisory Control and Data Acquisition (SCADA) systems. Another method is to modify the wireless sensor network node in order to gain network access or divert network traffic. Spoofing can corrupt the signals or messages sent from sensors to the controller [17]. A replay attack is a post-attack that follows a pre-attack in which the attacker watches, reads, and stores a set of data for retransmission. As a result, the retransmitted signal or data may induce malicious activity on sensors or controllers [19]. This replay assault was used as an advanced persistent threat to Iranian nuclear plants' SCADA systems. The assault is referred to as the Stuxnet worm [20, 21]. Similar attacks might be used to target additional critical infrastructures and industrial systems in the future.

Data storage threats

The majority of data storage operations for DT applications occur in the cloud. Stored data is sensitive and vulnerable to a range of dangers. When cloud computing is hacked, data breaches occur. There are various trust and privacy problems involved with data storage, especially in the public cloud, where the service provider organisation has total authority. However, data may also be stored in distributed file systems using methods such as IPFS (Interplanetary File System).

Threats to data storage

The majority of data for DT and triplet applications is stored on the cloud. Stored data is sensitive and vulnerable to a range of dangers. When cloud computing is hacked, data breaches occur. There are various trust and privacy problems involved with data storage, especially in the public cloud, where the service provider organisation has total authority. However, data may also be stored in distributed file systems using methods such as IPFS (Interplanetary File System).

DIGITAL TWIN USE CASES IN THE MEDICAL DOMAIN

The Patient's DT is designed to capture continuous data from the individual, including vital signs, medical status, reaction to treatment, therapy, and the surrounding environment. Each patient's data is kept in the Azure or AWS public clouds and sent to the DT platform. The ML system uses each patient's past and real-time data to forecast future health difficulties. The concept uses chronic diabetes patients' lifestyle, daily eating habits, and blood sugar data to alert them to prescriptions, dietary habit changes, physician consultations, and so on. Thus, DT uses a large quantity of rich data from numerous IoMT devices and AI-powered models to produce more tailored and effective treatment plans [28]. Each patient's unique DT helps them choose the appropriate prescription, anticipate the outcome of a procedure, and manage their chronic condition by harnessing insights from past data. Consider the following scenario: a patient with heart failure requires Cardiac Resynchronisation Therapy (CRT) through a pacemaker implant. Few people do not respond to the treatment because their hearts differ. Furthermore, for the right patients, the placement must be correct to avoid future issues. A DT of the patient's heart is created by combining the patient's MRI, ECG, and blood pressure data, allowing cardiologists to define the position of leads and virtually experiment with their placement before to intervention surgery. Another example is cancer treatment decision assistance, which assists in selecting the proper therapy. The DT, which incorporates the patient's imaging data, genetic data, and laboratory results, helps the practitioner determine the optimal treatment choice, whether surgery, radiation therapy, or hormone therapy. To treat chronic disease in a large population, DT examines physiological and behavioural data to identify chronic disease early.

FUTURE DIRECTIONS OF DIGITAL TWIN TECHNOLOGY IN HEALTHCARE

AI collects and evaluates data, which is subsequently recorded on blockchain. Nowadays, technological twinning is becoming increasingly hybridised. However, digital twinning has a number of problems that jeopardise its widespread adoption, including the handling of private and sensitive data, as well as networked devices, which are a popular target for hackers. As a result, governments and policymakers must examine both legal and regulatory factors while developing more secure data-sharing methods. Because information is the foundation of DTs, quality assurance methods must be implemented in real-world physical structures to integrate data with replicated processes (twins) and assure correct DT mode operation. The adoption of DT technology will enable future productivity improvements while also reducing risk in a variety of situations, such as those involving actual things, data, and virtual models, as well as the most complicated challenges in an artificial environment. DT technology allows for the analysis of physical and real-time photographs, as well as the improvement of therapeutic suggestions. In the future, however, there are other limits, including the usage of widely available data, which may serve as a baseline and change with time. This quick research demonstrates that the emerging notion of DTs in healthcare offers enormous promise during the COVID-19 pandemic. The broad use of DT technology in everyday clinical practice impedes the advancement of clinical processes and patient care in healthcare institutions. The makers of 'Cardio Twin' expect that their technology may be able to prevent heart disease (IHD) and stroke in the future [23]. As DT technology advances in the medical field, we may anticipate everyone on the planet to be able to receive highly tailored medical treatment and care at a fair cost [20, 21]. DT is currently in its early stages of development in the agriculture business.

DT can be used in agriculture for:

1. Storing and collecting data,
2. Categorising actions in complex workflows,
3. Automated data analysis,
4. Learning and measuring soil content and capacity,
5. Simulating crop outcomes,
6. Predicting weather, and
7. Recognising resource stress caused by factors such as invasive plants and animals, soil quality, pollution, and so on [23].

As space technology advances, engineers and scientists must make these trips more sustainable so that humans may fly deeper into space. The Commonwealth Scientific and Industrial Research Organisation (CSIRO) [26], Australia's national science agency, which has been working on DT solutions for mining operations, plans to develop DTs to aid mining processes in future space exploration by collaborating with Australian and international space agencies to make space operations more sustainable. More and more national and regional authorities are interested in constructing DTs in their cities. Cities with their own DT will benefit from better planning and management. The government will be able to better serve its constituents and handle concerns faster. These cities' DTs provide an added benefit in the case of natural disasters such as earthquakes, cyclones, and tsunamis, among others. Cities' DTs can be valuable in times of emergency, such as global pandemics, because several cities can swiftly communicate their local plans and status via DT [27]. In the future, DT technology can be used with other technologies to obtain better results; for example, mixed reality and DT technology can be utilised to improve DT visualisation and remotely supervised inspections [27]. Aside from that, DT is being used in the educational sector. Sepasgoza [27] demonstrated how combining DT with augmented and virtual reality (AR/VR) can be used to develop digital pedagogy for architecture, engineering, and construction students, which can be useful for educators delivering remote classes during emergencies such as pandemics or as part of regular online learning.

Humanome

The Humanome is the Copenhagen Institute for Futures Studies' notion of a medical digital triplet. The Humanome model is a personal health profile and data bank based on statistics from the government and private sectors. The individual is at the centre, surrounding by a virtual assistant. Four circles represent groups with specific data that, to varying degrees, impact health status. The top circle represents personal behaviour, which includes information about social media use, physical activity, and eating habits. Biology is the suitable category for data points such as genomes, other omics, and traditional biomarkers. The lowest category contains social components such as population, education, and employment, which include data.

The left circle represents environmental aspects such as climate, pollution, and noise. The outermost circles contain data controls and contracts, as all data movements in accordance with the Humanome must adhere to specific criteria. They cover transparency, traceability, and responsibility for data transit and treatment, as well as interoperability, security, and data safety. Data contracts cover secondary usage, anti-lock-in procedures, permission, donation, data sharing, and data recording. These critical data management safety considerations enable individuals trust companies and each other in a variety of settings. The Humanome is not intended to be a comprehensive database of all existing types of data. It is intended to inspire the kind of data currently available from the human body and its surroundings. Furthermore, the individual is not expected to collect, analyse, and assess all of the Humanome data on their own. A virtual assistant, such as artificial intelligence or a digital interface, might recognise and display both clinical and non-clinical sources of individual data.

CONCLUSION

A DT or triplet is a virtual replica of an actual entity that may be tracked, investigated, and enhanced. When a material thing is represented digitally, it becomes 'live' and 'dynamic', implying that the fundamental item can alter at any time. DT technology dramatically enhances patient care by allowing people to get reliable medical advice, book appointments with skilled medical professionals, electronically transfer drugs to pharmacies, and see doctor's notes and video appointment recordings online. DTs may make it simpler to adapt medical treatments to people based on their genetic composition, physiology, family history, past behaviours, and other aspects. Transportation, energy, and even defence systems will benefit from DTs since they rely heavily on IoT and need decision assistance. It is quite likely that various sorts of DTs will communicate with their physical counterparts as well as with one another. Maintaining the security of these systems is critical, as abuse can cause delays and difficulty in decision-making, with catastrophic repercussions. The safe implementation of DTs across various infrastructures is a key challenge. Such infrastructures are comprised of multiple technologies that are susceptible to a variety of attack vectors. The majority of possible threats provide a considerable danger to security and safety. However, these problems may be handled in a number of ways, as shown in this paper. Metaverse, which mixes VR goggles and other technology with a digital equivalent, is gaining popularity. The security of the metaverse should also be investigated. Further research will concentrate on in-depth threat mitigation and the creation of a comprehensive security architecture for the DT and triplet. Blockchain and smart contracts for metaverse security will also be studied.

BIBLIOGRAPHY

1. Ying Liu, Lin Zhang, Yuan Yang, Longfei Zhou, Lei Ren, Fei Wang, Rong Liu, Zhibo Pang, and M. Jamal Deen. "A novel cloud-based framework for the elderly healthcare services using digital twin." *IEEE Access* 7 (2019): 49088–49101.
2. Haya Elayan, Moayad Aloqaily, and Mohsen Guizani. "Digital twin for intelligent context-aware IoT healthcare systems." *IEEE Internet of Things Journal* 8, no. 23 (2021): 16749–16757.

3. W. Kritzinger, M. Karner, G. Traar, J. Henjes, and W. Sihn. "Digital Twin in manufacturing: A categorical literature review and classification." *IFAC-Papers OnLine* 51 (2018): 1016–1022.
4. F. Caputo, A. Greco, M. Fera, and R. Macchiaroli. "Digital twins to enhance the integration of ergonomics in the workplace design." *International Journal of Industrial Ergonomics* 71 (2019): 20–31.
5. Kalyanasundaram Subramanian. "Digital twin for drug discovery and development—The virtual liver." *Journal of the Indian Institute of Science* 100, no. 4 (2020): 653–662.
6. K. Sivalingam, M. Sepulveda, M. Spring, and P. Davies. "A review and methodology development for remaining useful life prediction of offshore fixed and floating wind turbine power converter with digital twin technology perspective." In *Proceedings of the 2nd International Conference on Green Energy and Applications (ICGEA)*, Singapore, 24–26 March 2018; pp. 197–204.
7. S. Haag and R. Anderl. "Digital twin–proof of concept." *Manufacturing Letters* 15 (2018): 64–66.
8. S. Boschert and R. Rosen. "Digital twin—The simulation aspect." In: Hehenberger, P., & Bradley, D. (eds.), *Mechatronic Futures*. Cham: Springer, 2016, pp. 59–74. doi: 10.1007/978-3-319-32156-1
9. Philippe Moingeon, Marylore Chenel, Cécile Rousseau, Emmanuelle Voisin, and Mickael Guedj. "Virtual patients, digital twins and causal disease models: paving the ground for in silico clinical trials." *Drug Discovery Today* 28 (2023): 103605.
10. F. Tao, J. Cheng, Q. Qi, M. Zhang, H. Zhang, and F. Sui "Digital twin-driven product design, manufacturing and service with big data." *The International Journal of Advanced Manufacturing Technology* 94 (2018): 3563–3576.
11. F. Tao, H. Zhang, A. Liu, and A. Y. C. Nee, "Digital twin in industry: State-of-the-art." *IEEE Transactions on Industrial Informatics* 15, no. 4 (April 2019): 2405–2415.
12. C. R. Monsone and J. Jósvai. "Challenges of digital twin system." *Acta Technica Jaurinensis* 12, no. 3 (2019): 252–267. doi: 10.14513/actatechjaur.v12.n3.514
13. V. Souza, R. Cruz, W. Silva, S. Lins, and V. Lucena. "A digital twin architecture based on the industrial internet of things technologies." In *Proceedings of the IEEE International Conference on Consumer Electronics (ICCE)*, 2019; pp. 1–2. doi: 10.1109/ICCE.2019.8662081
14. F. Tao, F. Sui, A. Liu, Q. Qi, M. Zhang, B. Song, ··· A. Y. Nee. "Digital twin-driven product design framework." *International Journal of Production Research* 57, no. 12 (2019): 3935–3953.
15. X. Lou, Y. Guo, Y. Gao, K. Waedt, and M. Parekh. "An idea of using Digital Twin to perform the functional safety and cybersecurity analysis." In *INFORMATIK 2019: 50 Jahre Gesellschaft für Informatik – Informatik für Gesellschaft (Workshop-Beiträge)*. Bonn: Gesellschaft für Informatik e.V., 23–26 September 2019, pp. 283–294. Standardization of Industry 4.0 Automation and Control Systems. Kassel. doi: 10.18420/inf2019_ws32
16. Q. Qi, F. Tao, T. Hu, N. Anwer, A. Liu, Y. Wei, ··· A. Y. Nee. "Enabling technologies and tools for digital twin." *Journal of Manufacturing Systems* 58 (2019): 3–21. doi: 10.1016/j.jmsy.2019.10.001
17. L. Hu, N. T. Nguyen, W. Tao, M. C. Leu, X. F. Liu, M. R. Shahriar, and S. N. Al Sunny. "Modeling of cloud-based digital twins for smart manufacturing with MT connect." *Procedia Manufacturing* 26 (2018): 1193–1203. doi: 10.1016/j.promfg.2018.07.155
18. F. Tao, M. Zhang, and A. Y. C. Nee. *Digital Twin Driven Smart Manufacturing*. Academic Press, 2019.

19. A. Riku. *Sensor Data Transmission from a Physical Twin to a Digital Twin*. Master, Aalto, 2019.
20. R. Cupek, M. Drewniak, A. Ziebinski, and M. Fojcik. "“Digital twins” for highly customized electronic devices – Case study on a rework operation." *IEEE Access* 7 (2019): 164127–164143.
21. Jaime Ibarra Jimenez, Hamid Jahankhani, and Stefan Kendzierskyj. "Health care in the cyberspace: Medical cyber-physical system and digital twin challenges." In: Farsi, M., Daneshkhah, A., Hosseinian-Far, A., Jahankhani, H. (eds.), *Digital Twin Technologies and Smart Cities. Internet of Things*. Cham: Springer, 2020. doi: 10.1007/978-3-030-18732-3_6
22. A.K. Srivastav and P. Das. "Digital twins in agriculture." In: *Biotechnology and IoT in Agriculture and Food Production*. Berkeley, CA: Apress, 2025. doi: 10.1007/979-8-8688-1469-3_24
23. Y. Maddahi, M. Kalvandi, S. Langman; N. Capicotto, and K. Zareinia. "RoboEthics in COVID-19: A case study in dentistry." *Frontiers in Robotics and AI* 8 (2021): 612740.
24. Kamel Boulos, N. Maged, and Peng Zhang. "Digital twins: from personalised medicine to precision public health." *Journal of Personalized Medicine* 11, no. 8 (2021): 745.
25. W. Shengli. "Is human digital twin possible?" *Computer Methods and Programs in Biomedicine Update* 1 (2021): 100014.
26. Commonwealth Scientific and Industrial Research Organisation (CSIRO), *Digital Twin*, n.d. [Online]: https://www.csiro.au/en/research/technology-space/robotics/Digital-Twin
27. K. Ahmed, P. Pathmanathan, S. Kabadi, J. Doren, N. Kruhlak, A. Lumen, M. Martinez, T. Morrison, P. Schuette, and M. Tegenge. "Successes and opportunities in modeling & simulation for FDA. *US Food and Drug Administration Report*, 2022. https://www.fda.gov/media/163156/download
28. V. Soni, "Digital twin – Top use cases in healthcare," *eInfochips*, March 5, 2021 [Online]. Available: https://www.einfochips.com/blog/digital-twin-top-use-cases-in-healthcare

Chapter 9

Employing deep learning paradigms for fire and smoke detection

Swathi Gowroju, B. Spandana, Kota Harshitha, Jason Das, Umar Faaruk, and Harsh Davey

9.1 INTRODUCTION

Effective detection of fires and smoke is the linchpin for safety and disaster risk mitigation in forests, industrial premises, and residential areas. Conventional techniques, such as smoke identification and temperature measuring sensors, are mostly slow and relatively deficient in the aspects of dynamism and high-risk environments, causing the delayed reactiveness towards any sign of fire, hence relating to lesser reliability. To address this situation, the paper presents an advanced fire and smoke detection system based on the YOLOv11 algorithm that is at the cutting edge of object detection technology.

YOLOv11 is famous for its unprecedented improvement in speed and accuracy and runs multiple kinds of object identification within the same frame, making it suitable for real-time applications.

The system involves video frames from high-quality cameras and utilizes prominent architecture for accurate localization and classification of threats, such as smoke and fire, drawing precise bounding boxes around the area detected. Given its characteristic architecture, it consists of three specific parts: a preprocessing unit, the YOLOv11 detection model, and a postprocessing unit. During preprocessing, the unit is responsible for the input frame, adjusting it through normalization and resizing operations to correspond to the YOLOv11 model. Detection models carry out highly accurate tests for the identification of smoke and fire, while the results are communicated by a postprocessing unit, which creates user alerts in assorted notification forms and plays real-time video with areas regarding detections highlighted.

This top-of-the-line detection system presents a strong and complete solution to the fire and smoke detection challenge. Real-time warnings and rapid approach in case of emergencies mean lower damage, better safety, and improved surveillance within high-stakes environments, a remarkable propulsion of safety technology in modern times.

DOI: 10.1201/9781003634560-9

9.2 RELATED WORKS

The challenges associated with fire detection and smoke detection have gained the most attention from various traditional and modern perspectives. Traditional recognition methods include the use of smoke detectors and many other temperature sensors which have also enjoyed wide acceptance only to be limited by being very dependent on changes in the environmental surroundings concerning heat or density of particles. These have a tendency of small feedback time and therefore can be easily persuaded to make false alarms under dynamic conditions or risky places, such as forests or industrial sites. To confound such challenges, researchers have shifted their focus of attention for later years into the domain of computer vision and deep learning-based detection methods. Many works sought to apply CNN model for fire and smoke detection. One such instance is where CNN architecture has been shown to offer improved accuracy when trained with reasonable and well-balanced data sets of labelled images of fire and non-fire. These systems are nonetheless challenged by how much computational performance they require and the necessarily lengthy assumptions in real time.

YOLO is one of the most widely used real-time object detection algorithms that has popularized this method with high accuracy. Using YOLOv10 in fine-tuning, experiments such as data augmentation, Excitation Attention Mechanism, and momentum optimization based on Stochastic Gradient Descent have been performed by Trong Thua Huynh et al. [1]. The model maintains a reasonable trade-off between speed and accuracy in its predictions, thereby making it viable for time-critical applications.

In their earlier forms, YOLO models have been applied in fire and smoke alarm-type applications, showing good performance under static backgrounds, while not being very good in managing complex and dynamic conditions. The recent trend involves putting greater attention measures and optimization methods to attain improved performance of the models with increased accuracy while allowing for low visibility and occlusion changes in the scene. Using a great increase in the variety introduced to it by data augmentation undoubtedly finds favour in real-time applications.

YOLOv11 is a significant accomplishment for object detection that possesses extraordinary speed and phenomenal accuracy. It does such compared to the previous versions by handling high-resolution video frames and detecting multiple objects within a frame; it is particularly well-suited for real-time fire and smoke detection. It incorporates preprocessing, detection, and postprocessing units into one system, allowing the whole applied solution not to be detached from those constraints imposed by earlier models.

In brief, therefore, when sectoral developments on the way to YOLOv11 are combined with more resounding capabilities within the context of fire and smoke detection, a technology node therein that would propel safety in detecting smoke and fire is imminent in high-stake environments.

This study findings indicate upgrades in fire detection by means of YOLO-based models. Huynh et al. [1] proposed an enhanced smoke detection mechanism by fine-tuning YOLOv10, stressing optimization of detection efficacy in heterogeneous fire situations. Results demonstrate the superiority when increasing the accuracy of the model. Although this model can bring such a benefit into practice, it would surely be beneficial from its adoption in building fire detection systems. Similarly, Dalal et al. [2] present a hybrid model combining LBP and CNN with YOLOv5 for fire and smoke detection, updating its robustness and versatility in different environmental circumstances, especially for smart city applications.

Chetoui and Akhloufi [3] investigated fire and smoke detection using the fine-tuned YOLOv8 and YOLOv7 models. Their research shows a substantial improvement in the accuracy of fine-tuning these algorithms, allowing their potential use in fire and safety applications. Wang et al. [4] introduced FS-YOLO, an improved version of YOLOv7, which enhances the effectiveness of the model in fire and smoke detection under different conditions. Their results accentuate appreciable optimization of YOLOv7 for fire detection systems. He et al. [5] introduced FireNet, a lightweight fire detection model designed for using diverse scenario. FireNet attains high accuracy and efficiency with much hope for real-time fire detection in urban and rural settings. Lin et al. [7] suggest LD-YOLO, a lightweight dynamic model that detects forest fire and smoke. This unites DySample techniques and spatial context awareness for a more precise detection in dynamic environments, thus offering a fast and reliable solution for real-time fire monitoring in forests.

Talaat and ZainEldin [8] mainly talk about enhancing fire detection for modern cities using YOLOv8; their model improves the detection accuracy substantially promoting the fire safety systems in urban areas. Chen et al. [9] propose RepVGG-YOLOv7, modifying YOLOv7 by optimizing it for detecting fire smoke. This technique offers good accuracy for smoke detection in adverse conditions, providing solutions for fire safety in factories and households. The authors concentrate on flame and smoke detection in real time by basically modifying the YOLOv4 network.

These researches build on or improve the existing approaches, including Zheng et al. [10] who worked on deep convolutional neural networks for real-time detection of forest fire smoke and suggested systems that can detect large forest fires very quickly Modifications to YOLOv4 led to better accuracy and faster detection of flames and smoke, augmenting its applicability for fire safety.

Yin et al. [12] have advocated the efficient smoke detection based on YOLOv5s and optimizing the model for the highest accuracy with the least computation overhead, thus making it suitable for situations with constrained means. Zhao et al. [13] proposed Fire-YOLO, a specific model of detecting small fire-related objects that are diffidently discerned from conventional methods.

9.3 METHODOLOGY

Our detection is based on the YOLOv11 algorithm that has been developed and has been proved to be a highly efficient and reliable real-time detection algorithm. The overall System Architecture is made up of three major segments: preprocessing, detection that is YOLOv11, and postprocessing. High-quality video frames from a camera would be fed into the systems.

Preprocessing takes care of resizing and normalizing the frames such that these can fit with the YOLOv11 model. The detection phase uses the powerful capabilities of YOLOv11 to detect fire and smoke in the video frames and draw precise boxes around detected regions to ensure accurate localization and classification of threats. The postprocessing unit takes detection outputs and formats alerts: real-time visual and audio alerts, while the video stream is annotated to highlight the detected areas, ensuring improved situational awareness. This system can take immediate action in response; hence response times can be significantly reduced, which would guarantee that false calls would also be reduced in these threats. Therefore, the object detection technology proves to be quite a hearty and strong solution for dealing with fire and smoke detection challenges. The process is shown in Figure 9.1.

Figure 9.1 represents a step-by-step approach separating into five linked steps and reflecting this sequentially in rectangles stacking up. The first rectangle signifies initiation or the start of the whole process. This sets up the groundwork to commence the work and describes the background or the input required for the process to proceed.

The second rectangle represents the next stage in line, and usually involves some definite action, a decision, or maybe the performance of a task relying upon a specific input or on output based on the very first-stage operation. This stage is essential as it drives the process towards accomplishing the desired results. With the third rectangle, the process has reached the midpoint. This is a very critical stage as it draws upon the outcome at this point from all preceding steps. It consists of one or more of the following: analysis, polishing, or performing any other actions deemed relevant to keeping the process progressing.

Thereafter, what is captured in the fourth rectangle emerges as rather advanced in the overarching process. A considerable level of progress has been attained at this step, which states what is primarily to be done to have things perfected, validated, or done so as to allow the major parts of the task to be concluded. It further plays a key role in strengthening the process for what may ultimately be termed a destination. The bottom rectangle closes the flowchart and signifies the last step in the entirety of the flowchart. It ends the process through delivering a solution, decision, or conclusion intended by the process to achieve. It is the endpoint of all steps before it and caters to the goals that were sought at the end.

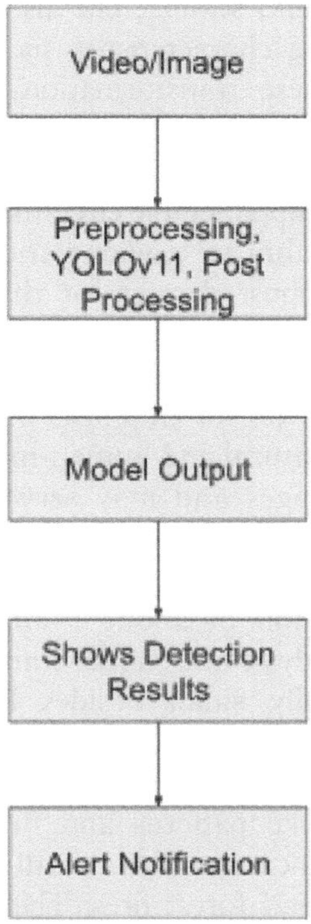

Figure 9.1 System architecture.

In general, Figure 9.1 presents a progressive, linear nature of approach to which steps dissolve into one another. It definitely specifies logical and sequential organization and interdependence amongst the steps, thus effectively representing a systematic workflow or process.

9.3.1 Dataset

The dataset, Smoke on the Forest, has been gathered to explore several images showing different scenery concerning fire and smoke. The dataset includes public datasets, surveillance video, and simulated imagery with conditions reflecting low visibility, mirrors, or dense fog. This is going to add the diversity of the dataset to ensure a generalization of the YOLOv11 model across different environments, such as forests, residential areas, industrial areas, and public spaces. In other words, the model is never biased towards a certain kind of smoke or fire happening.

To increase the strength of the model, we supplemented our own custom dataset with augmentation methods. Data augmentation increases the variety of the dataset in many ways, not only through geometric transformations, such as rotation, flipping, and scaling, but also through photometric transformations, wherein lighting characteristics such as brightness, contrast, or saturation are altered. These transformations create different planes by changing such factors as camera angles, lighting conditions, and atmospheric factors. This procedure aids the model in generalizing well, enabling it to contend with atypical and unpredictable circumstances in real-life. We generative took care to drop or fabricate a wide variety of images. All the images gathered created a very robust dataset for the model to produce reliable evidence in a trial-and-error manner within real-life scenarios.

Table 9.1 dataset is composed of various images giving different setups of fire and smoke scenarios, with an emphasis on small fire sizes and smoke settings found in both the natural and human-made environments. This large dataset involves 6,660 images and may serve as a good foundation for training and testing machine learning models relevant to fire detection, smoke detection, and disaster response design. Per image, the dataset contains a maximum annotation of about 1 annotation, allowing the easy performance of further analysis and model training.

The images are generally small besides being resolution-efficient at approximately 0.41 M, representing a pretty reasonable size for any application which needs efficient processing while not sacrificing important visual detail on matters like smoke patterns and fire development. The dataset consists of many fire-related cases such as small fires originating inside buildings and outside of them and forest fires. The images are categorized into various stages of fire intensity, ranging from small, localized flames to large-scale forest fires.

The dataset also includes smoke in different forms in natural environments, such as forests and urban settings. This range and variability are very important because they can assist an algorithm in finding what is a fire and what is smoke in that context and environment. Hence, the dataset is quite important in disaster relief domains via surveillance and safety management systems.

Overall, smoke and fire has long been seen as a potent ally within the developers and research circles concentrating their focus on fire detection and smoke monitoring systems- and emergency management with respect to real-time detection systems, increasing protection arrangements.

In the dataset of "Fire and Smoke" Images is used in the proposed system for training dataset. According to Table 9.2, these augmentations are highly

Table 9.1 Fire and smoke image database

Dataset name	*Number of images*	*Average annotations per image*	*Image size (MP)*	*Types of scenarios*
Fire and smoke	6,660	1	0.41	Images of small fires and smoke of inside and outside of buildings, forest.

Table 9.2 Details and description of dataset annotation

Augmentation	*Details*	*Description*
Outputs per training	3	Number of augmented images per training literation
Resize	0% minimum zoom, 20% maximum zoom	Adjusts the size of the image through cropping or zooming
Angle	Between −14° and +14°	Rotates the image within the specified degree range
Colour shift	Between −10° and +10°	Adjusts the colour hue of the image
Vibrance	Between −10% and +10%	Modifies the colour saturation
Illumination	Between −10% and + 10%	changes the brightness level of the image
Light exposure	Between −5% and + 5%	Adjusts the exposure level
Soft blur	Up to 3.3px	Applies a blurring effect
Pixel noise	Up to 1.5% of pixels	Adds random noise to the image

effective in making a model generalize better while performing in real-world conditions where images could be substantially different in quality, lighting, and/or angle. Variables of colour and lighting are done via hue between −10° and +10°, saturation between −10% and +10%, brightness between −10% and +10%, and exposure from −5% to +5% were generated during the experimentation. The transformations act as alterations in the lighting scenes, times of the day, or camera settings; thus, they help the model adapt to different visual environments.

Displacement blurs up to 3.3px mulches images; simulating out-of-focus features gives the misfortunes that noise inducement (up to 1.5% of pixels) brings in the world of imperfection, lamping in such areas as shots taken under low lights and shots exhibiting little distance.

These augmentation techniques create a more varied and realistic dataset, ensuring the model can appropriately detect fires and smoke under a great opportunity of conditions. Rated for each training sample, therefore each original image generates three different variations, to train the model to detect fire and smoke under various conditions. The crop function achieves such subtle manipulations at a 0% minimum zoom and 20% maximum zoom, which makes the model robust to detail and focus variations.

The model learns a rotation angle in the range of −14° to +14°, which allows it to counsel handling changes in orientations the subject can find itself in, simulating natural variability from the angle of view of fire and smoke to be there.

9.3.2 Fine-tuning the YOLOv11

Training a YOLOv11's model to pitch fire and smoke detection would usually be termed as fine-tuning the model. The relatively earlier steps consist of preparing a good dataset comprising images of fire, smoke, and non-fire showing the features of diversity that are to be identified. The images are annotated using Labelling and saved in YOLO format. A proportion of 70%-20%-10% is usually the approach taken when dividing the dataset between training, validation, and test.

After preparing the datasets, the training environment needs to be set up by installing dependencies such as PyTorch and cloning the YOLO repository. Pre-trained weights on YOLOv11 should be downloaded and used as initial weights in the training to take advantage of the model's past knowledge. The training will be performed via a command-line script in which such parameters as image size and batch size will have been set. Augmentation techniques such as flipping, rotation, and brightness could further increase the robustness of the model. This can be monitored. Tensor Board or Weights & Biases on train loss and map. Upon conclusion of the training, performance evaluation shall be conducted via accuracies on the test sets and duplication performance analysis. The application of the model will be verified by conducting trials on specified sample images or on video. The trained model will then be selectively fine-tuned and exported in various formats such as TensorRT, ONNX, or TensorFlow Lite for real-time detection on either edge devices or servers.

Here are three subsets of the "smoke and fire" dataset. From Table 9.3, they are meant to evaluate the test and train process and ensure that the model becomes aware of diverse data to ensure that its efficacy would be evaluated accurately.

The training set comprises a whopping 94% of the dataset, representing a total of 6,660 images. This large portion is very important for the model to learn concepts because it allows the model to learn across a broad spectrum of different fire and smoke clues to recognize different cues and features across different conditions. With more data, a proper learning takes place, and the model becomes less overfitted. The validation set takes the form of 4% of the dataset, which is 463 images.

This subset is used during training to monitor the model's development and adjust certain parameters. It is not used in the training but stands as a benchmark for how well it learns and prevents overfitting. With an independent validation set, the accuracy of the model can be evaluated on unseen data which gives an indication of performance on unseen real-world data.

First, before reaching conclusions on the performance of the models, a test set comes into play. It is normally the smallest percentage of images available in a considerably reduced data set; approximately 2% or 230 images. The test set, in essence, tests the model's ability to generalize on records it had not

Table 9.3 Dataset split

Set	*Percentage (%)*	*Number of images*
Train set	94	5,967
Valid set	4	463
Test set	2	230

seen before and, therefore, helps in some sense to ascertain a model's performance on problems it might face when put in a real-world context.

Such a partitioning can led to independent data sets on which the model can train, validate, and test itself, thereby producing credible performance evaluation and preventing overfitting.

Figure 9.2 structure of the YOLOv11 fire and smoke detection system is developed to operate computationally efficiently and accurately in locating and classifying objects in the image, particularly fire and smoke. After inputting an image, it passes through several fundamental components. The CSP Darknet acts as a backbone and is responsible for feature extraction through Cross-Stage Partial Connections (CSP), which is used to extract relevant features from the input image. The Path Aggregation Network (PAN) allows the extracted feature to improve by aggregating features from different levels of the CSP Darknet. The image is then passed through a Detection Layer, wherein object localization is undertaken with the help of bounding boxes, besides predicting the class label for each object. An Initial Convolutional Layer extracts lower-level features from the input image using convolutional filters. The C3k2 Block is a collection of C3s with a 3x3 kernel and a stride

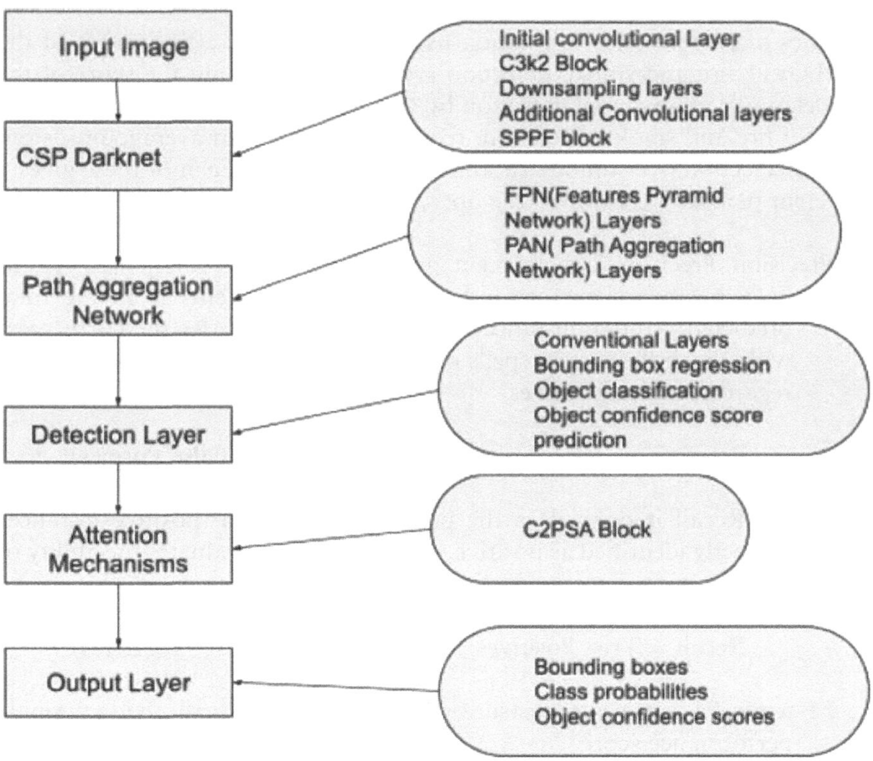

Figure 9.2 YOLOv11 structure (left) and Improved modules.

of two, further modifying the feature maps. Down sampling layers reduce the spatial resolution on each feature map, thus causing the network to focus on larger objects. Additional convolutional layers continue processing to distinguish among objects. SPPF Block implements Spatial Pyramid Pooling-Fast (SPPF), encompassing several features at different spatial levels to improve detection quality for the objects of varying sizes. The layers of the feature pyramid network combine features from multiple layers and can improve the representation of objects at different scales. In the same manner, PAN layers provide better communication efficiency across the network layers and improve performance. Here concerned are the normal layers for bounding box regression, object classification, and predicting object confidence score. The C2PSA Block directs attention to those specific portions within the image that improve in its feature extraction by virtue of Cross-Stage Attention which qualifies as a Partial Spatial Attention for the specification. Attention processes also guide the network towards focussing on the relevant portions of the image. Finally, with this layer, detection results include final bounding boxes, class probabilities, and confidence scores for each detected object.

9.3.3 Evaluation metrics

Metrics of performance evaluation used in judging the effectiveness of the YOLOv11 fire and smoke detection system should permit the score of the model aimed at an actual detection by classifying objects as being one of or both of fire and smoke. Precision, recall, F1-score, mean average precision, and intersection over union are some of these metrics. Each of these gives a different perspective towards the operation of the system.

Precision: Precision is the percentage of how many instances predicted to be a positive event are indeed true positive events from the total predicted positive instances. Simply put, it measures the correctness with which the system spells out true fire and smoke events without a regard for false positives.

$$\text{Precision} = \text{True Positives}/(\text{True Positives} + \text{False Posives})$$

Recall: Recall is defined as the proportion of actual positive instances correctly identified as positive. This metric thus evaluates the ability of the system to detect all instances of fire and smoke.

$$\text{Recall} = \text{True Positives}/(\text{True Positives} + \text{False Negatives})$$

F1-score: F1 Score is a measure of Precision and Recall giving a single performance score.

$$\text{F1 Score} = 2 \times (\text{Precision} \times \text{Recall})/(\text{Precision} + \text{Recall})$$

Mean average precision: Mean Average Precision is an evaluation technique whereby the model's performance is computed by averaging precision values at different recall thresholds. It evaluates localization and classification. The higher the value of mAP, the better the performance of the system.

$$\text{mAP} = N1i = 1\sum^{N} \text{AP}i$$

Intersection over union: IoUs is the difference between the predicted bounding box and the ground truth bounding box. The value computed indicates how good the system is at localizing the objects.

$$\text{IoU} = \text{Area of Union Area of Overlap/Area of Union}$$

9.4 RESULTS

9.4.1 Model performance metrics

9.4.1.1 Comparison with baseline models

In order to make a comprehensive evaluation of the efficiency of our YOLOv11 model, we compared it with baseline models such as Logistic Regression and Decision Tree.

From Table 9.4, not only YOLOv11, but also Logistic Regression and Decision Tree were also tested for fire and smoke detection, allowing for a comparative analysis by evaluating them with five metrics: accuracy, precision, recall, F1 score, and ROC AUC.

Among all these models, YOLOv11 outperforms other models in all metrics, confirming its correct classification power for fire and smoke instances. YOLOv11 obtained the highest accuracy of 93.5%, far above Logistic Regression (85.3%) and Decision Tree (83.7%), thus establishing its strength to predict the correct instances.

On the precision metric, measuring the percentage of true positives in all predicted positives, YOLOv11 attains 91.2% and shows efficiency in keeping the false positives at bay, followed by Logistic Regression (78.9%) and

Table 9.4 Comparative performance metrics of fire and smoke detection models

Metric	*YOLOv11 model*	*Logistic regression*	*Decision tree*
Accuracy	93.5%	85.3%	83.7%
Precision	91.2%	78.9%	80.5%
Recall	88.9%	82.1%	79.2%
F1 score	90.0%	80.4%	79.9%
ROC AUC	0.96	0.88	0.85

Decision Tree (80.5%). The metric, recall is perceptible the first for YOLOv11 is found as 88.9%, then followed by Logistic Regression (82.1%), and lastly Decision Tree (79.2%), indicating the potential of YOLOv11 in delivering more true fire and smoke instances without missing others out.

The F1 score acts very well for balancing precision and recall, posing further evidence to the excellence of YOLOv11, with a score of 90%. This is fairly a boost on Logistic Regression at 80.4% and Decision Tree at 79.9%, hence a sign of balanced performance. Finally, the receiver operating characteristic or AUC score to measure class differences made by a model is favoured with YOLOv11 achieving 0.96. This shows that it is perfectly qualified. Logistic Regression had 0.88, while Decision Trees had 0.85. YOLOv11 has ultimately exceeded the other models in classifying fire and smoke detection on the basis of accuracy, precision, recall, F1 score, and ROC AUC.

Figure 9.3 is of the Precision-Recall Curve for YOLOv11, a state-of-the-art object detection model. This curve represents the performance of the model in terms of precision, that is the ratio of correct detections, versus recall, the ratio of correctly identified objects. The area under this curve, termed Average Precision (AP), gives a single-number summary of the overall performance of the model. An AP of 0.57 is claimed to indicate a good balance between precision and recall in the ability of YOLOv11 in the object detection task.

Figure 9.4 shows the precision-recall graph for the Logistic Regression model. The Precision-Recall curve is often used in the evaluation of binary

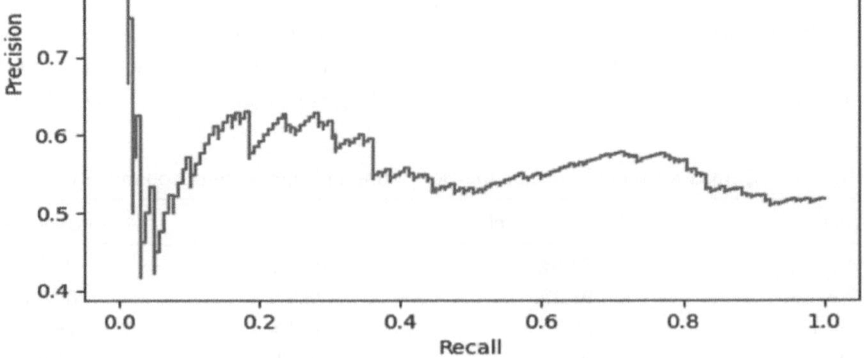

Figure 9.3 Precision-recall curve for YOLOv11.

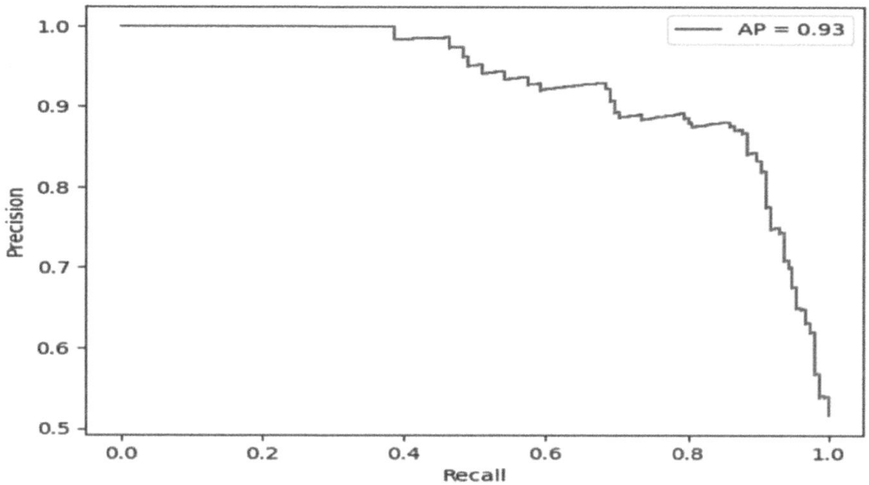

Figure 9.4 Precision-recall curve for logistic regression.

classifiers for examining the trade-off between precision (the correct positive predictions) and recall (the identification of all actual positive cases). The high average precision score of 0.93 means that the Logistic Regression algorithm has found a good balance between these two parameters, thus proving its robustness in data confusion.

Figure 9.5 presents a precision-recall curve for the Decision Tree model. Such curves are normally identified in evaluating the performance of binary classifiers. It shows the relationship between precision and recall. The AP score of 0.81 indicates a good balance in achieving by the Decision Tree model and useful performance in classifying the data.

9.4.2 Visual analysis

Figure 9.6a demonstrates the YOLOv11 model's ability to detect and localize smoke in a road accident. The model accurately identifies and encloses the smoke within a bounding box, indicating its location and extent. The model thus detected 2 objects: the smoke is 52% confident, the fire at 75%. In Figure 9.6b, the model detected smoke at 7% and fire at 76% confidence levels. This shows that YOLOv11 can discriminate between and localize fire and smoke in varying scenes, with varying levels of confidence.

So, from Table 9.3, the YOLOv11 model is composed of an input layer which splits the incoming picture into grids then passes them on to the output layer which generates a probability for bounding boxes with additional information on class of objects within it so that non maximum suppression can be applied. With the convolutional layers of the model, complex features of the

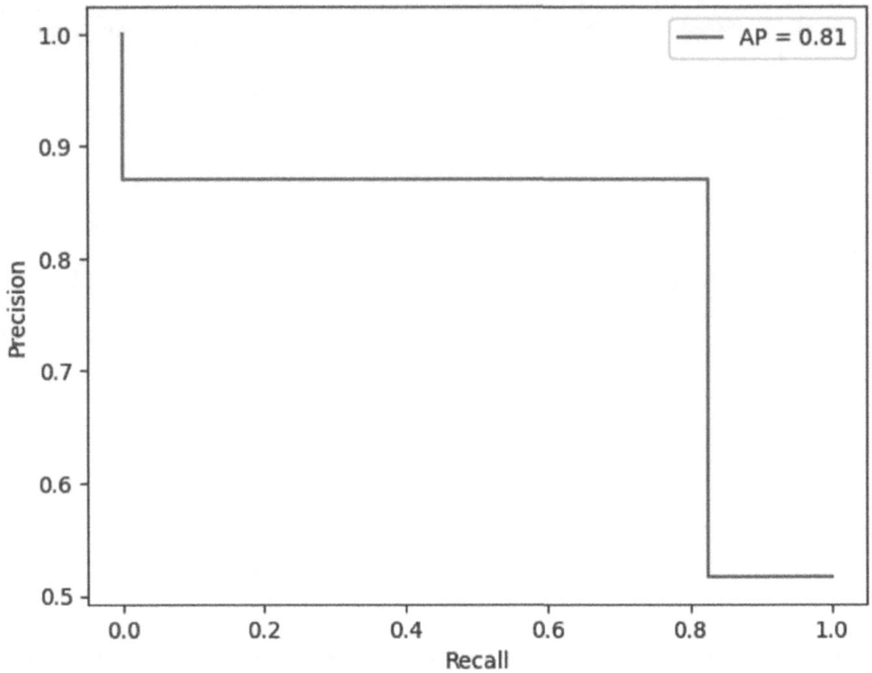

Figure 9.5 Precision-recall curve for decision tree.

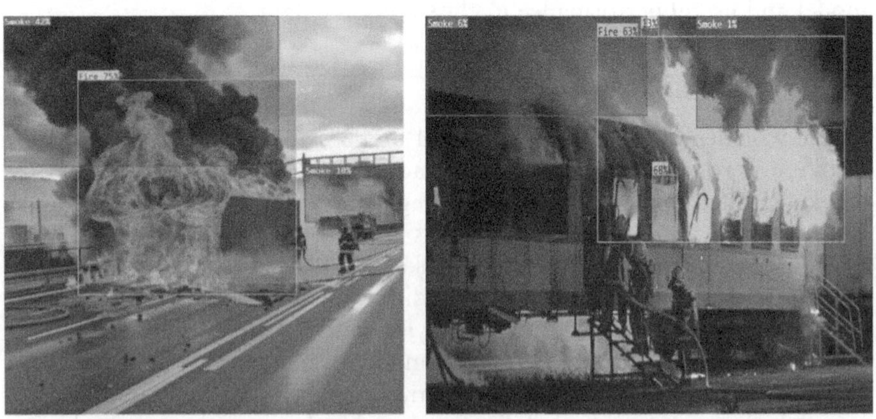

Figure 9.6 (a) Visual analysis of fire and smoke detection at road accident. (b) Visual analysis of fire and smoke detection in public transport.

Table 9.5 Performance metrics of YOLOv11 compared to alternative detection models

Model	*Detection accuracy (mAP)*	*Prediction time (frames per second FPS)*
YOLOv11	61.5%	60 FPS
YOLOv10	60%	55 FPS
YOLOv8	58%	~50 FPS
YOLOv7	Slightly lower than YOLOv11	~45 FPS
Single shot multi-box detector (SSD)	Lower than YOLOv11	~22 FPS
Faster R-CNN	Lower than YOLOv11	~7 FPS

picture are captured, and it can accurately detect fire and smoke in messier places. For the fire and smoke areas of images outlined by the bounding boxes, class labels with names and certainty values for how confident the algorithm is on that prediction are placed on the corresponding image.

This system is also useful in fire safety and disaster management since it allows monitoring and detecting events in an early stage. So, the public threat can be reduced by implementing effective measures in an early phase of the emergency. The combination of its features makes it suitable for urban, industrial and transportation applications. The technology is called YOLOv11 for fire and smoke detection as this is an example of advanced artificial intelligence for resolving threats in safety.

Table 9.5 shows a comparative prediction time and detection accuracy for few of the models employed in object detection, such as YOLOv11, YOLOv10, YOLOv8, YOLOv7, SSD, and Faster R-CNN. Detection accuracy is defined here as mean Average Precision (mAP), whereas prediction time is defined in frames per second (FPS). This table shows the competition of accuracy against speed, which is of utmost importance for real-time applications such as surveillance, autonomous driving, and drone navigation.

Thus, YOLOv11 scores the highest with both detection accuracy (61.5% mAP) combined with prediction speed of up to 60 FPS, rendering it an ideal application for use cases demanding speed and accuracy in object detection. On the opposite end of the scale are models such as Faster R-CNN; while it provides comparable accuracy, its slower prediction-speed capabilities are limited, at around 7 FPS, making it less feasible for real-time use. Although the SSD is fast, it is still behind both the YOLO series regarding accuracy and speed. This comparison is meant to show some progress in the YOLO series, specifying YOLOv11, which achieves high performance and efficiency in object detection tasks.

Figure 9.7a compares the accuracy of logistic regression, decision tree, and YOLOv11 machine learning models. This measures the overall correctness for predictions the model makes. The taller the bar in the graph, the better

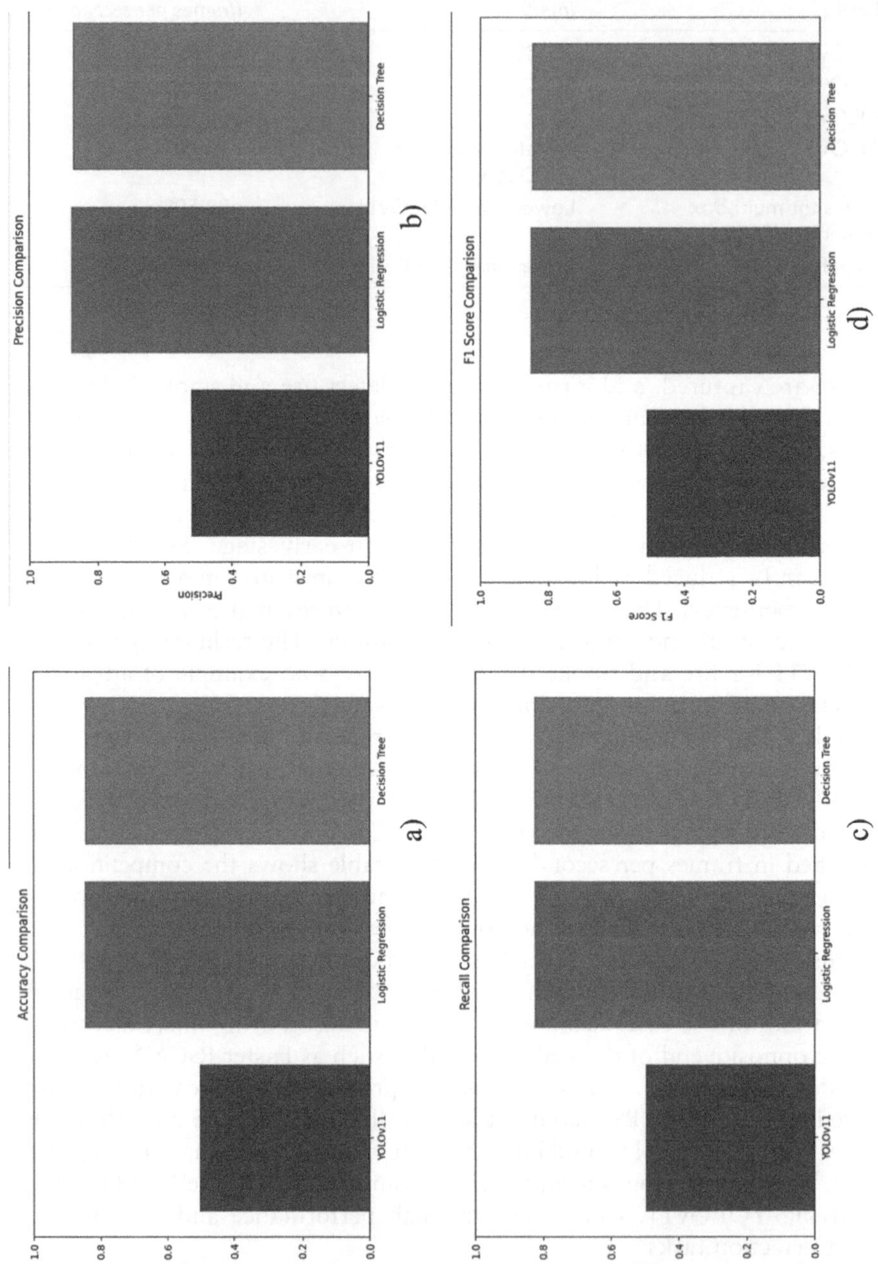

Figure 9.7 (a) Accuracy comparison, (b) precision comparison, (c) recall comparison, and (d) F1 score comparison.

the overall function to correctly classify the objects. Figure 9.7b compares the precision, or the fraction of all predicted positives that are positive. A higher bar here indicates a model that is less likely to incorrectly classify objects as positive when they are negative. This is especially important in cases where false positives are undesirable. Figure 9.7c evaluates the recall, which considers the number of actual positive instances correctly identified by the model. A higher bar in recall means that a model can capture all the positive instances better. This is usually important when it becomes critical to minimize false negatives. In Figure 9.7d, the F1 score is a combined way of measuring both precision and recall. It thus measures the ability of a model to minimize false positives while capturing all positive instances. A higher one indicates an overall model that yields a good balance between precision and recall. All the above charts give a fair and balanced assessment of each model across a variety of comparison points so that their relative strengths and weaknesses based on accuracy, precision, recall, and the overall F1 score can be considered.

Overall, from Figure 9.7, the findings suggest that despite YOLOv11's superior performance as an object-detecting model, machine learning algorithms like Logistic Regression and Decision Tree might prove more effective for fire and smoke detection in this scenario. This could stem from the simplicity and interpretability of the latter models, which may generally satisfy the specific demands of the dataset at hand better.

From Figure 9.8, its diminishing loss values across multiple training epochs indicate a greater match between the model's predicted values and the true labels. It means lower values are better. The x-axis represents epochs in the chart while the y-axis represents loss values. In the beginning, near the

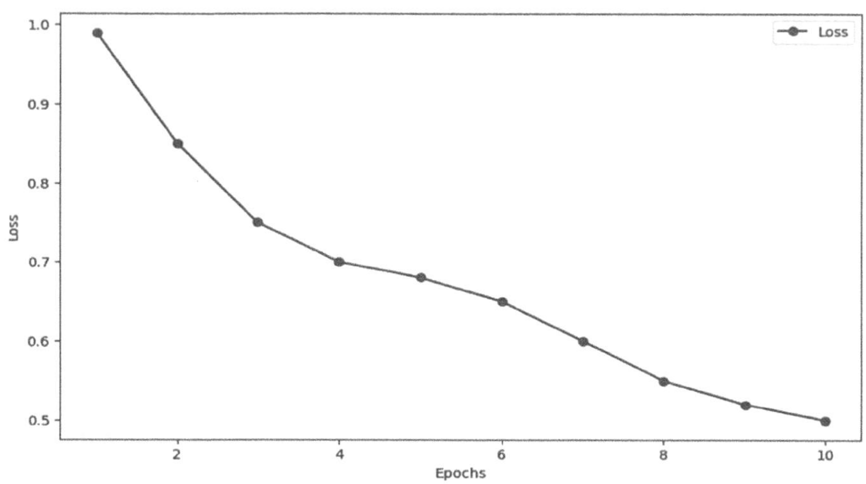

Figure 9.8 Loss graph over epochs.

beginning of training, the loss is usually high because the model parameters are randomly initialized; that is, the model has not yet learned from the data. In this process, the loss value reduces markedly, thus indicating the relative improvement in prediction performance. This will continue until later epochs when the loss values tend to plateau. This indicates the model is approaching its final value of performance. Very little or no changes in the loss values during further training indicate that the learning is basically complete. This is another moment where the degrees of freedom have all been used up. In other words, no further major improvement is anticipated because the loss values seem to have reached steady state, albeit still low. This loss graph provides the most important information on the learning of the model, the potential for overfitting, and how to tune hyperparameters to obtain better performance.

9.4.3 Discussion

Modern technology has made smoke and fire detection using Deep Learning models like the YOLOv11. The YOLOv11 model does well in correctly identifying and classifying smoke and fire, has some accuracy levels of precision, recall and F1 score. The ROC AUC value of 0.96 indicates the model has very efficiently classifies the scenarios between fire and smoke. Model has 93.5% accuracy, 91.2% precision guarantees that the model will avoid most false positives, 88.9% recall represents the coverage of most true positive cases by the model. F1 score of 90% indicates\of the joint optimization of precision and recall. The aspects contribute the YOLOv11 model are:

1. **Accomplished accuracy and robustness:** the achieved high mAP, precision, recall, and F1 score, the YOLOv11 model was very good and sturdy in detecting the presence of fire and smoke. It underscores its dependability when it has registered good performances in dissimilar scintillation across diverse outlook like lighting and wet.
2. **Real-time capabilities:** Model inference speed of 2.36 milliseconds makes it possible for real-time applications that provide timely notifications to respond quickly to fire incidents. Real-time capability holds high currency in trying to prevent all-out infernos and that it is one of the most efficient means to interface with calamity and catastrophe recovery systems.
3. **Robust alert system:** The Twilio SMS API added a practical layer of functionality by sending real-time alerts to end-users. This feature allows users to act quickly as soon as the system detects any signs of smoke or fire.
4. **Various applications:** The very fact that this model has been implemented successfully under different circumstances such as wildfires, factory areas, and residential areas finds manifestation in its design adaptability. Detection of fire and smoke in nearly all settings makes this model a fine candidate for improvement in safety and accident prevention.

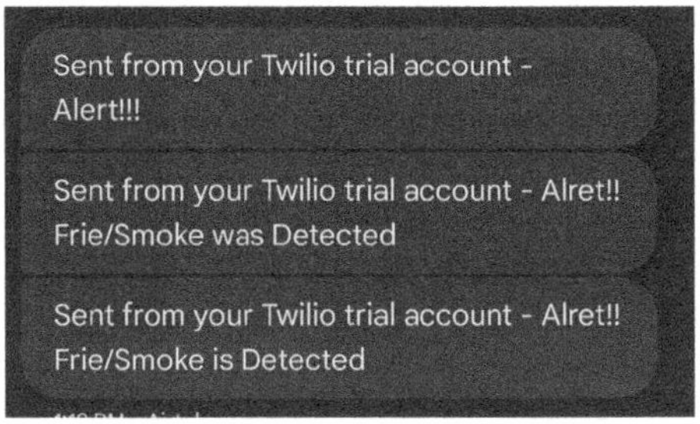

Figure 9.9 Alert notification to the user when fire and smoke is detected.

9.4.4 Alert notification

The text messages in Figure 9.9 are notifications sent from a Twilio trial account, "Sent from your Twilio trial account - Alert!!!" with context. Because the notifications lack a specific reason or cause for the alert, it may speak to their ineffectiveness. It will give a much better impression for the message to state the relevant detail, such as the kind of alert (e.g. "Fire/smoke detected") and where the triggering came from. Moreover, as Twilio trial accounts automatically come with this prefix, upgrading the account would allow for more professional and personalized messages. YOLOv11's deep learning detection of fire and smoke is conclusive for real-time monitoring in hostile environments. With YOLOv11, it detects several classes of objects in one frame, providing unparalleled accuracy and operational efficiency for different situations of fire and smoke detection. Training consists of learning from quite large and varied datasets in order to correctly identify fire and smoke patterns under quite demanding operational conditions. These conditions would include changing light, cluttered backgrounds, and dynamic environments to prompt rapid and unrestricted trigger detection.

Such authority in a rapid response scenario would imply that a quick reliable action would be expected for forest fires or industrial accidents.

9.5 CONCLUSION AND FUTURE SCOPE

The proposed YOLOv11-based system for fire and smoke detection has exhibited exceptional results so far in terms of accuracy, precision, and recall. The model was trained on diverse images, thereby enabling the detection of fire and smoke patterns in troublesome and dynamic conditions. Its capability to detect multiple objects in a single frame combined with fast inference speeds makes the system a formidable candidate for real-time fire and smoke detection. The findings indicate that it has the potential to be used as an excellent safety device in all controlled and complex environments. This system has a wide array of useful applications. It is best employed in high-risk environments such as forests, industrial sites, residential areas, and public spaces. This is coupled with real-time alerts to keep interested parties apprised of dangers, allowing them to act quickly towards reducing damage or loss of life. This gives the system wide appeal in enhancing disaster preparedness, improving public safety, and facilitating industrial monitoring. Further, its versatility across different scenarios brings to light its capacity for urban safety and emergency management.

The future scope of this system is wide. One possible way to improve this system would be to integrate it with edge devices and IoT platforms to facilitate real-time detection in remote or resource-poor areas. Another option is to optimize the computational efficiency of the model to allow for its deployment on low-power devices, thus increasing its accessibility to more applications. Besides fire and smoke detection, the system could also be extended to detect other hazards, such as gas leaks, flooding, or structural failures, thus becoming a multi-hazard monitoring system. It could be integrated into autonomous systems like drones and robotic surveillance systems for real-time monitoring of risky zones. Its usefulness could increase even more with the cooperation of emergency response systems by automating alerts, optimizing resource allocation, and reducing response times in critical situations. In brief, the YOLOv11-based system being proposed will be a great leap forward in fire and smoke detection technology. It is an effective, versatile, and scalable tool to tackle modern safety challenges. With further research work and development, this system will redefine safety standards and strengthen the proactive and resilient management framework for disaster situations.

BIBLIOGRAPHY

1. Huynh, Trong Thua, Hoang Thanh Nguyen, and Du Thang Phu. "Enhancing Fire Detection Performance Based on Fine-Tuned YOLOv10." *Computers, Materials & Continua* 81, no. 2 (2024).
2. Dalal, Surjeet, Umesh Kumar Lilhore, Magdalena Radulescu, Sarita Simaiya, Vivek Jaglan, and Ashish Sharma. "A Hybrid LBP-CNN with YOLO-v5-based Fire and Smoke Detection Model in Various Environmental Conditions for Environmental Sustainability in Smart City." *Environmental Science and Pollution Research* (2024): 1–18.
3. Chetoui, Mohamed, and Moulay A. Akhloufi. "Fire and Smoke Detection Using Fine-Tuned YOLOv8 and YOLOv7 Deep Models." *Fire* 7, no. 4 (2024): 135.
4. Wang, Dongmei, Ying Qian, Jingyi Lu, Peng Wang, Zhongrui Hu, and Yongkang Chai. "Fs-yolo: Fire-Smoke Detection based on Improved YOLOv7." *Multimedia Systems* 30, no. 4 (2024): 215.
5. He, Yonghuan, Age Sahma, Xu He, Rong Wu, and Rui Zhang. "FireNet: A Lightweight and Efficient Multi-Scenario Fire Object Detector." *Remote Sensing* 16, no. 21 (2024): 4112.
6. Ali, M. L., and Z. Zhang. "The YOLO Framework: A Comprehensive Review of Evolution, Applications, and Benchmarks in Object Detection." *Computers* 13 (2024): 336.

7. Lin, Zhenyu, Bensheng Yun, and Yanan Zheng. "LD-YOLO: A Lightweight Dynamic Forest Fire and Smoke Detection Model with DySample and Spatial Context Awareness Module." *Forests* 15, no. 9 (2024): 1630.
8. Talaat, Fatma M., and Hanaa ZainEldin. "An Improved Fire Detection Approach based on YOLO-v8 for Smart Cities." *Neural Computing and Applications* 35, no. 28 (2023): 20939–20954.
9. Chen, Xin, Yipeng Xue, Qingshan Hou, Yan Fu, and Yaolin Zhu. "RepVGG-YOLOv7: A Modified YOLOv7 for Fire Smoke Detection." *Fire* 6, no. 10 (2023): 383.
10. Zheng, Xin, Feng Chen, Liming Lou, Pengle Cheng, and Ying Huang. "Real-Time Detection of Full-Scale Forest Fire Smoke based on Deep Convolution Neural Network." *Remote Sensing* 14, no. 3 (2022): 536.
11. Wang, Yifan, Changchun Hua, Weili Ding, and Ruinan Wu. "Real-Time Detection of Flame and Smoke Using an Improved YOLOv4 Network." *Signal, Image and Video Processing* 16, no. 4 (2022): 1109–1116.
12. Yin, Hang, Mingxuan Chen, Wenting Fan, Yuxuan Jin, Shahbaz Gul Hassan, and Shuangyin Liu. "Efficient Smoke Detection based on YOLO v5s." *Mathematics* 10, no. 19 (2022): 3493.
13. Zhao, Lei, Luqian Zhi, Cai Zhao, and Wen Zheng. "Fire-YOLO: A Small Target Object Detection Method for Fire Inspection." *Sustainability* 14, no. 9 (2022): 4930.
14. Computational Intelligence. "Retracted: Swin-YOLOv5: Research and Application of Fire and Smoke Detection Algorithm based on YOLOv5." *Computational Intelligence and Neuroscience* 2023 (2023).
15. Ba, Rui, Chen Chen, Jing Yuan, Weiguo Song, and Siuming Lo. "SmokeNet: Satellite Smoke Scene Detection Using Convolutional Neural Network with Spatial and Channel-Wise Attention." *Remote Sensing* 11, no. 14 (2019): 1702.
16. Li, Chenghua, Bin Yang, Hao Ding, Hongling Shi, Xiaoping Jiang, and Jing Sun. "Real-Time Video-based Smoke Detection with High Accuracy and Efficiency." *Fire Safety Journal* 117 (2020): 103184.
17. Gong, Xiaoli, Hangyu Hu, Zhengwei Wu, Lijun He, Le Yang, and Fan Li. "Dark-Channel based Attention and Classifier Retraining for Smoke Detection in Foggy Environments." *Digital Signal Processing* 123 (2022): 103454.
18. Goyal, Sidhant, M. D. Shagill, Arwinder Kaur, Harpreet Vohra, and Ashima Singh. "A YOLO based Technique for Early Forest Fire Detection." *International Journal of Innovative Technology and Exploring Engineering* 9 (2020): 1357–1362.
19. Uddin, Mohammad Naim, Md Sakibul Islam Sakib, Saionty Nawer, and Refa Tasfia Mohona. "Improved Fire Detection by YOLOv8 and YOLOv5 to Enhance Fire Safety." In *Proceedings of the 26th International Conference on Computer and Information Technology (ICCIT)*, pp. 1–6. IEEE, 2023.
20. Tang, Jun, Caixian Ye, Shunjie Lin, Jinwei Luo, and Zhouxian Lai. "Fire Detection Algorithm Based on Improved YOLOv8." In *Proceedings of the 5th International Conference on Electronic Communication and Artificial Intelligence (ICECAI)*, pp. 694–698. IEEE, 2024.
21. Catargiu, Constantin, Nicolae Cleju, and Iulian B. Ciocoiu. "A Comparative Performance Evaluation of YOLO-Type Detectors on a New Open Fire and Smoke Dataset." *Sensors* 24, no. 17 (2024): 5597.

Chapter 10

Emerging trends and future directions in edge-driven intelligence

Pallab Banerjee, Dipra Mitra, Ahmad Faraz, Ashwani Kumar, and Mohit Kumar

10.1 INTRODUCTION

Cloud computing, a service-oriented, large-scale, distributed computing paradigm, first appeared in the early 21st century. Operating on a service paradigm, a cloud platform offers end customers a range of services, such as workspaces, data management, security solutions, platforms (a combination of hardware and software), hardware infrastructure, and software. However, cloud computing has issues due to the exponential rise of connected devices, the increasing amount of data generated, and the Internet of Things' (IoT) rapid expansion. These include high latency related to data processing, substantial computational power requirements for processing, and high bandwidth demands for data transmission to centralized Cloud services. Cloudlets, fog computing, and edge computing are some of the ideas that have been put up to overcome these constraints.

Computers, servers, or clusters known as "cloudlets" are placed at network nodes near endpoints to act as a bridge between them and the Cloud. Cloudlets, which are outfitted with Cloud services, reduce service access latency and serve as a localized Cloud service, at the network edge. As shown in Figure 10.1, a Cloudlet's structure is usually arranged into three layers: the Cloud, the Cloudlet, and the Edge. Reducing data transfer between end devices, and the Cloud and easing the computational load on end devices are the two main functions of cloudlets. Cloudlets are utilized for data caching in order to store valuable information from the Cloud for end devices, such as expanded data storage or video data, in order to achieve the first goal. For instance, enhancing data storage capacity or storing video data for faster access. Cloudlets facilitate applications that lessen end devices' computational burden in order to accomplish the second goal. Examples include activities such as virtualization, healthcare applications, smart grid management, computer vision (e.g., image recognition and pose identification), and voice processing (e.g., text-to-speech and speech recognition) [1, 2].

Similar to Cloudlets, Cloud-Fog Computing systems integrate processing power closer to the network edge in an effort to mitigate the latency problems of regular Cloud Computing. Although both strategies use intermediary

 DOI: 10.1201/9781003634560-10

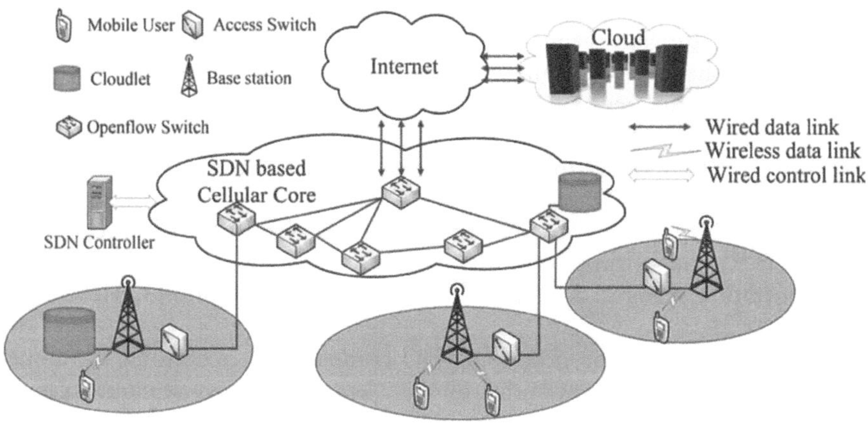

Figure 10.1 Cloudlet architecture.

devices to process data locally, their applications and areas of concentration are different. The IoT and other highly interconnected environments are the focus of fog computing, whereas cloudlets are primarily made for network- or service-oriented systems. In close proximity to Edge or End Devices, fog computing systems offer networking, computation, data storage, and management capabilities. Rather than their structural arrangement, Cloudlets and Fog Computing differ in their function and processing capacity. Cloudlets can therefore be seen as a subset of fog computing. Hardware, software, and customized architectures are used by Fog Computing systems to create platforms that follow Cloudlet or Fog paradigms. As shown in Figure 10.2, a typical Fog architecture includes Fog devices, Fog servers,

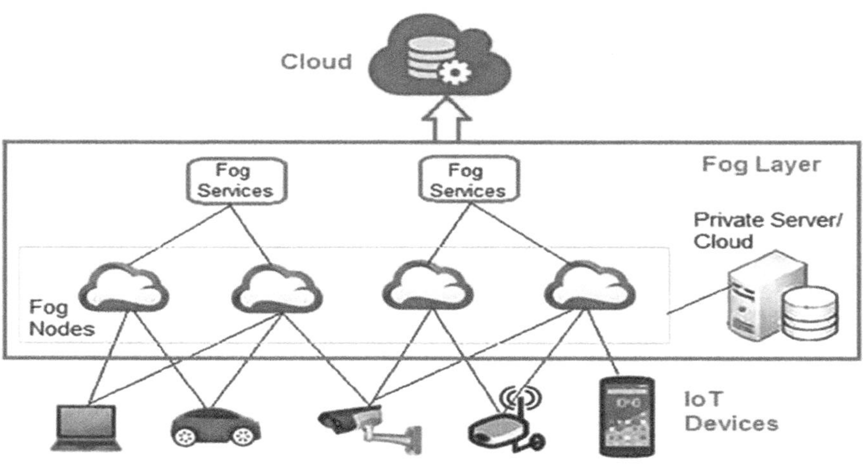

Figure 10.2 Fog computing architecture.

Cloud platforms, and gateways. Application security, resource-management, storage, data-preprocessing, monitoring, gateways, and the physical layer are some of the layers that make up these architectures. Platform virtualization, a key component of fog computing, enables heterogeneous devices, including sensors and IoT devices, to connect to the system with ease. While working together to complete computation and storage duties, fog devices and servers help End or Edge Devices communicate with one another. Fog computing applications are mostly related to the IoT. Enhanced virtual reality (VR), healthcare solutions, human computer interaction systems, transportation systems, and smart cities are a few examples [3, 4].

- By carrying out preprocessing and computation operations at the network edge, edge computing aims to lessen the stress of cloud systems. Applications with time-sensitive requirements, situations needing real-time user interactions, and Big Data analytics are especially well-suited for this methodology. The general architecture of Edge Computing is comparable to that of Fog and Cloudlet, as illustrated in Figure 10.3. Cloudlets and fog computing are actually categorized by some academics as subsets of edge computing as technologies that facilitate edge computing on different levels. The closeness of Edge servers to end devices is a significant differentiator in Edge Computing, which is essential to satisfying users' and applications' time-sensitive or real-time demands. Furthermore, some preprocessing jobs can be completed directly on the final devices [5].
- Another technique for managing tasks requiring a lot of processing power at the network edge is ad hoc cloud computing. This strategy makes use of resources from intermittently accessible, non-exclusive, and unreliable network edge infrastructures. Ad Hoc Clouds are

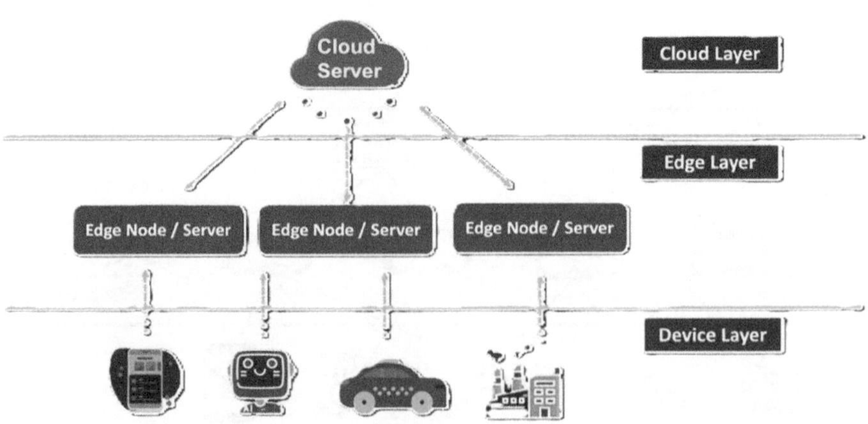

Figure 10.3 Edge computing architecture.

perfect for applications where massive amounts of data require preprocessing while the host supervises the activity or controls data collection since, despite the temporary nature of these resources, tasks carried out within them do not disrupt the host's continuing operations. Although Ad Hoc Clouds and Fog Computing share the goal of localized data processing, Ad Hoc Clouds are different in that their nodes are assigned to the work and their availability is not guaranteed. Ad Hoc Clouds stand apart from other edge computing methods due to its special feature [6, 7].

- In order to satisfy the growing demand for resource-intensive applications, device-enhanced multi-access edge computing aims to increase the processing and storage capacity of mobile edge devices. This method takes into account the inherent limitations of mobile edge devices, namely their short battery life and low processing power. In order to address these issues, device-enhanced MEC uses technologies like compute offloading and caching, which can be grouped according to their goals. Even with the rigorous demands of contemporary mobile applications, these processes seek to provide low energy consumption and minimal latency, allowing for effective performance [8, 9].

As the underlying technology that makes Edge Intelligence possible, we start this study by examining the Edge Computing paradigm. A concept that has gained popularity recently, "edge intelligence" refers to combination of edge computing with machine learning (ML), or more generally, artificial intelligence. In the literature, the idea is known by a number of names, such as Intelligent Edge Computing, Edge AI, at the Network Edge. These terms are used interchangeably throughout this chapter.

In the context of Edge AI, end devices process, analyze, summarize, or convert data using ML algorithms in addition to acting as data generators. These operations take place on the devices themselves in some situations as well as within network edge nodes.

In addition to Edge Computing's benefits, ML capabilities at the network edge offer the following advantages:

1. By reducing data dimensionality and collecting contextual information that can be transmitted to the Cloud for more in-depth analysis, preprocessing raw data at the edge minimizes bandwidth consumption.
2. It mitigates the computational load on cloud systems by enabling sensor data fusion, at the edge, as shown in surveillance-scenarios.
3. Especially in Big Data settings, using the processing capacity of edge devices and nodes improves the effectiveness and responsiveness of distributed ML algorithms.

But there are drawbacks to the Edge Intelligence ecosystem as well: ML techniques need to be modified for distributed computing and storage systems.

1. It's crucial to manage memory and processing power while training ML models and using them to draw conclusions.
2. Different time scales and data granularities require different ML methods.
3. To successfully incorporate ML into Edge Computing, structured solutions and standards must be created.

10.2 LITERATURE REVIEW

The combination of Edge Computing with Artificial Intelligence (AI), known as Edge Intelligence, has become a crucial paradigm for overcoming the drawbacks of centralized computing models, particularly in situations that call for real-time processing, low latency, and effective resource use. The fundamental ideas of edge computing, how it integrates with AI, and the developments, difficulties, and uses in this field are all covered in this overview.

Early in the 21st century, cloud computing emerged, bringing with it large-scale, centralized systems for data processing and storage. Nevertheless, the exponential growth of IoT devices and the requirement for real-time processing, particularly in relation to high latency, bandwidth consumption, and scalability, exposed the limitations of cloud computing. To solve these problems, paradigms such as Cloudlets, Fog Computing, and Edge Computing were developed.

- Cloudlets, which are mini data centers located near end devices, are used to reduce latency and offload computational responsibilities from both the Cloud and end devices. Applications include video caching, computer vision, and healthcare solutions.
- Cloud services are brought closer to the network edge by fog computing, which focuses on IoT-centric applications like smart cities and transportation systems. It uses a tiered architecture to offer computation, storage, and connectivity among several devices.
- The wider idea of Edge Computing, which emphasizes real-time processing at the network edge, enables applications like Big Data analytics and time-sensitive systems. To meet strict latency and energy requirements, Edge Computing places a higher priority on proximity to endpoints than Fog and Cloudlets do.

Edge Intelligence integrates Edge Computing infrastructure with ML techniques to handle data locally or at the network edge. This paradigm overcomes the limitations of transferring large volumes of raw data to the cloud, enabling context aware processing and efficient resource utilization.

The following are some main advantages of incorporating AI into edge computing:

1. Data preprocessing optimizes data transfer to the cloud by reducing dimensionality and locally extracting contextual knowledge while using less bandwidth.
2. Real-time aggregation and analysis of data from many sources is made possible via sensor data fusion, which is essential for applications involving monitoring and surveillance.
3. Accelerated ML Algorithms: Distributed ML models, especially in Big Data settings, can improve responsiveness by utilizing edge resources.

Many architectures and frameworks have been proposed to enable Edge Intelligence. These techniques aim to address a number of problems, including resource constraints, distributed model training, and heterogeneous device integration. Among the significant advancements are:

- Device-improved multi-access edge computing, which maximizes energy efficiency while enhancing edge devices' processing and storage capabilities to handle demanding workloads.
- Ad Hoc cloud computing, which uses intermittently accessible edge infrastructure for task execution and preprocessing.

Despite its potential, Edge Intelligence has a lot of obstacles to overcome:

- Algorithm adaptation: ML algorithms must be tailored for devices with limited resources and distributed contexts.
- Resource management: Making effective use of memory and processing power for inference and training is still a major concern.
- Heterogeneity: Standardized frameworks are necessary to integrate various devices and preserve interoperability.
- Scalability: There are technical challenges in managing fluctuating workloads and guaranteeing scalability in edge contexts.

Applications for edge intelligence have been discovered in a number of fields:

- Healthcare: AI-enhanced wearables for real-time monitoring and diagnosis.
- Smart cities: Solutions for public safety, energy efficiency, and traffic control.
- Industrial IoT: Manufacturing process optimization and predictive maintenance.
- Intelligent video analytics for monitoring and security is known as surveillance.

By overcoming the drawbacks of centralized computing paradigms, the combination of edge computing and AI holds revolutionary promise for a variety of businesses. Despite the notable advancements, issues with standardization, resource management, and algorithm optimization still exist. More reliable, effective, and scalable Edge Intelligence solutions will be made possible by ongoing research and development in this field.

10.3 AN OVERVIEW OF EDGE COMPUTING

Edge Computing is designed to do computing and data preparation tasks closer to the network edge rather than relying on remote service providers as standard Cloud Computing does. This approach ensures data integrity and confidentiality, allows for real-time answers, and reduces the amount of time and effort needed for data processing from the moment it is generated. For instance, studies show that Edge Computing can save energy consumption by roughly 40% by doing away with the need for communication.

By performing computations at the edge and removing the need to transmit data over insecure channels (such Wi-Fi and Bluetooth), which are commonly used in cloud systems, this design reduces the risk of data breaches and guarantees increased security. Additionally, masking or removing private or superfluous data during preprocessing before sharing it with external devices helps reduce the risk of sensitive information leaks.

Furthermore, Edge Computing provides an abstraction layer that makes it possible to aggregate complementing data from diverse endpoints. By simply converting and distributing relevant data for data fusion at the edge, this layer lessens the computational load that would otherwise be required on centralized Cloud servers.

The primary disadvantage of edge computing, however, is the hardware and processing capacity of endpoints at the network edge. These gadgets usually lack the processing power and large battery capacity necessary to support complex data processing algorithms because of their physical constraints. Finding a balance between processing speed and energy consumption is still very challenging.

Despite edge computing, cloud computing and related ideas like fog computing are still required. Since the network edge serves as a layer in a hierarchical data processing structure, tasks are preprocessed or processed closer to the edge, which has sufficient resources to finish the task.

Mobile Edge Computing (MEC) is a noteworthy use of Edge Computing, especially in the telecom industry. By placing edge computers in mobile base stations, MEC expands on Edge Computing by gathering and processing real-time network data while drastically cutting down on latency. With the extra advantage of location awareness, this model makes use of the same concepts as Edge and Fog Computing, allowing developers, content providers, and consumers to utilize location-specific data for a variety of purposes. In order to gather real-time network data and improve overall system performance, Nokia Networks created the first MEC system in 2012, integrating processing and storage capabilities into common telecommunications equipment.

10.3.1 Examples of edge computing applications

When low latency is essential and cloud computing might not be enough, edge computing, fog computing, and MEC are especially useful. Several important application areas are listed below:

- Autonomous driving: Safe navigation in autonomous driving depends on prompt decision-making. To reduce latency, raw data must be processed at the vehicle itself because even minor delays can have hazardous consequences. At 100 km/h, for instance, a 0.1-second latency would need the car to move almost 3 meters before the outcome is calculated. Research emphasizes how crucial quick data processing is for self-driving cars. By preprocessing raw data to extract point cloud features, frameworks such as F-Cooper, which was proposed in, leverage Edge Computing to fuse data and enhance object detection. The advantages of local data processing to extract pertinent aspects such object shape and movement are further demonstrated by pedestrian detection techniques employing LiDAR sensors. See for a detailed discussion of these techniques [10–12].
- Solutions for security: Edge computing can greatly improve security systems, including surveillance applications, in which cameras or edge devices locally process data to fuse information or infer outcomes. It can be used, for example, to identify known criminals before they do deadly acts. Edge Computing was used to track vehicle speed on highways in, with positive outcomes. To identify and lessen IoT security threats, Edge Computing incorporates security features including Edge-based Authentication, Authorization, and collaborative architectures in the context of distributed networks like the IoT. Furthermore, Edge Computing and Blockchain can guarantee energy efficiency and privacy in vehicle-related security [13–15].
- IoT applications: As the number of IoT sensors increases, Edge Computing can be used to locally preprocess data before transmitting it to cloud servers, which lowers latency and bandwidth. The WuKong framework, for example, supports smart home systems by fusing data from heterogeneous sensors for activity identification using Edge Computing. In a similar vein, processing data produced by dispersed sensors is made possible by the incorporation of Edge Computing into smart city projects. Frameworks for trusted domains, device-centric security designs, and end-to-end security are examples of security solutions for Edge Computing in the context of the IoT that safeguard data privacy across heterogeneous Edge devices.
- Location services: Location-based services like smart parking can benefit from the use of edge computing. For instance, Fog Computing can optimize car distribution in metropolitan areas by determining parking space availability in conjunction with Edge and Cloud systems.

In order to improve the overall service, edge devices can also employ location data to give contextual information prior to transmission. In, parking spot detection and license plate recognition were accomplished by using Deep Learning (DL) algorithms with Edge Computing. Bluetooth Low Energy (BLE) and Ultra-wideband (UWB) positioning systems at the network edge are used for patient tracking in hospitals and interior navigation, among other location-based applications.

- Network functions: Network functions, which were previously implemented in hardware, can now be integrated onto Edge devices through the use of Network Function Virtualization. This method offers real-time responses while improving privacy and lowering latency. To enhance system performance, a number of communication protocols were put into place at the network edge in. With high alarm prediction accuracy, Edge Computing also supports network applications including performance monitoring, physical impairment assessment, and alarm message filtering. Furthermore, by using containers to deploy ML models efficiently, Edge Computing can lower bandwidth usage while improving resource management and system security.

Although Edge Computing provides significant advantages in many fields, its efficacy hinges on the proper combination of specialized hardware and software. We examine the present software platforms and hardware architectures supporting Edge Computing in the part that follows, offering more in-depth analyses of their pertinent aspects.

10.3.2 Software and architectures for edge computing

When feasible, Edge Computing seeks to process data at the source device. However, specialized processing units in Edge Computing devices are necessary because CPUs sometimes lack the computational capacity needed to manage complicated tasks under real-time limitations. Facebook researchers, for instance, have shown that a large portion of the inference process in their apps is done directly on end devices, such tablets and smartphones. Alternatives like integrating co-processors, like Graphics Processing Units (GPUs), or adding several CPUs for parallel processing are frequently utilized to increase the computing capabilities of Edge devices.

For Edge Computing devices, several studies have proposed modular designs that allow control of both real-time and non-real-time units responsible for memory management and communication protocols, while ensuring real-time processing. In these configurations, a central core runs an operating system to manage the device's resources and decide where to execute tasks inside the global process. The gadget should also be updateable so that new features and improvements can be added. Scalability is another important factor; devices must be aware of the capacities of their neighbors in order to provide efficient network resource management. Communication protocols should enable communication with Fog or MEC nodes in addition to Edge devices for seamless information transit across the network.

To reduce latency, it separates the input data into three layers:

- Data that needs to be calculated instantly is processed by the real-time layer.
- Batch layer: Processes historical data to preprocess it and create batches.
- Serving layer: Offers access to the generated data and displays and conveys the calculated results.

A processing pipeline for Edge Computing is emphasized in both systems, which have a similar structure. Data collection, data preprocessing (including homogenization, filtering, and privacy masking), result calculation, result storage, and system interface are the stages that are usually included in this pipeline.

10.4 EDGE INTELLIGENCE

Edge AI, or Edge Intelligence, is the term used to describe the fusion of Edge Computing with AI. The primary goal of this technology is to bring AI capabilities closer to the network edge. Edge AI devices must have enough processing capacity to execute AI inference algorithms that process data in a timely manner and, in some situations, support learning algorithms in order to be effective. Because of this, Edge AI systems' performance measures are different from those of conventional AI systems that use high-performance computer resources. The following crucial elements need to be taken into account for Edge AI performance:

- Energy consumption: Controlling energy consumption is essential because Edge devices usually operate as separate nodes in a dispersed network without direct access to the electrical grid.
- Real time or soft real time constraints: The system must react quickly to inputs in order to satisfy the temporal requirements of AI services.
- Communication frequency: How often devices rely on the central network to process data is determined by how frequently they communicate with other nodes.

Because Edge AI devices have limited resources, AI algorithms need to be modified to function well in a low-power, distributed setting. Memory access should be improved to minimize redundant operations, memory bottlenecks, and needless energy consumption in order to improve AI performance.

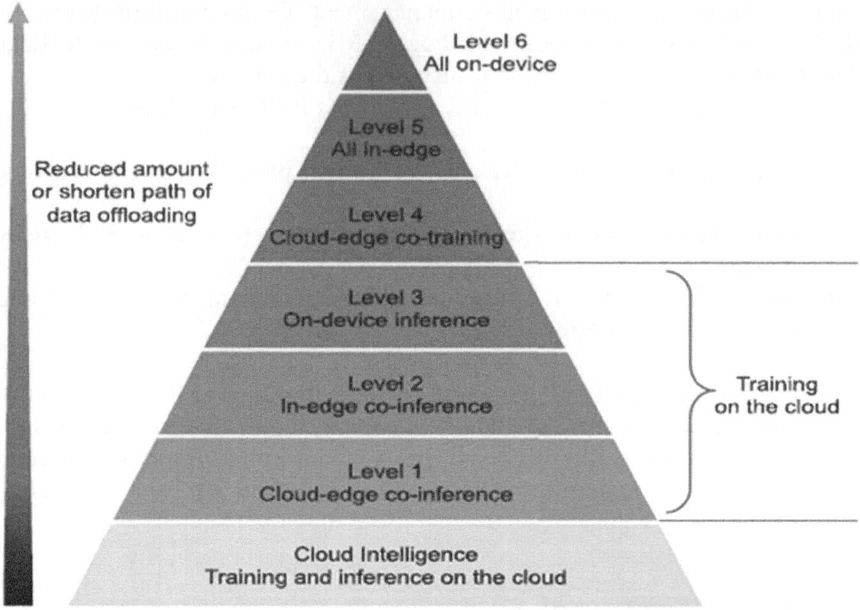

Figure 10.4 Levels of edge intelligence implementation [16].

Figure 10.4 illustrates the many degrees of Edge Intelligence implementation that were suggested in. The degree of migration of ML algorithms from the cloud to the network edge is represented by these levels.

Current developments and applications mainly concentrate on ML, especially DL, even though Edge Intelligence is made to execute a variety of AI algorithms at the network edge. As a result, Sections 10.4.1 and 10.4.2 offer a thorough analysis of cutting-edge AI methods designed to lessen the processing burden on edge devices. While Section 10.4.2 explores state-of-the-art DL approaches, Section 10.4.1 provides a general overview of ML techniques.

10.4.1 Machine Learning Algorithms for Edge Computing

The idea of Intelligent Agents has already been used to adapt and implement ML techniques at the network edge. An autonomous creature that senses its surroundings and chooses actions to accomplish a goal based on internal representations, recent (and occasionally historical) observations, a set of predetermined rules, or an AI model inference engine is known as an intelligent agent.

Reducing the length of AI models to accommodate low-resource devices while preserving speed is necessary when running AI algorithms at the network edge. Decision Jungle, which uses decision trees, is one example of this methodology. An ensemble of rooted decision directed acyclic graphs that are taught level by level, while maximizing an objective-function based on the graphs' structure make up a decision jungle. This technique has produced successful compression outcomes on a number of datasets. For example, the size of the Faces dataset was decreased from 7.17 MB to 1.72 MB, while the Decision Jungle for the Kinect dataset was decreased from 80 MB to 9 MB while preserving state-of-the-art accuracy [17, 18].

Random Forests (RF) have been subjected to similar methods. Each decision tree, is pruned to satisfy a global resource limitation while maximizing performance during the training and pruning phases of the RF compression process. Cutting-edge compression techniques are surpassed by the trimmed RF algorithm. After features were extracted from the data, RF was employed for human activity recognition, at the network edge. Depending on the volume of data, the accuracy ranged from 94% to 98%. Similar to Decision Jungle, this method offers excellent accuracy and is scalable to huge datasets.

Another well-liked technique in Edge AI is the k-Nearest Neighbors (kNN) classifier. One notable modification that condenses clusters to fit the limitations of low-resource devices is ProtoNN. This technique projects the complete dataset into a lower-dimensional space by using feature selection and dimensionality reduction. ProtoNN may be used on devices with as little as 16KB of RAM and provides state-of-the-art accuracy across a range of benchmarks.

Additionally, Edge AI applies ML methods to particular fields, including computer vision. For example, for tasks like human detection, feature extraction from images utilizing methods like edge gradient and histogram of gradient orientation has been applied, followed by classification approaches. This was illustrated in by achieving state-of-the-art results in human detection using Support Vector Machines (SVM) on the MIT pedestrian database. Similarly, suggested utilizing linear SVM classification in conjunction with Histogram of Oriented Gradients (HOG) for monocular vision-based smart car detection. This method produced positive results when evaluated in a variety of settings, including cities, roads, and occlusion situations.

Natural voice recognition also makes use of ML methods, as Nuance's Dragon Naturally Speaking system demonstrates. In addition to these methods, ML algorithms have been used for tasks like prediction and regression at the network edge. For example, it demonstrated how to train ML models at the network edge directly utilizing gradient descent techniques (e.g., SVM, K-means, and linear regression) without relying on external cloud servers. By employing numerous edge devices to do ML tasks concurrently, this technique leverages a distributed network to get around the processing limitations of individual devices. A final edge device gathers the results and preprocesses or processes the data for adaptation before forwarding it for further processing. This approach was tested with three Raspberry Pi3 devices and a laptop as edge devices, yielding nearly state-of-the-art results with SVM, K-means, and linear regression. All of these algorithms have the disadvantage that time complexity increases with data growth, notwithstanding their effectiveness. When dealing with large datasets, DL models may offer superior solutions.

10.4.2 Deep learning at the network edge

Artificial neural networks (ANN), which are made up of several layers of artificial neurons that process data to provide a result, are the foundation of DL. Before the final layer produces the classification or feature, data is transferred through each layer, where matrix multiplications calculate the input for the layer after it. A network is called a Deep Neural Network (DNN) when it has hundreds of layers. A variety of DNN structures have been created for particular uses, such as Recurrent Neural Networks (RNNs) for time-series processing, which use loops in the internal neuron connections to store previous inputs, and Convolutional Neural Networks (CNNs) for image and video processing, which perform convolutional filter operations in addition to matrix multiplications.

Cloud computing has historically been used for both training and inference because of the high processing power needed to train DL models. However, Edge Computing is currently being used due to growing time and security restrictions in applications like healthcare and driverless cars. Training the DNN using traditional Cloud Computing and transferring the inference process to the edge device (as illustrated in Figure 10.5b) or doing

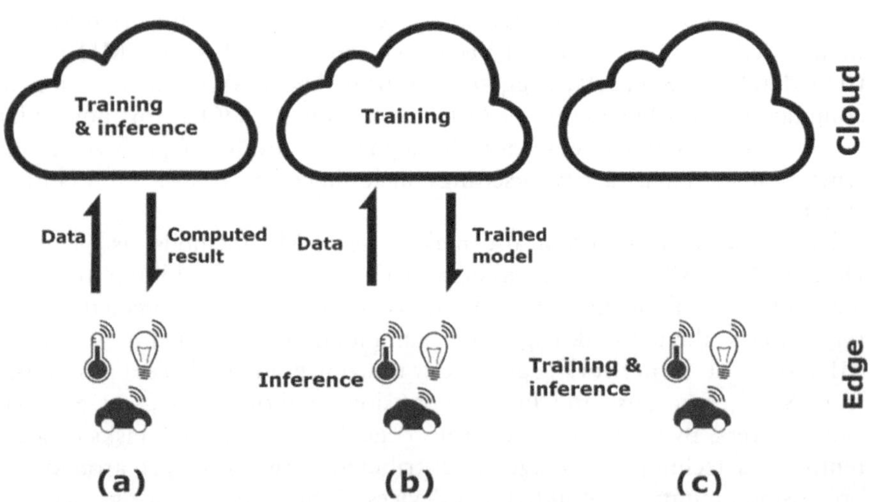

Figure 10.5 Different methods for training and interfernce. (a) Cloud-based training and inference. (b) Cloud training with edge inference. (c) Edge-based training and inference.

both training and inference directly on the edge device (as illustrated in Figure 10.5c) are two new methods for DL at the network edge. The edge device's resource needs vary according to the strategy selected.

When training takes place at the edge, the device needs to be highly computationally capable and have enough memory to hold the training data. Since just the trained model needs to be saved, the memory need is lower if inference is the only process carried out.

Researchers have created a number of methods to lower memory footprints and boost training speeds on low-resource devices in order to make it easier to train DL models on edge devices:

- Pruning: This method, which is modeled after synaptic pruning in real brains, eliminates unnecessary connections between neurons to minimize the amount of computation needed to process new information. It is also possible to exclude neurons with low weight values in relation to the DNN's global environment. Pruning produces DNNs that are smaller, quicker, and use less memory, which makes them appropriate for deployment on edge devices [19, 20].
- Weights quantization: This method collects related weights and quantizes them into integers or smaller values that take up fewer bits, as opposed to storing each weight as a separate value. While this lowers memory consumption, the accuracy of the model may be marginally impacted. A recursive process where the weights are continuously improved and measured results from the weights being re-adjusted during training.
- Federated-learning and model partition: Federated learning provides a distributed method for complicated tasks or big datasets, in which data is divided and delivered to several edge devices for local training. Active learning at the edge is made possible by each device's contribution to the DNN's training portion. This idea is expanded upon during inference by Model Partition, in which distinct devices compute each DNN layer, dividing the effort and enhancing scalability.
- Transfer-learning: This method uses previously trained models and transfers what they have learnt to a different field. While the subsequent layers of a DNN are retrained for the particular application, the first layers, which extract general information, are kept. By using an established structure, this minimizes training time and resource consumption, which makes it perfect for situations where there is not enough data to train a model from scratch.
- Knowledge distillation is a type of Transfer Learning in which knowledge is transferred from a big, highly skilled DNN (the teacher) to a smaller, more effective DNN (the student). By using strategies like pruning, the student network is trained to produce outcomes that are comparable to those of the instructor network while requiring less computing power.

- Gossip-training: This method uses randomized gossip algorithms to expedite training on edge devices. Each device trains on a subset of the data in this asynchronous, decentralized paradigm. Devices exchange results during random communication events, leading to the formation of a consensus. Active learning at the network edge is made possible by this technique, which divides the task among several devices.

These methods overcome the resource limitations usually found in low-power devices, enabling the effective training and inference of DL models on edge devices.

10.4.3 Evaluation and discussion

At the network edge, a range of algorithms, such as Speech Recognition, Computer Vision, Intelligent Agents, and Decision Jungles, have been created to address different applications. However, due to the enormous volume of data generated at the network edge and the need for fast processing, DL models have outperformed conventional methods. DL can readily manage large amounts of data for tasks like regression and classification. DL has long been employed in the cloud for both training and inference due to its superior processing capability. However, as applications that demand low latency have gotten more popular, Edge Computing—in particular, Edge Intelligence—has emerged as a more successful tactic.

The DL algorithms in use today are not made for edge devices; rather, they are made for high-resource devices. In order to modify these DL models for the network edge, researchers have been creating new methods. As a result, methods that drastically shrink DL models and make them suitable for edge devices have emerged, including quantization, federated learning, knowledge distillation, and pruning. Even though these methods have many benefits, not all applications may benefit from them. Pruning and quantization, for example, should be used carefully when high accuracy is required because they can lower accuracy. To find the method that works best for a given application, these approaches must be tested as part of the iterative DNN design process.

Table 10.1 offers a preliminary reference for choosing the best methodology by contrasting the previously discussed methods to show their primary distinctions. As demonstrated, the majority of these techniques concentrate on lowering the memory footprint of DL models in order to make them appropriate for network edge devices with limited resources. However, because some connections or settings are changed, precision is frequently sacrificed in the process. Federated learning, on the other hand, preserves the key components of the DL model while optimizing efficiency by distributing it across several devices. A pretrained DL model, which forms the basis of the reduced model, is a prerequisite shared by all of these methods.

The majority of research that use an Edge Intelligence approach concentrate on the middle tiers of the Edge AI framework (Figure 10.5), where

Table 10.1 Comparing methods for modifying deep learning models for edge intelligence gadgets

Method	*Memory reduction*	*Maintain accuracy*	*Original DNN*	*Multiple devices*	*Reduced datasets*
Pruning	Needed	Not needed	Needed	Not needed	Not needed
Quantization	Needed	Not needed	Needed	Not needed	Not needed
Federated learning	Needed	Needed	Needed	Needed	Not needed
Transfer learning	Not needed	Needed	Needed	Not needed	Needed
Knowledge distillation	Needed	Needed	Needed	Not needed	Needed
Gossip learning	Needed	Needed	Not	needed	Needed
Not needed					

inference is either done in a hybrid edge-cloud collaborative method or gradually moved to the network edge while training still takes place in the Cloud. Due to the constraints of edge devices, including their limited power and compute capacity, this trend has not yet been fully realized despite continuous research targeted at moving both training and inference procedures to the network edge.

10.5 CONCLUSION

With an emphasis on the most recent developments in Edge AI frameworks and devices, this survey offers a thorough examination of the enabling technologies for Edge AI.

There has been discussion of recent advancements in edge computing, emphasizing new software and hardware advances intended to solve the problems that cloud computing encounters in the modern world. Numerous application examples, including as autonomous driving, security solutions, IoT applications, location awareness systems, and network management, have illustrated the importance of these developments. The incorporation of additional modules and layers that facilitate process parallelization is what defines hardware advancement. Software developments, meanwhile, focus on increasing system security and speeding up data processing. For a better understanding, these elements have been shown and contrasted using a variety of tables.

The survey also emphasizes the rise of Edge AI devices and their potential advantages in other research fields, including computer vision, VR, IoT, and natural language processing. The present status of Edge AI devices and frameworks has been appraised based on their salient features in accordance with Edge Computing research, allowing for comparison to evaluate their applicability for different applications.

REFERENCES

1. Julien Gedeon, Jeff Krisztinkovics, Christian Meurisch, Michael Stein, Lin Wang, and Max Mühlhäuser. 2018. A Multi-Cloudlet Infrastructure for Future Smart Cities: An Empirical Study. In *Proceedings of the 1st International Workshop on Edge Systems, Analytics and Networking (EdgeSys'18)*. ACM, New York, pp. 19–24. https://doi.org/10.1145/3213344.3213348
2. Z. Pang, L. Sun, Z. Wang, E. Tian, and S. Yang. 2015. A Survey of Cloudlet Based Mobile Computing. In *Proceedings of the International Conference on Cloud Computing and Big Data (CCBD)*, pp. 268–275. https://doi.org/10.1109/CCBD.2015.54
3. R. K. Naha, S. Garg, D. Georgakopoulos, P. P. Jayaraman, L. Gao, Y. Xiang, and R. Ranjan. 2018. Fog Computing: Survey of Trends, Architectures, Requirements, and Research Directions. *IEEE Access* 6(2018), 47980–48009. https://doi.org/10.1109/ACCESS.2018.2866491
4. M. Kumar, A. Kumar, S. Verma, P. Bhattacharya, D. Ghimire, S. H. Kim, and A. S. Hosen. 2023. Healthcare Internet of Things (H-IoT): Current Trends, Future Prospects, Applications, Challenges, and Security Issues. *Electronics* 12(9), 2050.
5. Partha Pratim Ray, Dinesh Dash, and Debashis De. 2019. Edge Computing for Internet of Things: A Survey, e-healthcare Case Study and Future Direction. *Journal of Network and Computer Applications* 140(2019), 1–22. https://doi.org/10.1016/j.jnca.2019.05.005
6. Ana Juan Ferrer, Joan Manuel Marquès, and Josep Jorba. 2019. Towards the Decentralised Cloud: Survey on Approaches and Challenges for Mobile, Ad Hoc, and Edge Computing. *ACM Computing Surveys (CSUR)* 51(6), 1–36.
7. Gary A. McGilvary, Adam Barker, and Malcolm Atkinson. 2015. Ad Hoc Cloud Computing. In *Proceedings of the IEEE 8th International Conference on Cloud Computing*. IEEE, pp. 1063–1068.
8. Mahshid Mehrabi, Dongho You, Vincent Latzko, Hani Salah, Martin Reisslein, and Frank HP Fitzek. 2019. Device-Enhanced MEC: Multi-Access Edge Computing (MEC) Aided by End Device Computation and Caching: A Survey. *IEEE Access* 7(2019), 166079–166108.
9. A. Pratap, A. Kumar, and M. Kumar. 2021, May. Analyzing the Need of Edge Computing for Internet of Things (IoT). In *Proceedings of Second International Conference on Computing, Communications, and Cyber-Security (IC4S'20)*, Singapore, pp. 203–212.
10. Mingyue Cui, Shipeng Zhong, Boyang Li, Xu Chen, and Kai Huang. 2020. Offloading Autonomous Driving Services Via Edge Computing. *IEEE Internet of Things Journal* 7(10), 10535–10547.
11. Lei Liu, Chen Chen, Qingqi Pei, Sabita Maharjan, and Yan Zhang. 2021. Vehicular Edge Computing and Networking: A Survey. *Mobile Networks and Applications* 26(3), 1145–1168.
12. Shaoshan Liu, Liangkai Liu, Jie Tang, Bo Yu, Yifan Wang, and Weisong Shi. 2019. Edge Computing for Autonomous Driving: Opportunities and Challenges. *Proceedings of the IEEE* 107(8), 1697–1716.
13. Ganesh Ananthanarayanan, Paramvir Bahl, Peter Bodík, Krishna Chintalapudi, Matthai Philipose, Lenin Ravindranath, and Sudipta Sinha. 2017. Real-time Video Analytics: The Killer App for Edge Computing. *Computer* 50(10), 58–67.
14. M. Kumar, P. Mukherjee, S. Verma, Kavita, M. Kaur, S. Singh, ... and M. F. Ijaz. 2022. BBNSF: Blockchain-based Novel Secure Framework Using RP2-RSA and ASR-ANN Technique for IoT Enabled Healthcare Systems. *Sensors 22*(23), 9448.

15. Khan Muhammad, Salman Khan, Vasile Palade, Irfan Mehmood, and Victor Hugo C. De Albuquerque. 2019. Edge Intelligence-Assisted Smoke Detection in Foggy Surveillance Environments. *IEEE Transactions on Industrial Informatics* 16(2), 1067–1075.
16. Z. Zhou, X. Chen, E. Li, L. Zeng, K. Luo, and J. Zhang. 2019. Edge Intelligence: Paving the Last Mile of Artificial Intelligence With Edge Computing. *Proceedings of the IEEE* 107(8), 1738–1762. https://doi.org/10.1109/JPROC.2019.2918951
17. Jamie Shotton, Toby Sharp, Pushmeet Kohli, Sebastian Nowozin, John Winn, and Antonio Criminisi. 2013. Decision Jungles: Compact and Rich Models for Classification. In *Advances in Neural Information Processing Systems*, p. 26.
18. Feng Nan, Joseph Wang, and Venkatesh Saligrama. 2016. Pruning Random Forests for Prediction on a Budget. In *Advances in Neural Information Processing Systems*, pp. 2334–2342.
19. Hu Zhang Chiliang Guan Yingda Tao, and Ye Zuochang. 2019. Accelerating Convolutional Neural Networks with Dynamic Channel Pruning. In *Proceedings of the Data Compression Conference (DCC)*. IEEE, pp. 563–563.
20. Ji Lin, Yongming Rao, Jiwen Lu, and Jie Zhou. 2017. Runtime Neural Pruning. In *Proceedings of the 31st International Conference on Neural Information Processing Systems*, pp. 2178–2188.

Chapter 11

Advancements in early detection of lung cancer

A comprehensive review of AI-based techniques

Takreem Fatima Khan and Swaleha Zubair

11.1 INTRODUCTION

The primary component of the human respiratory system is the lungs, which are air-filled organs located in the thoracic cavity (chest). Lung cancer is the most common cause of cancer-related deaths due to the possibility of malignant alteration in lung cells [1]. Permanent alterations in Deoxyribo Nucleic Acid (DNA) sequences are called mutation or uncontrolled tissue growth. Mutations may result from inherited genetic defects or environmental influences. Tobacco smoke compounds are the most common external influence, although there are many other potential carcinogens as well [2]. New tissue replaces typically damaged tissue, but when a malignant mutation is present, the growth of the new tissue is uncontrolled, which results in the formation of cancerous cells. Lung nodules are deformities that grow inside the lung and can be cancerous or non-cancerous, but most of them are non-cancerous, and some may indicate early-stage cancer.

According to recent studies, the 5-year survival rate for lung cancer is approximately 20% [3]. The World Health Organization (WHO) expects that by 2030, the percentage of deaths from cancer will rise to 45% [4]. Early diagnosis of lung cancer significantly increases lung cancer survival rate. Computed tomography (CT) scans are helpful for early identification of lung nodules [5]. The internal structure of the body is depicted in depth by the scanned images, which provide top, bottom, and front views, respectively. Compared to standard X-rays, more details regarding the blood arteries, soft tissues, and bones can be found in CT images. However, because lung nodules resemble other structures, such as blood vessels, it becomes challenging to locate them and identify potential cancerous lung nodules. Therefore, morphological analysis is crucial as the cancerous cells are distinguished morphologically by the irregular shape and size of the nucleus [6]. So, the analysis of benign and malignant nodules is commonly

DOI: 10.1201/9781003634560-11

done using morphological features found in CT images. The basic approach dramatically depends on highly qualified radiologists distinguishing between benign and malignant nodules. A comprehensive evaluation becomes challenging for radiologists due to the similarities in features of malignant and benign nodules. Therefore, there is an intense need to develop a computer-aided design system to identify cancerous nodules. AI-based methods have recently gained significant importance in the medical field, particularly for using medical databases to diagnose diseases [7]. These methods are used to improve medical diagnostics and predict diseases early, and they have shown promising results in the early detection of lung cancer. This intelligent method consists of techniques such as image processing, image segmentation, and classification algorithms using machine learning [8]. Machine learning enables computers to learn from training data and improve over time. Machine learning algorithms use statistical techniques to produce predictions by recognizing data patterns and learning from them. Machine learning applies various strategies, including supervised and unsupervised learning [9]. When a model is given a set of examples and their corresponding labels, it is said to be "supervised learning", in which the model learns to recognize the proper label. The most popular forms of supervised learning are classification and regression. On the other hand, unsupervised learning occurs when no input labels are provided. Using the similarity between the inputs, the model tries to predict the label as output between the inputs after learning how similar they are. Unsupervised learning uses the clustering technique to sort inputs into similar groups. A substantial increase in the use of supervised machine learning algorithms in the medical industry has been seen in recent years, significantly to predict diseases utilizing medical databases [10]. Supervised machine learning algorithms have shown promising results in classification problems such as the classification of lung nodules into benign and malignant. On the other hand, unsupervised machine learning algorithms play a significant role in image segmentation problems in finding the Region of Interest [11].

Different approaches have been proposed for lung cancer detection as depicted in Figure 11.1. However, these frameworks need more precision in detecting lung nodules. Therefore, the techniques employed in these frameworks must be further refined to address this limitation [12]. In this study, we have highlighted these gaps and discussed potential strategies to address them. In the next section, we conducted a comprehensive examination and analysis of recently developed approaches. The methodology for article selection is detailed in Section 11.3, followed by an in-depth analysis and discussion in Section 11.4. Section 11.5 outlines the identified limitations and future research directions, while Section 11.6 provides the conclusion of the study.

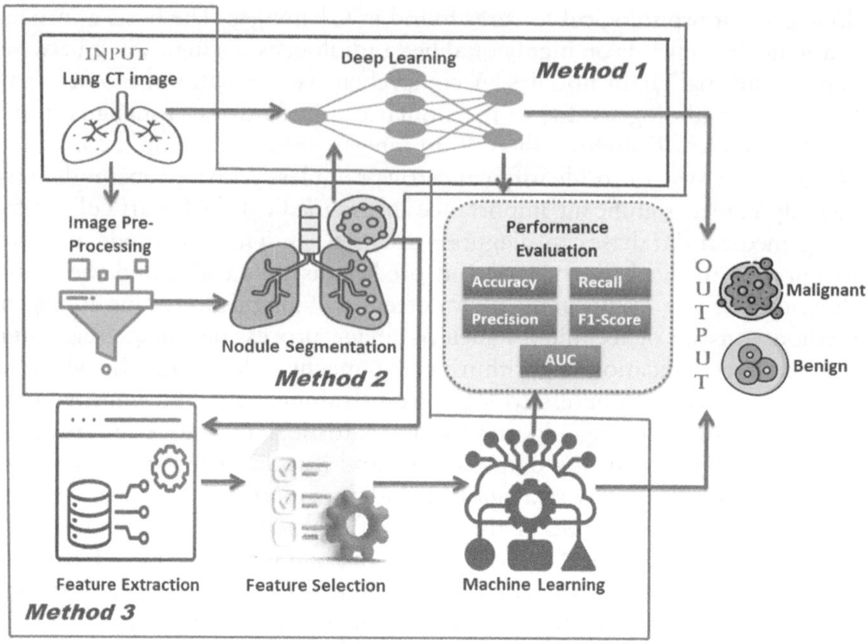

Figure 11.1 Different AI-driven methodologies have been proposed in the literature.

11.2 RECENT LITERATURE ON AI-BASED LUNG CANCER DETECTION

A number of researchers have proposed and developed different approaches for detecting lung cancer using AI-based methodologies as presented in Table 11.1. In the research conducted by Makaju et al. [13], instead of a Gabor filter, the Gaussian Filter and median filter are used as image enhancement techniques, which is followed by watershed segmentation to locate the lung nodule. Features like area, perimeter, centroid, diameter, eccentricity, and Mean intensity are extracted to train the classifier. Support Vector Machine (SVM) is used as the classifier in this model, giving 86.6% accuracy. In the work done by Venkatesh et al. [14], k means clustering is used to carry out the segmentation process. Convolutional Neural Network (CNN) is used for feature extraction and classification after Particle Swarm Optimization Techniques (PSO) is used to select the tumor-containing cluster among the six clusters. The accuracy provided by this model was 99.96%. Using an ensemble learning strategy, Gautam et al. [12] make use of deep transfer learning, namely ResNet-152, DenseNet-169, and EfficientNet-B7, three of the most advanced CNN models. There is a novel procedure for choosing and allocating weights to each base model to improve the performance of the ensemble method by combining the results of two standard

Table 11.1 Comparative analysis of AI-based techniques for early lung cancer detection

Reference	*Year*	*Dataset*	*Pre-processing*	*Segmentation*	*Feature extraction*	*Feature selection*	*Classification*	*Limitation*
Gautam et al. [12]	2024	LIDC-IDRI	–	–	ResNet 152, Dense Net 169, EfficientNet B9	–	Ensemble technique	To eliminate noise from the images, no image processing techniques were utilized.
Venkatesh et al. [14]	2023	LIDC-IDRI&Kaggle	Median filter	K-means clustering and PSO	CNN	–	CNN	Three input images are used in the model's testing, which is insufficient to verify the model's performance.
Maleki et al. [15]	2023	Taken from hospital in Tehran, Iran	Median Filter	Watershed Segmentation	Gabor, Sobel, Scharr, Prewitt, Gaussian and Roberts Edge Filter	PCA and LDA	RF and SVM	The lung section is just segmented rather than lung nodules, which could affect the model performance in terms of computational cost and time
Shafiet al. [4]	2022	LUNA16		CapsNet	CNN	–	SVM	Image denoising has not been employed to remove noise.
Bhattacharjee et al. [17]	2022	LIDC-IDRI	–	Adaptive Thresholding	–	–	Optimized RF	Nodules measuring more than or equal to 3 mm were only considered.

(*Continued*)

Table 11.1 (Continued)

Reference	*Year*	*Dataset*	*Pre-processing*	*Segmentation*	*Feature extraction*	*Feature selection*	*Classification*	*Limitation*
Nageswaran et al. [19]	2022	A collection of 83 CT scans from 70 patients	Geometric mean filter	K- means	–	LDA	ANN	The features that have been extracted out of the segmented region are not specified.
Priyadharshini et al. [2]	2021	LIDC-IDRI	–	FCM	DWT		BAT-CNN	The pre-processing technique for images is not well specified.
Kareem et al. [18]	2021	IQ-OTH/ NCCD	Bit-plane slicing, Gaussian Filter, Morphological Operations	Otsu's thresholding	Gabor and GLCM	–	SVM	The feature selection technique could also be used to achieve better results.
Vijh et al. [16]	2020	NCI lung cancer database	Median Filter	Global Thresholding	GLCM	WOA	SVM	Only a few samples of images are considered for research
Makaju et al. [13]	2018	LIDC/IDRI	Gaussian and median filter	Watershed segmentation	–	–	SVM	Feature selection technique is not applied, which can improve the model performance.

evaluation metrics, the F1-score and ROC-AUC score. The suggested ensemble attains 97.23% accuracy.

Maleki et al. [15] used four different approaches, and one of the more successful ones was the one that involved extracting specific features such as Gabor, Sobel, Scharr, and Robert. Then, dimension reduction techniques such as PCA and LDA are used. The model attained a 95% accuracy after applying classification algorithms such as Random Forest (RF) and SVM. Shafi et al. [4] have created a hybrid model that uses machine learning algorithms for classification and deep learning methods for segmentation and feature extraction. This hybrid model attained 94% of accuracy. To accurately detect lung cancer, Priyadharshini et al. [2] developed a model in which the learning rate is modified in CNN by BAT optimization technique. The CT scan image is segmented using the Discrete Wavelet Transform (DWT), which is utilized to split an image into four smaller bands; the Low (LL) band image was considered. In the experiment, 96.43% accuracy was achieved.

Vijh et al. [16] implemented the Gray Level Co-occurrence Matrix (GLCM) approach to extract texture and statistical features from the lung CT image. To select the best features for accurate results and building a strong model, Whale Optimization Algorithm (WOA) is employed. Using SVM for classification, the performance of the suggested model in terms of accuracy, sensitivity, and specificity are 95%, 100%, and 92%, respectively. In addition to a visualization tool demonstrating how the retrieved features are accountable for the malignant cluster, Bhattacharjee et al. [17] presented a well-defined method for detecting malignant nodules. A hybrid strategy based on an optimized RF classifier produces the best results, motivated by hyperparameter optimization. This experiment was conducted on the Lung Image Database Consortium (LIDC-IDRI) dataset, which achieved 92.14% accuracy by 10-fold Cross-Validation technique. Using image processing and computer vision techniques, Kareem et al. [18] suggested a framework for lung cancer detection. Image enhancement, image segmentation, and feature extraction approaches are the three preprocessing steps included in this. Finally, SVM is used to classify the instances. Performance evaluations are conducted with various SVM kernels and feature extraction methods. The best approach attained 89.89 % accuracy. Nageswaran et al. demonstrated image processing and machine learning techniques to classify and predict lung cancer accurately. The dataset for the experimental study had 83 CT scans from 70 different patients. During the preprocessing of images, the geometric mean filter is employed. The images are then segmented using the K-means algorithm. This segmentation is used to find the relevant portion of the image. Next, machine learning-based classification techniques are applied. Artificial Neural Network (ANN), K-Nearest Neighbor (KNN), and RF are a few machine learning approaches that were applied for the categorization. It was found that the ANN model can predict lung cancer with the highest accuracy [19]. Various performance metrics used by different researchers is presented in Table 11.2.

Table 11.2 Quality of service (QoS)

Reference	*Accuracy*	*Precision*	*Recall*	*F1-score*	*Specificity*	*Sensitivity*	*AUC*	*GM*	*FPR*
Makaju et al. [13]	✓								
Venkatesh et al. [14]	✓				✓	✓			
Gautam et al. [12]	✓	✓	✓	✓			✓		
Maleki et al. [15]	✓	✓	✓	✓					
Shafi et al. [4]	✓	✓	✓	✓					
Priyadharshini et al. [2]	✓	✓	✓	✓	✓	✓		✓	
Vijh et al. [16]	✓				✓	✓			
Bhattacharjee et al. [17]	✓	✓		✓	✓	✓			✓
Kareem et al. [18]	✓	✓		✓	✓	✓			
Nageswaran et al. [19]	✓				✓	✓			

11.3 METHODOLOGY

The primary goal was to collect pertinent articles that included the specified keywords "lung cancer", "deep learning", "machine learning", "ensemble technique", "detection", "hybrid approach", and "CT". The search was further limited by a date range that included publications from 2018 to 2024. A total of 630 articles were found in the first search, which were then filtered down by carefully examining their titles, abstracts, and keywords to ensure they were relevant. During the screening process, articles that did not directly pertain to the use of CT scans for lung cancer diagnosis or that did not employ pertinent methodologies such as ensemble techniques or hybrid

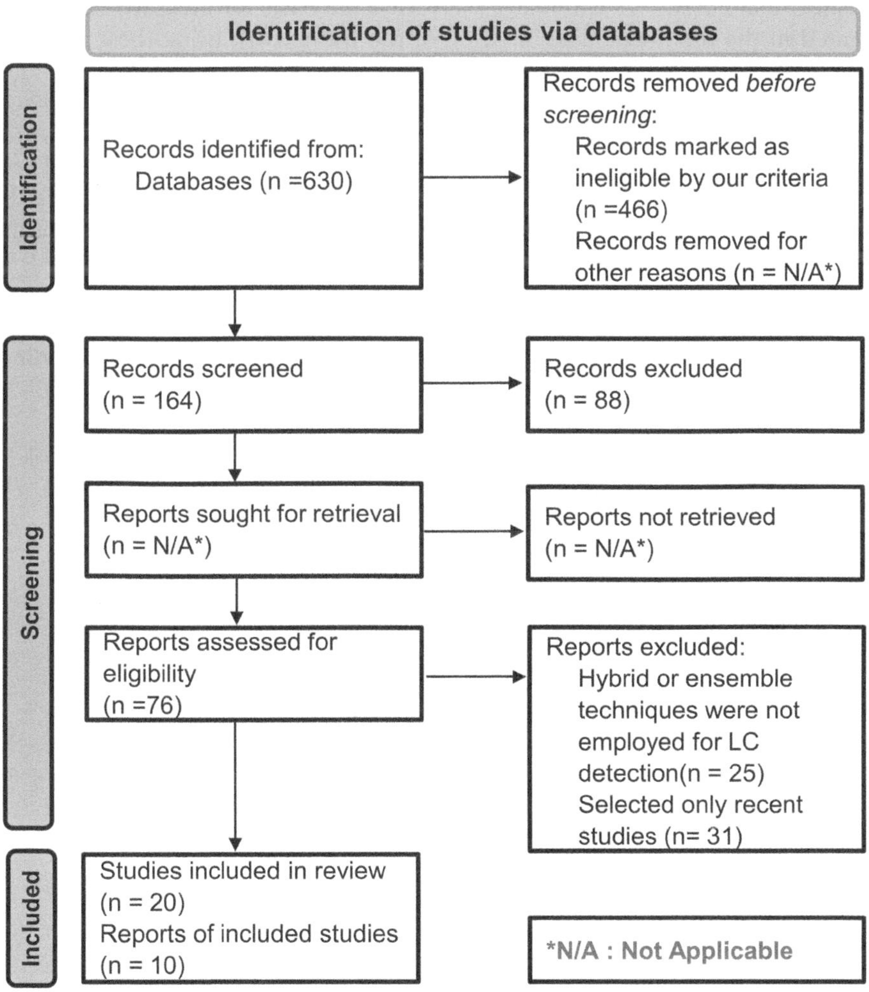

Figure 11.2 PRISMA diagram for the process of selection of articles.

models were eliminated. A final set of 20 papers for the literature review was acquired after this selection procedure, guaranteeing a varied representation of research addressing the convergence of AI approaches, lung cancer, and medical diagnosis. From the initial identification of publications to the final selection of research included in this review, the PRISMA diagram [20] in Figure 11.2 encapsulates the steps of our literature search. We have selected the ten most recent studies related to our required study.

11.4 ANALYSIS AND DISCUSSION

The main focus of this research study is the AI-based framework for lung cancer diagnosis. CT scan images served as the basis for most works investigated in the literature. The building of the framework using these CT scan images comprises a number of phases, the most crucial of which is the noise removal process [21]. This step is essential because in a lung CT image, various tiny spherical structures are surrounded across the lung region, which can be airways, blood vessels and lung tissues, as shown in Figure 11.3. These tiny structures can be falsely detected as lung nodules, which should be avoided and eliminated. As described in Table 11.1, we can see most of the researchers have used a median filter to remove noise [13–16, 19].

Subsequently, the lung region containing the tumor is segmented through segmentation techniques. Various techniques used in the existing research for segmenting lung nodule regions include Global Thresholding,

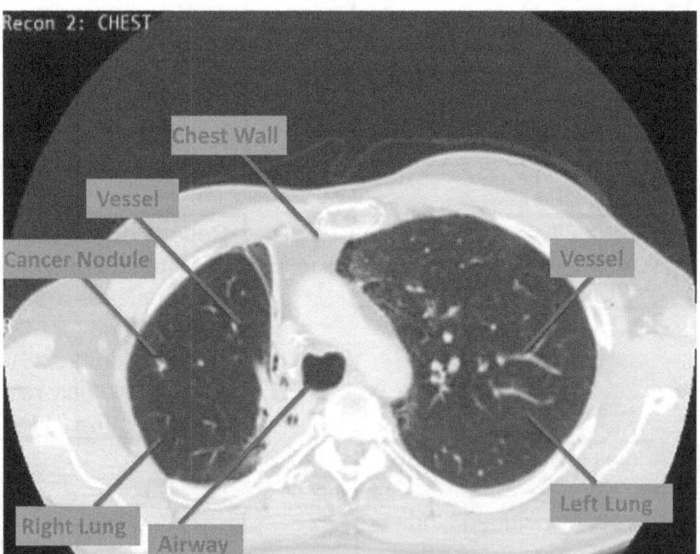

Figure 11.3 Description of a lung CT scan.

Otsu Thresholding, Watershed Segmentation, CapsNet, etc. In the subsequent step, feature extraction and selection techniques are implemented, followed by a classification algorithm in which CNN, ANN, SVM, and RF have produced the best results. Evaluation strategies are crucial for assessing the performance of these algorithms and figuring out how effective they are in detecting disease. As depicted in Figure 11.4, different evaluation metrics that are commonly used include Accuracy (ACC), Sensitivity (SE), Specificity (SP), Receiver Operating Characteristic curves (ROC), Area Under ROC Curve (AUC), Precision (P), Recall (R), F1-score (FM), False Positive Rate (FPR) and Geometric Mean (GM).

Based on the analysis of the research conducted by various researchers, hybrid model combining image processing, machine learning, deep learning, and meta-heuristic algorithms are proposed in most of the existing research [4, 14–16]. Different ways have been implemented to develop a hybrid model. Some researchers employed deep learning methods as a feature extractor, followed by machine learning methods for classification purposes. For instance, CNN is utilized as a feature extractor, and SVM is applied as a classifier after the flattening layer, as demonstrated in [4]. Some researchers have used Metaheuristic algorithms (WOA) as feature selection techniques, which helps in improving the performance of machine learning methods

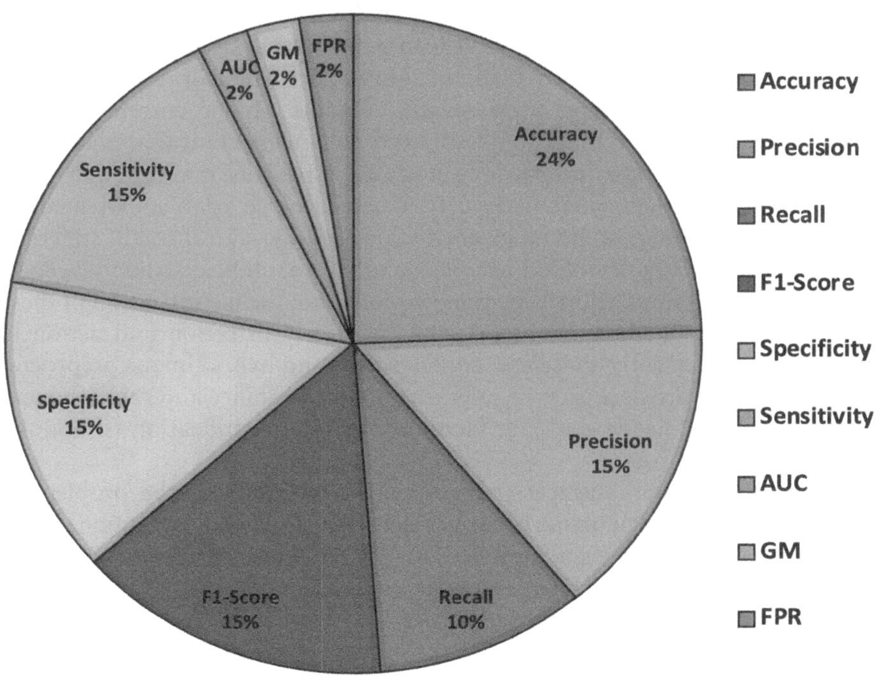

Figure 11.4 Evaluation criteria used by various studies.

used for classification [16]. Metaheuristic algorithms like PSO and BAT have also played a significant role in the segmentation process for selecting the optimal cluster that contains the lung nodule [2, 14]. These processed and segmented images are then given as input to deep learning techniques for the classification of segmented lung nodules into benign and malignant, which have resulted in robust models for lung cancer detection. Therefore, research has shown that in the detection of lung cancer, image processing techniques and the image segmentation method had a significant impact on the performance of the machine learning algorithm as well as deep learning algorithm [22].

Most of the examined studies primarily focus on the use of hybrid models. Additionally, some research explores ensemble approaches for the early detection of lung cancer, as ensemble techniques have shown promising outcomes in various image classification and pattern recognition applications. Ensemble techniques combine the predictions from multiple models [12, 23]. The fundamental concept is that the strengths of one model can offset the shortcomings of another by combining the outputs of different models, leading to an overall improvement in performance.

11.5 LIMITATIONS AND FUTURE DIRECTIONS

Despite the substantial progress made in lung cancer diagnosis through hybrid techniques and ensemble learning, our analysis has shown some major limitations that require further examination. These drawbacks underscore the necessity for ongoing research aimed at refining current methodologies, augmenting model robustness, and enhancing clinical applicability.

The precise identification of lung nodules, especially micro-nodules and those attached to adjacent tissues, is a considerable problem in medical imaging. In CT images, the lungs are surrounded by several small, spherical objects that may signify blood arteries or other anatomical structures, complicating the differentiation of genuine nodules. So, the identification of these nodules is very challenging and crucial for timely detection and action in lung cancer. To resolve this issue, sophisticated and hybrid image preprocessing techniques are necessary to augment nodule visibility and raise segmentation precision, hence enabling far more reliable identification of nodules in clinical applications.

The second major obstacle encountered in this study is the problem of dataset imbalance. The majority of publicly accessible and institutional lung cancer datasets demonstrate an imbalanced distribution of classes, characterized by a markedly reduced incidence of benign cases in comparison to malignant ones. This imbalance may result in biased model training, wherein the artificial intelligence system exhibits increased sensitivity to the majority class while encountering difficulties in accurately predicting instances of the minority class. Consequently, the performance metrics of the model, including sensitivity, specificity, and overall generalization may be influenced, thereby potentially constraining the clinical applicability of the proposed methodology. To reduce the effects of dataset imbalance, subsequent research efforts should investigate the incorporation of data balancing methodologies such as Generative Adversarial Networks (GANs) and synthetic data augmentation techniques. GANs possess the capability to produce high-quality synthetic lung CT images that closely resemble actual clinical cases. This process enhances the dataset and augments the representation of minority classes [24].

A significant problem in deep learning-based lung cancer diagnosis is the absence of model interpretability, as most deep learning architectures function as "black-box" systems with intricate, high-dimensional feature representations. In clinical practice, the reliance on and adoption of AI models depend on their capacity to deliver clear and explained decision-making processes that correspond with radiologist expertise. The inability to comprehend model predictions raises issues about bias, dependability, and potential misdiagnoses, consequently hindering the clinical acceptance and regulatory approval of AI-driven diagnostic tools. Future research should concentrate on incorporating Explainable AI (XAI) methodologies, such as Feature Importance Analysis and Shapley Additive Explanations, to improve model transparency and interpretability, hence rendering AI systems more applicable to real-world clinical settings [25].

Conventional AI models trained on single-institution datasets frequently exhibit restricted generalizability, since they fail to consider the inherent diversity in medical imaging across diverse demographics and clinical environments. Lung CT images might vary widely due to variations in patient demographics, imaging techniques, scanner manufacturers, and disease manifestations. These variances can induce dataset biases, resulting in AI models excelling on the training dataset while struggling to preserve accuracy when confronted with novel data from disparate sources. Federated learning (FL) presents an effective solution by enabling models to be trained on heterogeneous datasets from many medical institutions, without necessitating direct data exchange [26]. By facilitating decentralized training among hospitals or imaging centers, FL enables the model to learn from a wider array of lung CT images, encompassing variations in scanner configurations (e.g., slice thickness, contrast levels), population-specific disease presentations, and the annotation methodologies employed by radiologists. This will facilitate the development of a model that is more robust and adaptive to practical clinical environments.

11.6 CONCLUSION

Early detection of lung cancer is of critical importance enhancing patient outcomes with CT imaging functioning as an essential diagnostic tool. However, the manual interpretation of these images frequently exhibits inconsistencies, thereby necessitating the use of artificial intelligence-driven computer-aided diagnosis (CAD) systems. In this study, we conducted a comprehensive review of diverse artificial intelligence-based methodologies for the detection of lung cancer, highlighting their potential to improve both diagnostic accuracy and efficiency. Despite significant advancements in AI-assisted lung cancer detection, certain challenges still persist, such as data imbalance, model interpretability, and restricted generalization across varied datasets. Subsequent study ought to concentrate on augmenting segmentation accuracy, integrating explainability frameworks within AI models, and utilizing extensive and varied datasets to improve model generalization. Advancing these AI-driven approaches enables the medical community to get reliable early lung cancer detection system, hence reducing mortality rates and enhancing patient prognosis.

REFERENCES

1. D. M. Abdullah and N. S. Ahmed, "A review of most recent lung cancer detection techniques using machine learning," *Int. J. Sci. Bus.*, vol. 5, no. 3, pp. 159–173, 2021.
2. P. Priyadharshini and B. S. E. Zoraida, "Bat-inspired metaheuristic convolutional neural network algorithms for CAD-based lung cancer prediction," *J. Appl. Sci. Eng.*, vol. 24, no. 1, pp. 65–71, 2021.
3. J. Zhou and H. Xin, "Emerging artificial intelligence methods for fighting lung cancer: A survey," *Clin. eHealth*, vol. 5, pp. 19–34, December 2022.
4. I. Shafi, S. Din, A. Khan, I. D. L. T. Díez, R. D. J. P. Casanova, K. T. Pifarre, and I. Ashraf, "An effective method for lung cancer diagnosis from CT scan using deep learning-based support vector network," *Cancers (Basel)*, vol. 14, no. 21, p. 5457, November 2022.
5. L. Hussain, H. Alsolai, S. B. H. Hassine, M. K. Nour, M. A. Duhayyim, A. M. Hilal, … and M. Rizwanullah, "Lung cancer prediction using robust machine learning and image enhancement methods on extracted gray-level co-occurrence matrix features," *Appl. Sci.*, vol. 12, no. 13, p. 6517, July 2022.
6. B. R. Pandit, A. Alsadoon, P. W. C. Prasad, S. Al Aloussi, T. A. Rashid, O. H. Alsadoon, and O. D. Jerew, "Deep learning neural network for lung cancer classification: Enhanced optimization function," *Multimed. Tools Appl.*, vol. 82, no. 5, pp. 6605–6624, February 2023.
7. M. Kumar, S. Verma, A. Kumar, M. F. Ijaz, and D. B. Rawat, "ANAF-IoMT: A novel architectural framework for IoMT-enabled smart healthcare system by enhancing security based on RECC-VC," *IEEE Trans. Ind. Inf.*, vol. 18, no. 12, pp. 8936–8943, 2022.
8. A. Kumar, M. Kumar, V. P. Bhardwaj, S. Kumar, and S. Selvarajan (2024). A novel skin cancer detection model using modified finch deep CNN classifier model. *Scientific Reports*, *14*(1), 11235.
9. A. Kumar, M. Kumar, R. P. Mahapatra, P. Bhattacharya, T. T. H. Le, S. Verma, … and K. Mohiuddin, "Flamingo-optimization-based deep convolutional neural network for IOT-based arrhythmia classification," *Sensors*, vol. 23, no. 9, p. 4353, 2023.
10. K. Pradhan and P. Chawla, "Medical Internet of things using machine learning algorithms for lung cancer detection," *J. Manage. Anal.*, vol. 7, no. 4, pp. 591–623, October 2020.
11. R. Kishore, M. Satpathy, D. K. Parida, Z. Nussinov, and K. K. Sahu, "Detection of lung nodules using unsupervised machine learning method," *Adv. Intell. Syst. Comput.*, vol. 1108, pp. 463–471, 2020.

12. N. Gautam, A. Basu, and R. Sarkar, "Lung cancer detection from thoracic CT scans using an ensemble of deep learning models," *Neural Comput. Appl.*, vol. 36, no. 5, pp. 2459–2477, February 2024.
13. S. Makaju, P. W. C. Prasad, A. Alsadoon, A. K. Singh, and A. Elchouemi, "Lung cancer detection using CT scan images," *Proc. Comput. Sci.*, vol. 125, pp. 107–114, 2018.
14. C. Venkatesh, J. Chinnababu, A. Kiran, C. H. Nagaraju, and M. Kumar, "A hybrid model for lung cancer prediction using patch processing and deeplearning on CT images," *Multimed. Tools Appl.*, vol. 83, no. 15, pp. 43931–43952, 2024.
15. N. Maleki and S. T. A. Niaki, "An intelligent algorithm for lung cancer diagnosis using extracted features from computerized Tomography images," *Healthc. Anal.*, vol. 3, p. 100150, November 2023.
16. S. Vijh, D. Gaur, and S. Kumar, "An intelligent lung tumor diagnosis system using whale optimization algorithm and support vector machine," *Int. J. Syst. Assur. Eng. Manag.*, vol. 11, no. 2, pp. 374–384, April 2020.
17. A. Bhattacharjee, R. Murugan, and T. Goel, "A hybrid approach for lung cancer diagnosis using optimized random forest classification and K-means visualization algorithm," *Health Technol. (Berl)*, vol. 12, no. 4, pp. 787–800, July 2022.
18. H. F. Kareem, M. S. Al-Husieny, F. Y. Mohsen, E. A. Khalil, and Z. S. Hassan, "Evaluation of SVM performance in the detection of lung cancer in marked CT scan dataset," *Indones. J. Electr. Eng. Comput. Sci.*, vol. 21, no. 3, pp. 1731–1738, March 2021.
19. S. Nageswaran, G. Arunkumar, A. K. Bisht, S. Mewada, J. S. Kumar, M. Jawarneh, and E. Asenso, "Lung cancer classification and prediction using machine learning and image processing," *BioMed Res. Int.*, vol. 2022, p. 1755460, 2022.
20. M. J. Page, J. E. McKenzie, P. M. Bossuyt, I. Boutron, T. C. Hoffmann, C. D. Mulrow, . . . and D. Moher, "The PRISMA 2020 statement: An updated guideline for reporting systematic reviews," *Rev. Panam. Salud Publica/Pan Am. J. Public Heal.*, vol. 46, p. e112, 2022.
21. S. Alagarsamy, R. Raja Subramanian, T. Shree, S. Kannan, M. Balasubramanian, and V. Govindaraj, "Prediction of lung cancer using meta-heuristic based optimization technique: Crow search technique," in *Proceedings of the IEEE International Conference on Computing, Communication, and Intelligent Systems (ICCCIS'21)*, 2021, pp. 186–191.
22. T. Kadir and F. Gleeson, "Lung cancer prediction using machine learning and advanced imaging techniques," *Transl. Lung Cancer Res.*, vol. 7, no. 3, pp. 304–312, June 2018.
23. M. Sakib and T. Siddiqui, "Multi-network-based ensemble deep learning model to forecast ross river virus outbreak in Australia," *Int. J. Pattern Recognit. Artif. Intell.*, vol. 37, no. 10, p. 2352015, 2023.
24. A. Aggarwal, M. Mittal, and G. Battineni, "Generative adversarial network: An overview of theory and applications," *Int. J. Inf. Manag. Data Insights*, vol. 1, no. 1, p. 100004, 2021.
25. Y. Nohara, K. Matsumoto, H. Soejima, and N. Nakashima, "Explanation of machine learning models using shapley additive explanation and application for real data in hospital," *Comput. Methods Programs Biomed.*, vol. 214, p. 106584, 2022.
26. J. Wen, Z. Zhang, Y. Lan, Z. Cui, J. Cai, and W. Zhang, "A survey on federated learning: Challenges and applications," *Int. J. Mach. Learn. Cybern.*, vol. 14, no. 2, pp. 513–535, 2023.

Chapter 12

Fitness and nutrition planner driven by AI

M. Sirish Kumar, J. Sankar Babu, A. Jyothi Babu, and G. Laasyapriya

12.1 INTRODUCTION

In order to help people reach their fitness goals, a computer-based system that is powered by artificial intelligence can provide them with personalized exercise and nutrition recommendations. By analyzing a user's fitness data including their food intake, level of physical activity, and medical history these systems provide individualized recommendations on how to achieve their goals. In order to help people reach their fitness goals, this advice may include recommendations for diet, exercise (including what to eat and how much to exercise), and exercise intensity and duration. Based on the user's unique situation and objectives, the system employs AI to provide tailored recommendations. With this technology, everyone may reach their fitness goals faster and easier. Machine learning pipelines can be easily constructed with the help of Media Pipe, an open-source Python package. Making, training, and deploying machine learning models for different uses should be made easier using this. Classification, grouping, and regression are typically utilized machine learning problems, and it offers high-level abstractions for these problems. It also includes resources for assessing models, model selection, hyper-parameter optimization, and feature engineering. This is the framework that the rest of the article follows. The next section delves into the relevant literature. The suggested work, which comprises models for posture estimation and dietary recommendations, is discussed in Section 12.3. The results and relevant graphs are provided in Section 12.4. Section 12.5 wraps up the article and delves into its potential future developments.

12.2 RELATED WORKS

It is impossible to keep track of everyone and see how they are doing with the present system. Among the most visible examples of AI's impact on the health and fitness sector, AI- powered exercise machines stand out. People are inspired to finish and accomplish their exercise goals with their help, and

DOI: 10.1201/9781003634560-12

they also offer helpful information and direction [1]. Although present RFID-based systems are able to detect human activity, they are unable to identify the specific perpetrator. Because it can only identify acts and not the people who did them, efficient monitoring in a large group is useless [2].

The concept remains unchanged, even when this method is employed. With the use of a recommendation system, users will be able to tailor their diet and workout video suggestions to their specific requirements and tastes. A prototype platform for workout video recommendations, "Fitness that Fits," also does similar research. It takes a hybrid approach, combining fundamental ideas from neighborhood-based and content-based collaborative filtering systems, to provide end users with individualized fitness videos. It leverages 8 million videos from YouTube that depict fitness exercises [3]. This technology can be useful for doctor monitoring because it uses computer vision algorithms to detect critical limb posture abnormalities during exercise. The present setup only works with a single camera in two dimensions, but it can be upgraded to work in three. Utilizing a camera with a top-down perspective or a depth perception system [4]. By employing the problem recommendation strategy, which aims to improve student performance, students can improve their score on a particular exam. Like an examination, it could also verify the user's accuracy in performing the activity. The great performance of the trained RNN in predicting the test data is demonstrated by the MSE values, which are in the order shown [5].

The software standardizes data for different body types and use the Open Pose model to predict postures in exercise videos in order to evaluate crucial information such body component angles [6]. This paper delves into a number of yoga-related mobile apps that leverage AI techniques to give users personalized experiences and positive feedback [1]. It also presents a new concept for an AI-based yoga trainer that can remind, teach, guide, and motivate users to practice yoga or while doing yoga.

The chapter discusses established backbone architectures, loss functions, evaluation methods, and datasets utilized in human pose estimation utilizing deep learning and publicly available datasets. It also offers a complete summary of current achievements in this area. Also covered are the two main steps of pose estimation, which are finding relevant points and then combining them into a legitimate posture configuration [6]. Proposed in the article [3] was a knowledge tracing model based on Bayesian analysis. Using a Hidden Markov Model, it updates the likelihood that the student would understand the concept depending on her success on exercises, representing the student's understanding of the subject as a binary variable.

Since it operates at the notion level, this paradigm doesn't care about the connection between concepts. A recurrent neural network (RNN) based deep knowledge tracing (DKT) model was presented in the article [7]. By using students' knowledge states as latent variables, it achieves better performance than a Bayesian-based model [8]. Taking the semantics of exercises into account was suggested as a way to enhance DKT in the workplace [3]. Modeling the number of latent idea correlations was the goal of the study in [6]. A human position prediction model trained on the COCO datasets is utilized by the system. This model is a convolutional neural network (CNN). On the other hand, the authors suggest that incorporating exercise data to fine-tune the CNN model could improve its accuracy [4]. This approach can enhance exercise programs while decreasing the likelihood of harm [6]. A RNN model for DKT was suggested in the article. This model is superior to a Bayesian one that uses latent variables to represent students' knowledge states [8]. The most current instances make use of COCO and MPII as their default datasets. The learning process is often evaluated using the L2 loss function, with PCKh@0.5 being the most frequent evaluation metric [6].

In this research [9], we offer a method for making exercise suggestions using AI. This approach suggests activities that might significantly enhance learning for certain types of students. Students are able to get more done in the same amount of time when this strategy is used, according to experiments.

The report continues by exploring possible future improvements to the system [10]. The authors indicate that tweaking the CNN model for faster inference can boost the system's real-time performance. They also propose that adding a depth perception mechanism or using a top view camera can help extend the system to work in 3 dimensions [4].

The POSTURECHECK system uses a Microsoft Kinect camera to measure an individual's posture as they exercise in real-time, making it useful for physical therapists [11]. The system extracts distinct data from the data using Bayesian estimate and majority vote. The user's upper body and displays the results of a posture check. After detecting an incorrect posture, POSTURECHECK suggests ways to fix it [10].

12.3 PROPOSED WORK

12.3.1 System overview

An intuitive app that calculates body mass index (BMI) using the user's height, weight, and gender is the suggested effort. The user's dietary preferences (vegetarian, non-vegetarian, egg) and aspirations are also recorded. In addition to a weekly exercise plan and food advice chart, the app takes into account the user's BMI and their goal. Users can track their progress as they perform suggested exercises [11] (Figure 12.1).

The user's login or registration is the starting point of the system's overall flow, as shown in Figure 12.1. He or she inputs their own body statistics on the subsequent screen. After that, it asks what the end goal is. It creates a personalized plan for their diet and exercise routine based on the information they supply. Additionally, the user has the option to select a training routine from the provided selection.

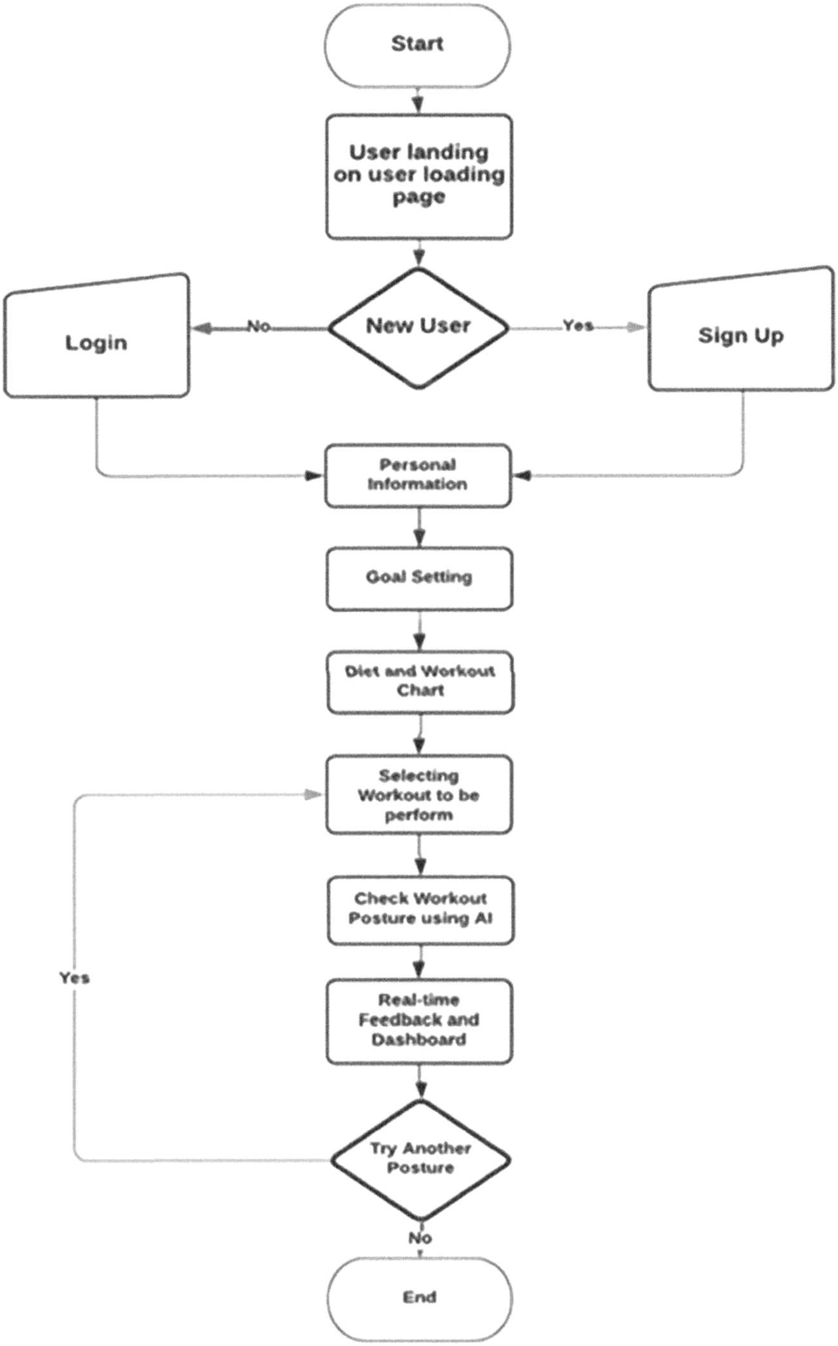

Figure 12.1 System flow diagram.

What the AI-enabled camera sees is interesting. Verify that the user has executed the exercise correctly by checking the posture and angles. In order to choose the next exercise, the user can simply repeat the methods. The Google Calendar API will send the reminder and progress update once the exercise is finished if the user has scheduled it for a specific time.

The proposed system doesn't necessitate any specific software or hardware for posture estimation or capture, but the device in question should have the capability to record and process media pipe for posture analysis as well as real-time video feeds.

12.3.2 Methodology

The proposed system will provide the user with an ongoing exercise guide. The user's training performance will be enhanced, and the hassle of searching for a suitable gym while on the go will be entirely removed. Also, the user won't have to waste time consulting with others for diet advice because the device would provide them with a personalized plan based on their fitness objectives. Here is an outline of the whole approach.

12.3.2.1 Algorithms used logistic regression

Using a collection of independent variables, logistic regression determines the probability of an occurrence, such voting or not voting.

12.3.2.1.1 Formula

The equation $g(y) = \beta o + \beta 1$ for weight gain, $\beta 2$ for weight loss, $\beta 3$ for muscle gain, $\beta 4$ for beginner, $\beta 5$ for intermediate, and $\beta 6$ for advance (12.1) can be paraphrased as follows:

$$g(y) = \beta_0 + \beta_1 x_1 + \beta_2 x_2 + \beta_3 x_3 + \beta_4 x_4 + \beta_5 x_5 + \beta_6 x_6 \tag{12.1}$$

where $g(y)$ is the log-odds of the user achieving their fitness goal, β_0 is the intercept, β_1,β_2,β_3 are coefficients for weight gain, weight loss, and muscle gain goals, β_4,β_5,β_6 are coefficients for beginner, intermediate, and advanced levels, and x_1 through x_6 are the corresponding input variables

12.3.2.1.2 CNN

The formula for the convolutional layer is

$$n*m \tag{12.2}$$

Completely linked layer:

$$(n+1)*m \text{ is the formula for this layer} \tag{12.3}$$

The output layer is defined as

$$(n*m*k + 1)*f \tag{12.4}$$

12.3.2.1.3 Posture analysis

The correct way to do push-ups should be defined first. Make sure your elbows are bent at a 90-degree angle when you lower them to perform push-ups. Inadequate squatting occurs when the angle of the elbow bend is more than 90° to 180°. According to mathematical notation, it can be expressed as:

$$\angle((xe - xf, ye - yf), (xe - xs, ye - yf))\angle 180o + \theta \tag{12.5}$$

In addition, as it is not feasible to instantly calculate the straight line of the waist, you should measure the height of the hand by sizing up the space between the fingers and the shoulder.

$$1 > \frac{|x_f - x_s|}{|(x_f - x_e)(y_f - y_e)|} > \tau \tag{12.6}$$

where (xe, ye), (xf, yf), (xs, ys) are the points of the elbow, fingers, and shoulder, and θ is the allowable error range.

12.3.2.2 Diet recommendation

The diet advice system is built on two datasets: food and nutrition distribution. Food databases include nutrient values and the optimal times to consume foods like eggs, broccoli, brown rice, and so on. The nutrition distribution databases, on the other hand, include calorie breakdowns depending on lipids, proteins, and other micro-nutrients. As we all know, counting calories is critical when it comes to meeting fitness objectives. These datasets, when combined, help to determine the right food items to add to the user's diet chart based on their fitness goals (Figures 12.2 and 12.3).

The BMI is calculated using a formula when the system is given the appropriate inputs, which include age, food type (vegetarian or not), weight, and height.

$$\text{BMI} = \frac{\text{Weight (kg)}}{\text{Height m}^2} \tag{12.7}$$

where:

- Weight is measured in kilograms (kg)
- Height is measured in meters (m)

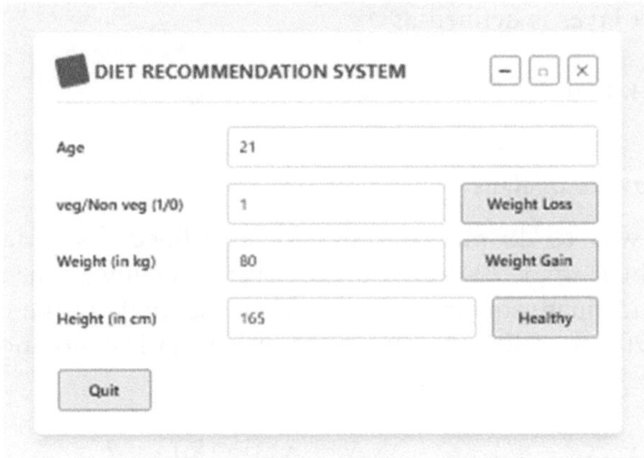

Figure 12.2 Input on dietary recommendations.

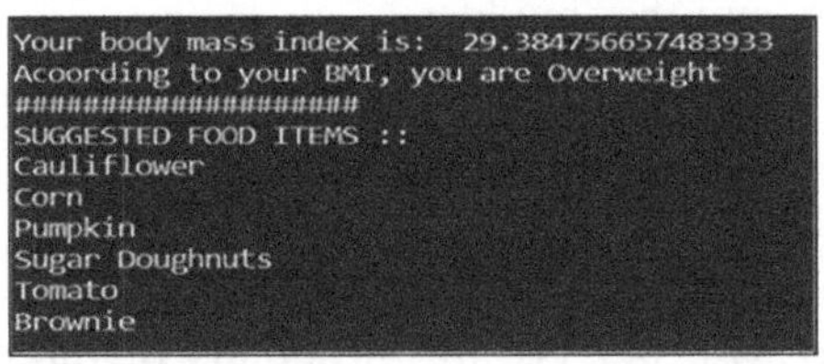
Your body mass index is: 29.384756657483933
According to your BMI, you are Overweight
######################
SUGGESTED FOOD ITEMS ::
Cauliflower
Corn
Pumpkin
Sugar Doughnuts
Tomato
Brownie

Figure 12.3 Advice on departure (results).

The results show if the person is overweight or underweight, for example. Now the user has a diet chart based on their goals and inputs from the recommendation system. To help the user better understand the diet and how to reach their goal, the Diet Chart breaks down each meal of the day into its own column for each day of the week.

Using the user's height and weight, BMI can be used to evaluate their weight status as overweight, underweight, or fit. Recommendations are not given to users who are already physically fit. When a person is underweight, recommendations are made to help them lose weight. When they are overweight, ideas are made to help them gain weight. When making recommendations for vegans and the system considers the user's dietary preferences, whether they are vegetarian or not.

12.3.2.3 Exercise monitoring using AI

The Media Pipe library in Python allows users to perform various human point evaluations. It has potential applications in object detection and classification in images, face feature and expression recognition in videos, and object and person tracking in still images. Relevant features can also be derived from audio signals through analysis. Media Pipe also lets developers classify emotions, objects, and data anomalies using Machine Learning models. With Media Pipe, a complete and versatile tool set is at your fingertips for easy human point detection in any video or image. Research has shown that using deep learning for exercise suggestions can help with respiratory difficulties, as mentioned in [12].

With the use of AI, activity-detecting wearable may deliver users tailored workout recommendations. Artificial intelligence apps can help users enhance their work and identify signs of weariness [6]. Media Pipe analyzes movements, shapes, and procedures in real-time using computer vision. To make its position estimates, distance calculations, and threshold increases, it use the Python Media Pipe library [4]. Figures 12.4 and 12.5 illustrate all the points.

It depicts every part of the human body, which can be seen clearly in the image up there. After that, the code is plotted using the points, and the

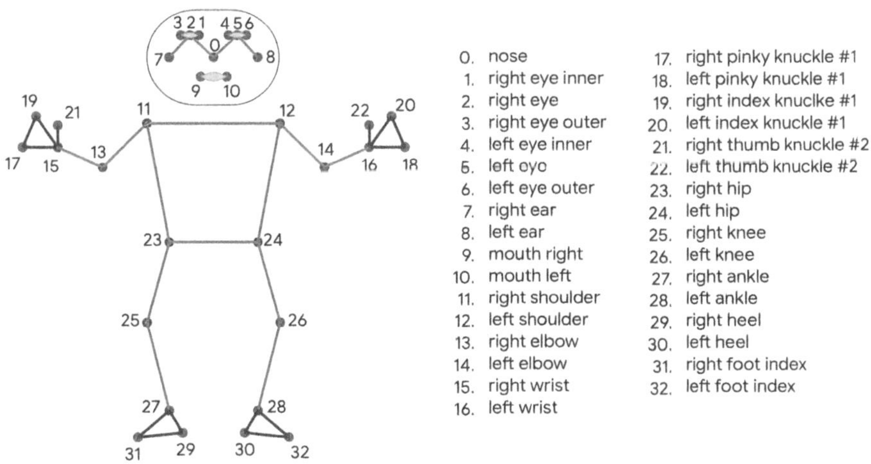

Figure 12.4 Artificial intelligence-defined human body points.

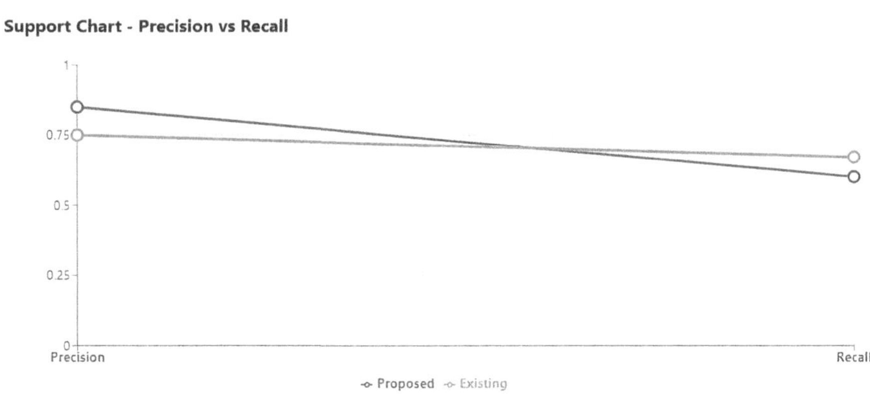

Figure 12.5 Nutritional assistance.

threshold limit is set to a certain value. Everything is derived from the Media Pipe Python package. Computer vision inference may be applied to any kind of sensory data, including audio and video, using an open-source technology called Media Pipe. As a network of interchangeable parts, Media Pipe allows for the construction of such a perception pipeline. Media Pipe v0 is now in its alpha stage.

12.4 RESULTS AND DISCUSSION

12.4.1 Diet recommendation

Knowledge systems, which are based on diet-related information, can be used [13]. Nonetheless, this case makes use of the Random Forest Classifier method. Classification and regression issues are best addressed using the machine learning method known as Random Forests. The purpose of a classifier model is to sort incoming data into predefined categories. The data used to train the many decision trees in a random forest algorithm is chosen at random.The need to handle two datasets (food data and nutrition distribution) and provide a combined result led to the selection of the Random Forest method to serve as a reference for diet recommendations. Random Forest Procedures Algorithm Procedures:

First, a collection of characteristics and pieces of information are selected for every decision tree within the Random Forest model. A dataset with k records is partitioned into n records at random and m features, in a nutshell. Decision trees are constructed independently for every sample.

Second, a result is produced by every decision tree.

Finally, either Averaging or Majority Voting is used to evaluate the final result in Classification and Regression.

Description of datasets are below:

1. *Food data set*:
   The 90 food items that make up the food data set are categorized according to the following: calories, lipids, proteins, sugar, salt, potassium, iron, calcium, carbohydrates, fiber, and sugar. The values given are per gram. Additionally, foods are categorized according to their vegetarian or non- vegetarian status and the optimal time to eat them.
2. *Nutrition distribution*:
   Calorie distribution as it relates to micro nutrients is the primary topic of this data set. A 160-calorie serving would have 15 grams of fat, 2 grams of protein, 0.55 milligrams of iron, etc. At least forty-five distinct patterns exist. Calorie counting and food product recommendations will be made easier with this breakdown of calories.

Table 12.1 The accuracy table of the algorithm

Algorithm	*Precision*	*Recall*	*F1 score*	*Support*
Logistic regression	0.75	0.65	0.62	30
Support vector machine	0.68	0.54	0.74	35
Naïve Bayes	0.82	0.64	0.62	40
CNN	0.83	0.72	0.63	52
YOLOv5	0.89	0.61	0.56	45

Decision Tree and Random Forest are the two algorithms that were compared in the previous description. Table 12.1 contains the values for each algorithm's Precision and Recall, which were used to produce a line chart. Above, you can see the accuracy achieved by using the Random Forest Algorithm, which is depicted in blue.

The percentage of nutrients in different food items are shown in Figure 12.6. Similar to how this Nutrients Value Chart can be generated with AI (as mentioned in [14]), the values are predicted using an appropriate Machine Learning Algorithm. The bar chart uses a number of color schemes to illustrate the contents, which provide a succinct description of the nutritional percentages and food item recommendations. Consumption of certain foods will be suggested in relation to the number of calories needed to reach the goal, with these suggestions being grounded in the micro nutrients.

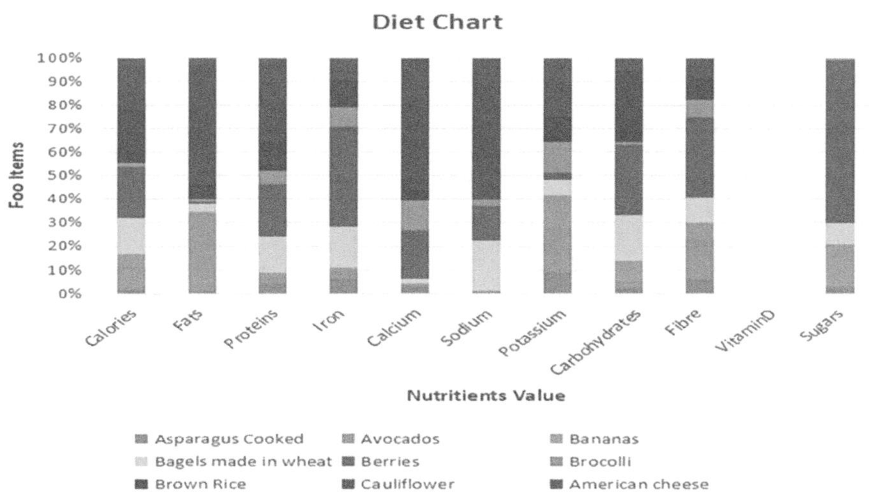

Figure 12.6 Visual guide to nutrients.

12.4.2 Workout monitoring

Here, appropriate AI monitoring is carried out utilizing Media Pipe Algorithms and angle measures, in addition to rehabilitation, which is used for posture correction [15].

As depicted in Figures 12.7–12.10:

- Significant red marks indicate an intermediate or inappropriate posture.
- Green marks: These marks indicate the final, correct position. When the user is prepared to do push-ups, as seen in Figures 12.7 and 12.8, the transition state is displayed by that scarlet mark. It changes to green

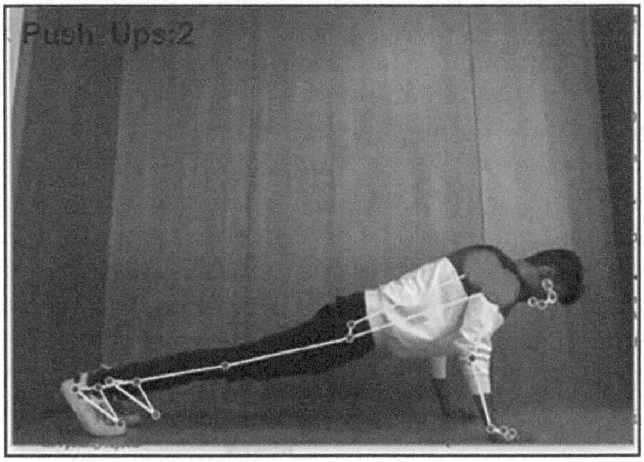

Figure 12.7 The transition state from the side.

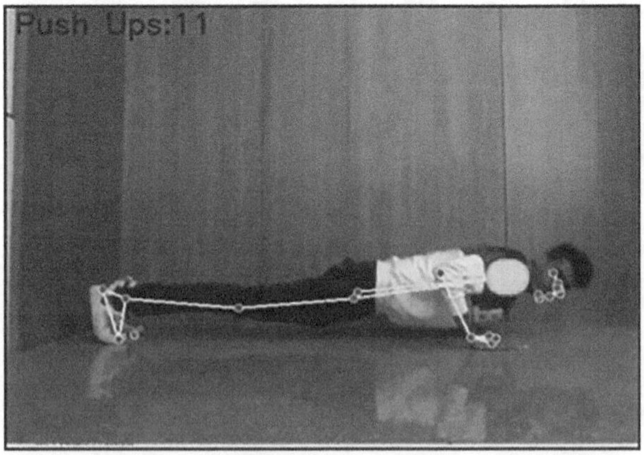

Figure 12.8 The success state from the view.

whenever the performer bends below a specified angle to complete the exercise, as seen in Figures 12.9 and 12.10. The user can perform the workout from any angle; the system can detect and evaluate posture from any perspective. With every successful green mark, the counter is also incremented. The number increases by one when the red mark becomes green. At the same time, the user has to be very precise while exercising so that they can get the number up and reach their objective. The majority of people experience this problem, and it's mostly due to the fact that their posture fluctuates over time without affecting accuracy or correctness.

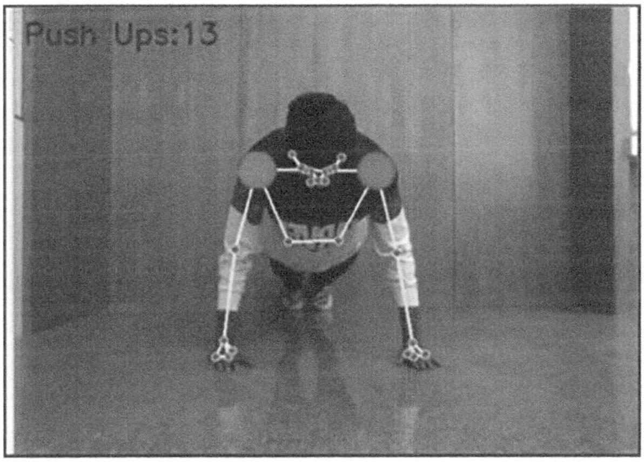

Figure 12.9 The transition state's front side.

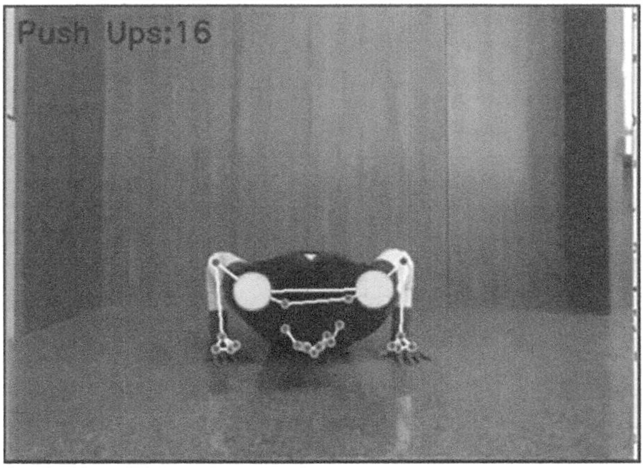

Figure 12.10 At a glance, the success state.

All of the study methodologies are listed in Table 12.1. YOLOv5, Logistic Regression, Support Vector Machine, Naive Bayes, and CNN were used. Support, F1 Score, Precision, and Recall are computed. In addition, you can see the line chart in Figure 12.10, which shows the different algorithm parameters graphically, using all of these values except Support. The support parameter for different methods is shown in Figure 12.11, which explains support, or the frequency of the truth value.

Some of the exercises' correctness is shown in Table 12.2 with respect to F1 Score, Support, Precision, and Recall. Squats, barbell bicep curls, bench presses, and Russian twists are shown in Figure 12.12, along with their corresponding accuracy charts. Figure 12.13's line chart displays the present technique (RNN [5]) as a dotted line and the suggested algorithm (CNN) as a solid line.

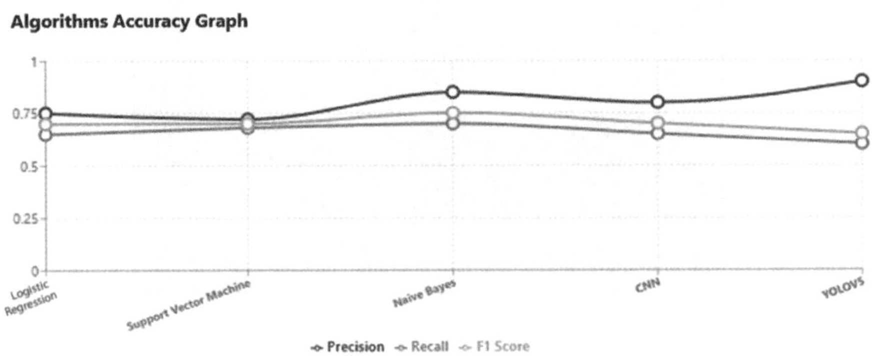

Figure 12.11 Algorithm with their accuracy.

Table 12.2 Workout's accuracy table

Workout	*Precision*	*Recall*	*F1 score*	*Support*
Squats	0.83	0.62	0.55	32
Barbell bicep curls	0.67	0.65	0.74	28
Bench press	0.86	0.54	0.59	26
Russian twist	0.75	0.64	0.41	41

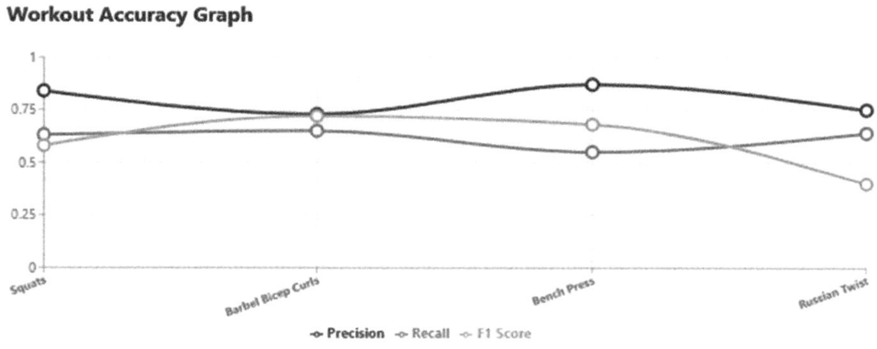

Figure 12.12 Workout accuracy.

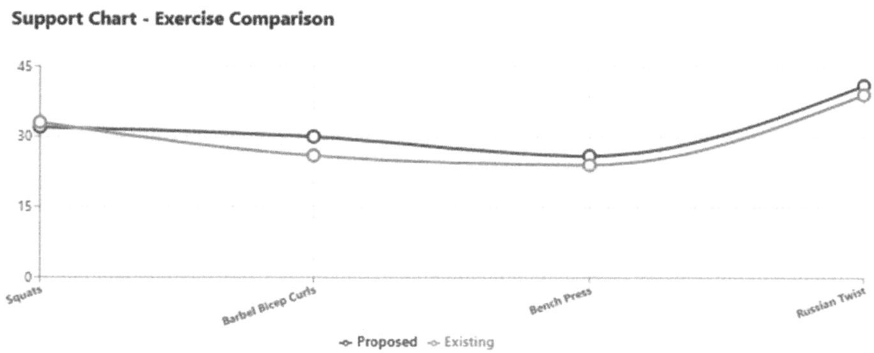

Figure 12.13 Workout support.

12.5 CONCLUSION

A gym trainer and food recommendation system powered by AI can help people who wish to get in shape. In order to tailor workout programs and dietary recommendations to each user's specific needs, this system analyzes their data and applies machine learning algorithms. The quantity of food items available for recommendations is one example of the limitations. There is also complete disregard for third-party supplements such as Wavy Protein, BCEE, etc. There are only a few of exercises that can be tracked when it comes to workout recommendations. Anyone wishing to enhance their health and nutrition can benefit from an AI-powered system that suggests meals and exercises. Advanced exercises, such as Yoga postures, and the external dietary supplement suggestions can be added to this method to make it even more effective.

REFERENCES

1. Vedangi Agarwal, Konark Sharma, and Abha Kiran Rajpoot, "AI based Yoga Trainer-Simplifying Home Yoga Using Mediapipe and Video Streaming," *Proceedings of the 3rd International Conference for Emerging Technology (INCET)*, pp. 1–5. IEEE, 2022.
2. Zijuan Liu, Xiulong Liu, and Keqiu Li, "Deeper Exercise Monitoring for Smart Gym Using Fused RFID and CV Data," *Proceedings of the IEEE Conference on Computer Communications (INFOCOM'20)*, pp. 11–19. IEEE, 2020.
3. Tewodros Legesse Munea, Yalew Zelalem Jembre, Halefom Tekle Weldegebriel, Lonbgiao Chen, Chenxi Huang, and Chenhui Yang, "The Progress of Human Pose Estimation: A Survey and Taxonomy of Models Applied in 2D Human Pose Estimation," *IEEE Access* 8 (2020): 133330–133348.
4. Amit Nagarkoti, Revant Teotia, Amith K. Mahale, and Pankaj K. Das, "Real-time Indoor Workout Analysis Using Machine Learning & Computer Vision," *Proceedings of the 41st Annual International Conference of the IEEE Engineering in Medicine and Biology Society (EMBC)*, pp. 1440–1443. IEEE, 2019.
5. Arash Golibagh Mahyari and Peter Pirolli, "Physical Exercise Recommendation and Success Prediction Using Interconnected Recurrent Neural Networks," *Proceedings of the IEEE International Conference on Digital Health (ICDH)*, pp. 148–153. IEEE, 2022.
6. Lei Yang, Yingxiang Li, Degui Zeng, and Dong Wang, "Human Exercise Posture Analysis based on Pose Estimation," *Proceedings of the IEEE 5th Advanced Information Technology, Electronic and Automation Control Conference (IAEAC)*, vol. 5, pp. 1715–1719. IEEE, 2021.
7. T. Tran, Jea-Won Choi, and Jong-Wook Kim, "Recommender System with AI for Fitness Assistance System," *Proceedings of the International Conference on Ubiquitous Robots (UR)*, pp. 489–492. IEEE, 2018.
8. R. Brunda, K. S. Preethi, Sushmitha N. Reddy, Khushi Aralikatte, and S. Manjula, "B-Fit: A Fitness and Health Recommendation System," *International Research Journal of Engineering and Technology (IRJET)* 9, no. 7 (2022): 1083–1087.
9. Zhizhuang Li, Haiyang Hu, Zhipeng Xia, Jianping Zhang, Xiaoli Li, Zisihan Wang, Xiaoke Huang, Shan Zeng, and Beixu Qiu, "Exercise Recommendation Method based on Machine Learning," *Proceedings of the International Conference on Advanced Learning Technologies (ICALT)*, pp. 50–52. IEEE, 2021.
10. Elham Saraee, Saurabh Singh, Ajjen Joshi, and Margrit Betke, "PostureCheck: Posture Modeling for Exercise Assessment Using the Microsoft Kinect," *Proceedings of the International Conference on Virtual Rehabilitation (ICVR)*, pp. 1–2. IEEE, 2017.
11. Fangzhe Ai, Yishuai Chen, Yuchun Guo, Yongxiang Zhao, Guowei Fu, and Zhenzhu Wang, *Concept-Aware Deep Knowledge Tracing and Exercise Recommendation in an Online Learning System*. National Natural Science Foundation of China, 2019.
12. M. Usharani Bhimavarapu Nalini Chintalapudi Sreedevi, and Gopi Battineni, "Physical activity recommendation system based on deep learning to prevent respiratory diseases," *Computers MDPI* 11, no. 10 (2022): 150.
13. Vishal Varma, Izhar Alam, Shreyas Arya, and Bharat Kapila, *Knowledge Based Expert Systems, Diet Recommendation System*. IEEE, 2020.
14. Thomas Theodoridis, Vasilis Solachidis, Kosmas Dinitropoulos, and Lazaros Gymnopoulos, "A Survey on AI Nutrition Recommender System," *Proceedings of the 12th ACM International Conference on Pervasive Technologies Related to Assistive Environments*, pp. 540–546, 2019.
15. Seung-Ho Han, Han-Gyu Kim, and Ho-Jin Choi, "Rehabilitation Posture Correction Using Deep Neural Network," *Proceedings of the IEEE International Conference on Big Data and Smart Computing (BigComp)*, pp. 400–402. IEEE, 2017.

Chapter 13

Introduction to AI and data science in healthcare applications

Raj Shekhar, Jaya Dash, Riwitika Gupta, Ashwani Kumar, and Ramesh Chandra Poonia

13.1 INTRODUCTION

Rapid advances in Artificial Intelligence (AI) and Data Science have transformed several sectors; surely, among them, the healthcare sector is one of the most promising. It not only streamlined the health care system but also revolutionized the approach that healthcare practitioners and researchers took toward diagnostics and the treatment and patient care they provided. AI and Data Science have delivered solutions revolutionary and innovative based on the tremendous quantity of data being generated within the healthcare system. Health care systems generate large amounts of data every day. These include patient records and medical images, clinical trials, and wearable devices. The majority of the data remains untapped due to its volume and complexity. AI and Data Science have arrived as a much-needed solution to process and interpret these datasets, extracting patterns and insights that were not known before. These discoveries give healthcare providers a basis for more informed decisions, better patient outcomes, and greater efficiency in operations.

Among the most critical roles of AI [1] in medicine will be the potential to enable precision medicine, predicting at least part of the risk and disease associated with making recommendations on tailored treatment, while data science methods are used for determining risk factors and patterns of diseases that lead to informing planning strategies for preventing them as well as public health policy.

13.1.1 Importance of healthcare innovation

Traditionally, direct care, paper records, and centralized facilities have been applied to deliver care in the world's healthcare systems. Although the systems have produced fantastic medical developments over the years, they do have some challenges that make them incapable of adapting to changing patient and healthcare needs. Imbalanced data security as the cost-effectiveness of the conventional medical system enhances [1]. Main challenges include access to care, since data management would be manual,

DOI: 10.1201/9781003634560-13

and therefore both time-consuming and error prone. Antiquated technology and infrastructure may restrict the ability to diagnose and forecast illness. Complex rules and regulations governing healthcare systems can stifle creativity and effectiveness [2]. AI-powered technologies are able to evaluate enormous volumes of data to help with diagnosis, forecast the course of diseases, and customize treatment regimens. By providing real-time health data, wearables such as fitness trackers and smartwatches enable proactive health management. Online consultations enhance access to care and lower geographic obstacles, especially in rural regions. EHRs make sharing, storing, and collecting data easier while guaranteeing that medical professionals have current, correct patient data. With AI stepping into the healthcare world, it will automate the procedure of prediction and diagnosis for an accurate result and data science's involvement in this process would make the management of the records and data more civilized and accessible.

Significance of advancements in healthcare

- **Improved patient outcomes:** Better patient monitoring, individualized treatment, and early disease identification are made possible by innovative healthcare technology, which enhance patient outcomes.
- **Enhanced efficiency:** Automation and AI-driven solutions streamline administrative processes, reduce paperwork, and optimize hospital workflows.
- **Cost reduction:** Innovations help in minimizing healthcare costs through efficient resource allocation, reducing hospital readmissions, and promoting preventive care.
- **Better access to care:** Telemedicine and AI-powered diagnostics allow remote and underserved populations to access quality healthcare services.
- **Advancements in medical research:** Data-driven approaches accelerate drug discovery, improve clinical trials, and enhance medical research efficiency.
- **Increased patient engagement:** AI-powered chatbots, wearable technology, and smartphone health apps enable people to actively manage their own health.
- **Enhanced decision-making:** AI and big data analytics support healthcare professionals in making data-backed, accurate decisions in diagnostics and treatment planning.
- **Tackling global health challenges:** Innovations address critical health challenges such as disease outbreaks, healthcare workforce shortages, and public health crises effectively.
- **Ethical and safe healthcare practices:** AI-driven tools ensure standardized procedures, reducing human errors and maintaining ethical medical practices.

- **Sustainability in healthcare:** Smart technologies promote environmentally friendly solutions, reducing waste and optimizing energy consumption in healthcare facilities.

13.1.2 Defining artificial intelligence and data science

In the twenty-first century, AI has emerged as a very significant technological advancement that affects many facets of our life, including finance, entertainment, healthcare, and transportation. Data science is the process of using statistical, machine learning (ML), and computational approaches to gain valuable perception from complicated information. These resources can be used by healthcare workers to make well-informed decisions, improve the precision of diagnoses, and improve patient care through the creation of customized treatment strategies. The marriage of AI and data science in healthcare is revolutionary because of the combination of the best of both worlds to tackle intricate medical issues [3]. AI algorithms improve clinical decision-making, automate time-consuming procedures, and allow for the creation of predictive models based on data science.

13.1.3 Scope of AI and data science in healthcare

The application of AI and data science has seen revolutionary advances in clinical settings to improve patient care and effectiveness in healthcare. AI intervention, computer vision, reads clinical images such as MRI, CT scans, and X-rays to identify abnormalities such as tumors, fractures, and neurological conditions. Data science enhances the precision of diagnosis and minimizes human error by providing aggregation and interpretation of imaging data. Telemedicine platforms based on AI improve real-time patient monitoring and remote consultations. Health markers are received by wearable sensors and devices, which are analyzed by data science tools to identify abnormalities and suggest immediate treatment. AI accelerates the drug discovery process by reviewing clinical and biological data to identify promising candidates. Through optimizing the design of clinical trials, data science models reduce the time and cost of bringing new therapies to market. AI and data science utilize genetic profiles and other patient data to create personalized treatment plans. Optimizing medication selection and dosage improves therapeutic outcomes and reduces side effects.

AI and data science improve hospital operations by optimizing patient flows, automating routine functions, and optimizing resource management. These technologies improve the overall patient experience [4] while decreasing costs and administrative workload. Robotic devices driven by AI like the devices, enable surgeons to carry out difficult procedures more accurately, less invasively, and more efficiently. By reviewing the results of robotic procedures, data science optimizes surgical techniques.

The scope of AI and Data Science in Healthcare are in following areas:

- **Predictive analytics:** AI models analyze patient data to predict disease risks, allowing for early intervention and prevention.
- **Medical imaging and diagnostics:** AI-powered computer vision enhances the accuracy and efficiency of radiology, pathology, and other imaging techniques.
- **Personalized medicine:** AI-driven algorithms assess genetic, environmental, and lifestyle factors to provide customized treatment plans.
- **Drug discovery and development:** AI accelerates drug research by analyzing vast datasets and identifying potential compounds for new medicines.
- **Virtual health assistants:** AI-based chatbots and virtual assistants provide basic healthcare guidance and support patient inquiries.
- **Remote monitoring and wearable devices:** AI-powered wearables help track patient vitals and detect anomalies in real time, improving chronic disease management.
- **Healthcare administration automation:** AI streamlines administrative tasks such as billing, scheduling, and electronic health record (EHR) management.
- **Epidemiology and public health:** AI and data science analyze population data to detect and predict disease outbreaks and health trends.
- **Surgical robotics:** AI-assisted robotic systems enhance surgical precision, reducing risks and improving patient recovery times.
- **Mental health support:** AI-based applications provide psychological assistance through chatbots and sentiment analysis tools.

13.2 OVERVIEW OF AI IN HEALTHCARE

13.2.1 Rise of AI in medicine

The integration of AI in medicine is a long way from its early concepts to current real-world applications that enhance the care of patients and operations of healthcare. This has gone through a long evolution from infancy back in the 1970s to current uses. AI concept was born during the 1950s; the term "Artificial Intelligence" was used for the first time in 1955 in the Dartmouth College Conference. However, a few drawbacks found in early models kept them away from general acceptance and its application to healthcare. In the 1970s, applications of AI were solving biomedical problems. MYCIN, an AI system that assisted in the identification of treatments for infections in the blood, and INTERNIST-1 that was one of the first artificial medical consultants, assisting with diagnostic decision-making, were some of the fruits of research during this period. The early 2000s were the beginning of the modern period, where the focus shifted from rule-based systems to data-driven ML algorithms. Its most significant advancements were in the 2010s, with the rapid explosion of deep learning and neural networks. Now this process has come a long way to a point in 2025 where it is integrated into all aspects of healthcare delivery and management. It accurately interprets radiological images, assisting in the early diagnosis of diseases, rapid drug development and predicts patient-specific treatment outcomes [5], AI-based chatbots and virtual assistants provide personalized assistance, huge investments in AI research aid with innovations in genomics, oncology, and wearable health technology.

13.2.2 Key AI technologies in healthcare

The healthcare industry has seen a paradigm shift with the emergence of AI, bringing in state-of-the-art technologies that transform diagnostics, therapeutic planning, and patient-centric care. Some of the most revolutionary AI technologies are ML, Deep Learning [6], Natural Language Processing (NLP), and Computer Vision, each being a cornerstone in transforming modern healthcare practices. ML is a core cornerstone of AI, where systems can process large datasets and identify patterns in order to make knowledge-driven decisions. It can be applied to predict disease outbreaks, plan personalized therapy, and detect medical claim fraud. Deep Learning is one of the areas of ML, which uses artificial neural networks for processing large datasets and identifying complex patterns. It helps us find images for diagnosis of diseases like cancer or fractures, process molecular data for finding new drugs, and find genetic markers in precision medicine [7]. NLP enables machines to understand and communicate with human language. NLP is used in the health sector to draw out meaningful information from unstructured data in EHR such as patient history and clinical notes. For interaction with patients, NLP has also been powering chatbots and virtual assistants. Computer Vision has become the central part of health care in understanding visual data. Its applications have been to understand radiological images for the disease diagnosis of fracture or cancer, to understand the skin disorders of dermatology, and to understand biopsy samples of pathology. This combination led to a future that is more personal, predictive, and precise patient care.

The AI Technologies in Healthcare are as follows:

- **Machine learning (ML)**: Used for disease prediction, patient risk assessment, and personalized treatment recommendations [8].
- **Natural language processing (NLP)**: Helps extract meaningful insights from clinical notes, patient records, and research literature.
- **Computer vision**: Enhances medical imaging diagnostics by improving accuracy in detecting abnormalities in radiology and pathology.
- **Robotic process automation (RPA)**: Automates repetitive administrative tasks such as billing, appointment scheduling, and medical coding.
- **Deep learning**: Advances in deep neural networks improve diagnostics, drug discovery, and medical image analysis.

- **Chatbots and virtual assistants:** Provide patient engagement, initial diagnosis, and mental health support.
- **Predictive analytics:** Uses AI models to forecast disease trends, hospital resource needs, and patient deterioration risks.
- **Edge AI and IoT integration:** Enables real-time monitoring of patient health data through connected devices and wearables.
- **Federated learning:** Ensures secure, decentralized AI training on sensitive healthcare data while maintaining patient privacy.
- **Genomic AI:** Analyzes genetic data for insights into hereditary diseases, precision medicine, and genomic research.

13.2.3 Applications of AI in healthcare

The different uses of AI in healthcare are extensive and far-reaching, from disease diagnosis and prediction to the application of individualized treatment protocols and the use of virtual health assistants. Technology can sometimes substitute or enhance human capability by providing quicker or more accurate means of detecting, treating or preventing disease. AI-based technologies are changing the way diseases are diagnosed, making it more accurate and faster. The other AI technology-the predictive analytics [9] evaluates patient data to predict the risk of any disease. For example, AI may predict the likelihood of heart attack or diabetes hence, interventions applied early to enhance outcomes. AI technologies enable clinicians to adjust therapy appropriately since they record patient response to treatment in real-time. This dynamic, data-driven process ensures that patients receive optimized care adapted to their situation, avoiding trial-and-error treatment. Virtual assistants can book appointments, remind patients to take medication, and respond to health-related queries. Some advanced systems can triage symptoms and recommend the appropriate course of action, thus reducing healthcare providers' workload. They also provide support in chronic disease management by monitoring symptoms and giving personalized health advice, thus enabling proactive patient care. These uses of AI in healthcare are a giant leap toward a future where medical services are not just more efficient and accurate but highly personalized [10].

The applications of AI in Healthcare are in the following:

- **Early disease detection:** AI-powered screening tools help in the early detection of diseases such as cancer, diabetes, and cardiovascular conditions.
- **Medical imaging analysis:** AI enhances radiology, MRI, and CT scan interpretations, reducing diagnostic errors.
- **Robotic surgery:** AI-assisted robots improve surgical precision and reduce recovery times.
- **Personalized treatment plans:** AI analyzes patient data to recommend tailored treatment strategies.

- **Electronic health records (EHR) management:** AI automates data entry, retrieval, and recordkeeping, reducing administrative burden.
- **Telemedicine and virtual healthcare:** AI enables remote consultations and diagnoses through chatbots and video conferencing.
- **Drug discovery and development:** AI accelerates research by predicting drug efficacy and reducing testing time.
- **Mental health support:** AI-based chatbots offer psychological assistance and therapy recommendations.
- **Healthcare fraud detection:** AI identifies fraudulent billing and insurance claims, ensuring financial security.
- **Public health monitoring:** AI predicts disease outbreaks and assists in pandemic response planning.

13.3 ROLE OF DATA SCIENCE IN HEALTHCARE

13.3.1 Data-driven decision-making

Data science has emerged as a major part of the healthcare industry. Data science has emerged as a major part of the healthcare industry to enhance patient care, streamline processes, and facilitate evidence-based decision-making. Since healthcare data is the foundation to develop insights and innovation in various medical disciplines, its importance cannot be underestimated. Healthcare data gives the providers information regarding patient populations, helps in tracing health trends, and indicates the risk factors, ultimately bringing about improved clinical outcomes. Data-driven decision-making [11] enables the healthcare professionals to make informed decisions on diagnosis, treatment plans, and patient management, thus offering a more personalized care process. Healthcare data can be broadly categorized into the following types: structured, unstructured, and semi-structured. Quantitative analysis and developing insights with algorithms and statistical methods require structured data. EHRs, demographical data, laboratory tests, and billing data are all examples of structured data that are structured and easily retrievable in databases. Unstructured data, however, is difficult to analyze as it does not have a fixed structure. Examples include clinical notes, imaging data such as X-rays and MRIs, and patient feedback. Semi-structured data falls between the structured and unstructured types and has some organizational features that allow it to be analyzed more easily but do not fit neatly into standard databases. Examples include emails, messages, and some health records.

13.3.2 Key data science techniques

With an explosion of health-related data in such an era, data science techniques offer a medium for turning a huge complex amount of data into meaningful insights. Predictive analytics, data visualization, and statistical modeling are amongst the most influencing techniques. Every one of them plays an important role in bringing insights out from unprocessed data. Among them, predictive analytics is at the forefront of the innovation that happens in healthcare. This technique allows doctors to foresee patient results, detect potential dangers, and prevent them from occurring by using past and present data. Predictive models, for example, can be applied in the identification of early warning signs of chronic diseases, predicting outbreaks of disease, and forecasting readmission rates of patients. Data visualization [12] is what connects the large data sets with actionable understanding. Tools such as dashboards, heatmaps, charts, and graphs enable healthcare professionals to quickly identify trends, anomalies, and patterns. For example, a hospital may employ visual dashboards for monitoring patient flow, allocation of resources, and follow-up of treatment results to optimize operational efficiencies. Statistical modeling lies at the heart of evidence-based medicine. The various models may assist researchers and practitioners to identify correlations of variables, make judgments on the effectiveness of therapies, or develop measures to quantify risks using regression analysis, hypothesis testing, and survival analysis.

Key data science techniques

- **Data mining:** It can extract meaningful patterns from large datasets in healthcare settings to find out trends, correlations, and suspected risk factors of certain diseases. Through it, early detection of diseases and information about the patients' demographics can be known.
- **Statistical analysis:** Statistical analysis applies statistical approaches to understand medical data, by which medical people can base medical decisions on relevant information. These include hypothesis testing, regression analyses, and prediction modeling that offer better clinical care.
- **Machine learning algorithms:** Artificially intelligent models through ML algorithms aid in predicting diseases, assessing risks, and automating diagnoses. These algorithms can help to identify abnormalities within medical images, predict deterioration, and personalize treatment.
- **Big data analytics:** Big Data Analytics: Healthcare produces large amounts of data in the form of EHR, genomic data, and patient monitoring logs. Big data analytics helps in analyzing these data for better management of hospitals, allocation of resources, and care for patients.
- **Data visualization:** The transformation of complex healthcare datasets into graphical formats such as charts and heat maps will allow doctors, researchers, and policymakers to read data more effectively. This will improve transparency and facilitate better decision-making in medical practices and public health initiatives.

13.3.3 Applications of data science in healthcare

Data science is going to be a very promising future in health care. It can be applied in medical imaging, pharmaceutical development, virtual assistance, engagement of patients and so on, predominantly in EHR analysis, Population health management, and Genomic data analysis. EHR analysis is the principle of modern health care data science. In the EHR systems, both organized and unstructured patient data such as lab results, diagnoses, treatments, and medical histories are stored. This makes the improvement of EHR analysis even greater with ML models by automating procedures such as medical coding, lowering the administrative workload, and minimizing errors. Population health management uses data science to tackle the broader health needs of communities and demographics. Aggregated health data can help healthcare organizations identify patterns in disease prevalence, resource use, and risk factors. Population health insights guide the distribution of resources and optimize systems for providing treatment [13]. Genomic data analysis is a transformative application of data science, driving advancements in personalized medicine. Researchers can find genetic markers associated with diseases and create tailored treatments by examining large genomic datasets. Techniques such as genome wide association studies and ML allow for the accurate identification of genetic predispositions, which opens up the possibility of tailored treatments. In a nutshell, the application of data science into healthcare has evolved into a new era of innovation, significantly transforming the way medical data is leveraged to address critical challenges.

The applications of Data Science in Healthcare are:

- **Electronic health records (EHR) analysis:** Data science enhances patient record management by improving organization, retrieval, security, and interoperability among healthcare institutions.
- **Disease prediction and prevention:** Predictive analytics utilizes patient data to assess risks of developing diseases and suggest timely interventions.
- **Genomic research:** Data science aids in analyzing genetic sequences, enabling the identification of hereditary disease risks and personalized treatment plans.
- **Clinical decision support systems (CDSS):** AI-powered systems assist healthcare professionals in diagnosing conditions and recommending treatment plans based on patient history and medical guidelines.
- **Patient monitoring and wearables:** Wearable technology integrated with data science allows continuous monitoring of patient vitals, helping in early detection of abnormalities.
- **Operational efficiency in healthcare facilities:** Big data analytics streamlines workflow, optimizes staff allocation, and enhances overall hospital management.

- **Fraud detection in healthcare:** Advanced analytics identify anomalies in billing, insurance claims, and medical records to prevent fraudulent activities.
- **Public health and epidemiology:** Large-scale health data analysis supports the detection, tracking, and mitigation of disease outbreaks and health crises worldwide.
- **Pharmaceutical research and drug discovery:** AI-driven data science accelerates drug discovery by analyzing vast amounts of biomedical literature, clinical trials, and patient outcomes data.
- **Medical imaging enhancement:** AI-powered imaging techniques help detect diseases like cancer at early stages, improving diagnostic accuracy and treatment effectiveness.

13.4 CHALLENGES AND LIMITATIONS

Despite the tremendous power of AI and Data Science [14–17] in healthcare, its adoption is fraught with several challenges and limitations. One of the major issues is data used, which is sensitive in nature. Breach of healthcare information or misuse can cause serious harm. HIPAA and GDPR compliance must be ensured to protect patient information; data fragmentation across several systems of healthcare is difficult to integrate and analyze information itself.

Bias in the AI algorithm. ML algorithms are based on historical data and may reflect biased data against people based on race, gender, or other aspects of socio-economic status. Biases might contribute to inappropriate and unequal predictions with respect to care for the patients. Overcoming these will take a team effort to create datasets that have wide representation among patient populations.

In addition, AI [18] and Data Science solutions for healthcare require heavy investment in infrastructure and workforce training for successful implementation. Most of the healthcare institutions lack the required computational power and expertise to fully utilize these technologies in resource-poor settings. Overcoming these barriers requires collaboration between healthcare providers, technology developers, and policymakers to create an ecosystem that fosters innovation while adhering to ethical and regulatory standards.

13.4.1 Technical challenges

- **Data quality and availability:** AI and data science models rely on huge volumes of high-quality data. However, the data available for healthcare is fragmented, incomplete, or inconsistent across different institutions, thereby becoming hard to analyze.

- **Interoperability issues:** Healthcare data exists in multiple formats across various systems, making integration and seamless data exchange between hospitals, clinics, and research centers challenging.
- **Algorithmic bias:** AI models rely on historical data, which may reflect existing biases in patient demographics, potentially leading to disparities in healthcare predictions and treatments.
- **Computational complexity:** Advanced AI models require significant computational resources, which may not be available in all healthcare institutions, especially in developing regions.
- **Real-time processing limitations:** AI-driven healthcare applications, such as medical imaging and predictive analytics, depend on real-time data processing. However, delays in processing can hinder timely decision-making and affect patient outcomes.
- **Model interpretability:** Many AI models, especially deep learning algorithms, function as "black boxes," making it challenging for healthcare professionals to comprehend and trust their decision-making processes.
- **Security and privacy concerns:** Highly sensitive patient information is vulnerable to breaches and cyberattacks. The biggest challenge is keeping AI models secure and ensuring they comply with HIPAA and GDPR rules.
- **Scalability and deployment:** Deploying AI solutions across diverse healthcare settings demands robust infrastructure, staff training, and ongoing monitoring to maintain optimal performance and ethical compliance.

13.4.2 Implementation barriers

Healthcare organizations generally rely on antique systems which were not designed to accommodate AI. Grafting AI onto such antique systems is a cumbersome and costly affair that would not disrupt existing processes or patient care. Major changes and a complete redesign of the current IT infrastructure are often required for AI integration. This may be financially and logistically challenging for healthcare organizations [19], especially the smaller or resource-constrained ones. These costs can be both upfront, or initial investment, and ongoing, or maintenance and scaling. This can influence the financial sustainability of healthcare organizations, especially those in low-resource settings.

- **High implementation costs:** Integrating AI and data science into healthcare demands substantial financial resources for infrastructure, hardware, and software. This expense can pose challenges, especially for smaller healthcare facilities.
- **Lack of skilled workforce:** Implementing AI in healthcare requires professionals proficient in both medical and data science domains, but such expertise is currently limited.

- **Resistance to change:** Many healthcare professionals hesitate to adopt AI-driven solutions due to unfamiliarity, skepticism, and concerns about potential job displacement.
- **Regulatory and ethical concerns:** Compliance with stringent regulations and ethical considerations slows down the deployment of AI-driven healthcare solutions.
- **Integration with legacy systems:** Many healthcare institutions still rely on outdated legacy systems that are incompatible with modern AI-driven technologies, making integration a complex and time-consuming process.

13.4.3 Future prospects and opportunities

AI in healthcare [20] is the future bright and holds significant promises for lower costs, more operational efficiency, treatment tailoring, and diagnostic capabilities. Most new technologies often require significant one-time investments in infrastructure, education, and research. Partnerships between the public and private sectors could be exploited to spread out the cost burden and stimulate more extensive utilization of innovative solutions. Cloud computing lowers the initial investment costs and makes the advanced technology accessible to small organizations as health care organizations pay for services according to consumption. To ensure that the health care data is accurate, complete, and up to date on a regular basis, develop strong data governance mechanisms. This includes the establishment of procedures for controlling data quality, strengthening data integrity, and improving data validation procedures. To ensure that these technologies are used effectively and ethically, there will be a need for cooperation between the patients, the developers of these technologies, regulators, and health care professionals. This will ultimately lead to a healthcare system [21] that is more patient-oriented, egalitarian, and efficient. Technologies such as AI, blockchain, the Internet of Things, robots, and telemedicine are changing healthcare about accessibility and cost, patient outcomes, and allowing patients to receive something tailored in treatment [22]. If used correctly, they should be able to finally address long-standing problems in healthcare delivery, such as inefficiencies, high prices, and unequal access, especially in resource-constrained environments.

13.5 CONCLUSION

Healthcare, as an industry, has become revolutionized through the integration of AI and Data Science with unprecedented advancements in diagnostics, treatment planning, patient care, and hospital management. These technologies enhanced medical decision-making, improved outcomes for patients, and optimized delivery of healthcare based on vast clinical data. AI-powered tools such as predictive analytics, ML algorithms, and big data analytics have enabled early disease detection, personalized medicine, and real-time patient monitoring. Moreover, automation of administrative processes through AI-driven tools has relieved the burden of healthcare professionals to focus more on patient-centric care.

Though AI and Data Science have such transformational potential, there is a lot more that needs attention for their practical deployment. There are issues in terms of data privacy, algorithmic bias, interoperability, and conformity to regulatory norms toward ethical and equitable deployment. This also comes at very high costs and requires professional personnel, and such requirements make them a bit difficult to handle for developing health systems. Cooperation between healthcare providers, data scientists, policymakers, and technology developers can help get past these obstacles.

Future of AI and Data Science in healthcare looks promising as it continues to improve research and innovation for a more advanced solution. Robotic-assisted surgeries to AI-based drug discovery is all set to open more avenues for applications of these technologies that improve efficiency, accuracy, and accessibility in healthcare. However, along with that come also balancing the technology with ethics-a safe and secure end for AI for all sections of society.

Further development in the healthcare industry will rely on embracing AI and Data Science, which will open the doors to a more efficient, cost-effective, and patient-centered approach to medicine. In this way, these technologies will become the basis for building future global healthcare systems if governed appropriately, continuously innovated, and responsibly implemented.

REFERENCES

1. Saif, Sohail, Debabrata Datta, Anindita Saha, Suparna Biswas, and Chandreyee Chowdhury. "Data science and AI in IoT based smart healthcare: Issues, challenges and case study." In *Enabling AI Applications in Data Science*, edited by Aboul-Ella Hassanien, Mohamed Hamed N. Taha, Nour Eldeen M. Khalifa, pp. 415–439. Cham: Springer International Publishing, 2021.
2. Yang, Yin, Keng Siau, Wen Xie, and Yan Sun. "Smart health: Intelligent healthcare systems in the metaverse, artificial intelligence, and data science era." *Journal of Organizational and End User Computing (JOEUC)* 34, no. 1 (2022): 1–14.
3. Sarker, Iqbal H., Mohammed Moshiul Hoque, Md Kafil Uddin, and Tawfeeq Alsanoosy. "Mobile data science and intelligent apps: concepts, AI-based modeling and research directions." *Mobile Networks and Applications* 26, no. 1 (2021): 285–303.
4. Khan, Z. Faizal, and Sultan Refa Alotaibi. "Applications of artificial intelligence and big data analytics in m-health: A healthcare system perspective." *Journal of Healthcare Engineering* 2020, no. 1 (2020): 8894694.

5. Agah, Arvin. "Introduction to medical applications of artificial intelligence." *Medical Applications of Artificial Intelligence* (2013): 19–26.
6. Shekhar, Raj, Deepak Singh Tomar, Bhagwati Sharan, and R. K. Pateriya. "Human activity recognition using deep learning techniques for healthcare applications." In *Proceedings of the 15th International Conference on Computing Communication and Networking Technologies (ICCCNT)*, pp. 1–6. IEEE, 2024.
7. Panesar, Arjun. *Machine Learning and AI for Healthcare*. Coventry, UK: Apress, 2019.
8. Shekhar, Raj, Deepak Singh Tomar, R. K. Pateriya, and Bhagwati Sharan. "Human activity recognition with smartphone using classical machine learning models." In *Proceedings of the 10th International Conference on Computing for Sustainable Global Development (INDIACom)*, pp. 85–90. IEEE, 2023.
9. Raparthi, Mohan, Srihari Maruthi, Surendranadha Reddy Byrapu Reddy, Praveen Thunki, Prabu Ravichandran, and Sarath Babu Dodda. "Data science in healthcare leveraging AI for predictive analytics and personalized patient care." *Journal of AI in Healthcare and Medicine* 2, no. 2 (2022): 1–11.
10. Shaheen, Mohammed Yousef. *Applications of Artificial Intelligence (AI) in Healthcare: A Review*. Berlin, Germany: ScienceOpen Preprints, 2021.
11. Sarker, Iqbal H. "Data science and analytics: an overview from data-driven smart computing, decision-making and applications perspective." *SN Computer Science* 2, no. 5 (2021): 377.
12. Amsini, P. "Data science in healthcare 4.0: An introduction." In *Cybersecurity and Data Science Innovations for Sustainable Development of HEICC*, edited by Thangavel Murugan and W. Jai Singh, pp. 1–15. Boca Raton: CRC Press, 2025.
13. Fatema, Nuzhat, and Jafar A. Alzubi. *AI and Machine Learning Paradigms for Health Monitoring System: Intelligent Data Analytics*. Singapore: Springer Nature, 2021.
14. Mehta, Nishita, Anil Pandit, and Sharvari Shukla. "Transforming healthcare with big data analytics and artificial intelligence: A systematic mapping study." *Journal of Biomedical Informatics* 100 (2019): 103311.
15. Bohr, Adam, and Kaveh Memarzadeh. "The rise of artificial intelligence in healthcare applications." In *Artificial Intelligence in Healthcare*, edited by Adam Bohr and Kaveh Memarzadeh, pp. 25–60. London: Academic Press, 2020.
16. Datta, Sudipto, Ranjit Barua, and Jonali Das. "Application of artificial intelligence in modern healthcare system." In *Alginates-Recent Uses of This Natural Polymer*, edited by Leonel Pereira. London: IntechOpen, 2019.
17. Liebowitz, Jay, ed. *Data Analytics and AI*. New York: CRC Press, 2020.
18. Santosh, K. C., Loveleen Gaur, K. C. Santosh, and Loveleen Gaur. "Introduction to AI in public health." In *Artificial Intelligence and Machine Learning in Public Healthcare: Opportunities and Societal Impact*, edited by K. C. Santosh and Loveleen Gaur. Singapore: Springer, pp. 1–10, 2021.
19. Jiang, Fei, Yong Jiang, Hui Zhi, Yi Dong, Hao Li, Sufeng Ma, Yilong Wang, Qiang Dong, Haipeng Shen, and Yongjun Wang. "Artificial intelligence in healthcare: Past, present and future." *Stroke and Vascular Neurology* 2, no. 4 (2017): 230–243.
20. Noorbakhsh-Sabet, Nariman, Ramin Zand, Yanfei Zhang, and Vida Abedi. "Artificial intelligence transforms the future of health care." *The American Journal of Medicine* 132, no. 7 (2019): 795–801.

21. Boulos, Kamel, N. Maged, Guochao Peng, and Trang VoPham. "An overview of GeoAI applications in health and healthcare." *International Journal of Health Geographics* 18, no. 1 (2019): 7.
22. Park, Chan-Woo, Sung Wook Seo, Noeul Kang, BeomSeok Ko, Byung Wook Choi, Chang Min Park, Dong Kyung Chang et al. "Artificial intelligence in health care: current applications and issues." *Journal of Korean Medical Science* 35, no. 42 (2020): e379.

Chapter 14

AI-driven prediction of drug-target interactions and binding affinity for drug discovery in healthcare

Tanya Liyaqat, Tanvir Ahmad, and Md Khalid Jamal

Advancements in technology, particularly artificial intelligence (AI), have revolutionized various scientific domains and industries, providing a solid foundation for research and innovation [1]. Among several areas, drug discovery stands out as a critical field benefiting immensely from technological progress. Drug discovery is a multidisciplinary approach that integrates principles of biology, chemistry, and pharmacology to identify new drug candidates for various diseases. The ultimate goal is to find compounds that are not only effective in treating specific conditions but also safe for human consumption [2]. However, this process is renowned for its high cost intensity as it exceed billions of dollars from initial discovery to market approval [3]. Despite the challenges and high costs associated with drug discovery, it remains an ongoing effort in the pharmaceutical industry. Companies continuously invest and engage in intricate operations involved in drug discovery to bring new medicines and vaccines to the market. Technological advancements such as high-throughput screening [4], computer-aided drug design [5], and molecular modeling [6] have significantly enhanced the efficiency and precision of drug discovery process. For instance, researchers employ innovative approaches to gain deeper insights into disease mechanism. By understanding the underlying mechanisms of diseases, drugs that specifically target these mechanisms are developed for improved treatment options [7]. These technological advancements have not only streamlined the drug discovery process but have also paved the way for the systematic identification and development of therapeutic compounds, laying the foundation for the intricate drug discovery pipeline.

14.1 DRUG DISCOVERY AND ITS PIPELINE

The process of discovering chemical compounds that can effectively treat, manage, and potentially cure diseases is called drug discovery. It is a multifaceted approach and is carried out in several phases that consist of the identification, synthesis, characterization, screening, and evaluation of potential drug

DOI: 10.1201/9781003634560-14

candidates for therapeutic efficacy. Upon successful outcomes in preliminary phases starting with target identification and validation to lead optimization, the promising molecules advance to the drug development phase which involves clinical trials and regulatory approval [8]. The detail of the phases involved in drug discovery pipeline is illustrated below.

14.1.1 Target identification and validation

- Identification of disease targets: In this phase, researchers identify biological targets that are made of nucleic acids. The targets are the proteins that play a major role in the progression of the disease. For example, BACE1 (β-site Amyloid preCursor protein cleaving Enzyme 1) is a protein responsible for Alzheimer's disease (AD) and hence a popular drug target for researchers due to its pivotal role in the pathogenesis of this disease [9].
- Validation of drug targets: Once potential targets are identified, they are validated to ensure that they are indeed relevant to the disease of interest and are suitable for therapeutic intervention. This phase involves conducting a series of experiments to affirm the role of identified target in disease pathology and to assess its potential as a therapeutic target.

14.1.2 Lead identification

Lead identification discovers promising chemical compounds or 'leads' that demonstrate potential therapeutic activity against the identified target. High-throughput screening (HTS) [10] and virtual screening [11] are two complementary approaches used for this purpose. HTS is a laboratory-based method that involves the testing of large number of compounds for their ability to modulate the activity of a target protein. Virtual screening, on the other hand, is a computational approach that uses modeling and simulation techniques to predict the likelihood of compound binding to a target protein. Virtual screening offers several advantages over HTS such as the ability to rapidly screen large chemical libraries and greater cost-effectiveness. Factors such as potency, selectivity, and various physicochemical properties, is pivotal at this phase and serve as the foundation for optimizing subsequent leads.

14.1.3 Lead optimization

Identified leads undergo several rounds of lead optimization that test compounds against various properties such as binding affinity, efficacy, solubility, toxicity, etc., and enhance their therapeutic potential. The primary objective is to retain favorable properties in lead molecules and eliminate any structural deficiencies [12]. To improve the potency and safety of lead compounds, researchers conduct structure-activity relationship (SAR) [13] studies to understand how changes in the chemical structure of lead compounds affect their biological activity.

14.1.4 Preclinical research

Preclinical research serve as a bridge between initial drug discovery and human clinical trials and provide insights into the expected biological action of a compound and its efficacy in patients. It also aims to identify and characterize any potential toxicities associated with the drug to enable informed risk assessment before proceeding to human trials. There are two primary types of preclinical trials: general pharmacology and toxicology. Pharmacology involves studying the pharmacokinetic and pharmacodynamic properties of a drug whereas toxicological testing assesses the potential toxic effects of a compound [14]. By conducting thorough preclinical evaluations, researchers generate data on the safety and efficacy of a potential drug candidate. The data is compiled into an Investigational New Drug application which is submitted to regulatory authorities such as the FDA (US Food and Drug Administration) to get approval for initiating trials in humans.

14.1.5 Clinical development

- Phase I clinical trials: Investigational drugs undergo Phase I clinical trials to evaluate their safety in healthy volunteers. These trials provide initial data on the tolerability, metabolism, and dosage of the drugs.
- Phase II clinical trials: Drugs that pass Phase I trials proceed to Phase II trials where they are tested for efficacy and safety in patients with the target disease. Phase II trials assess the drug therapeutic potential and optimal dosage regimen.
- Phase III clinical trials: Drugs that demonstrate efficacy and safety in Phase II trials advance to Phase III trials, which involve larger patient populations. Phase III trials provide conclusive evidence of the drug efficacy and safety.

14.1.6 Regulatory approval and marketing

Pharmaceutical companies submit detailed data from preclinical and clinical studies to regulatory agencies such as the FDA for review. If the drug meets the safety, efficacy, and quality standards, it is granted marketing approval. After approval, the drug undergoes post-marketing surveillance to monitor its safety and efficacy in real-world.

14.2 CHALLENGES IN DRUG DISCOVERY

Conventional experimental methods used in the drug discovery process are both costly and time-intensive [3]. For instance, the development of a new molecular entity can incur costs of approximately 2.6 billion dollars, and the journey from initial discovery to market approval typically spans a lengthy period of over 12 years [15, 16]. Despite remarkable progress in biotechnology and pharmaceutical research, the rate of new drug approvals by regulatory agencies has shown a decline in recent years. Reports indicate that FDA grants approval to only handful of pharmaceuticals annually, despite significant investments made in research and development [17]. This emphasize the need for more efficient and cost-effective drug discovery methods such as those facilitated by computational approaches to enhance the success rate and pace of bringing new medications to market. The challenges associated with each stage of drug discovery can be pointed as follows:

1. Target identification and validation: Identifying suitable drug targets with therapeutic potential while minimizing off-target effects is a significant challenge. Validating these targets experimentally can be time-consuming and resource- intensive.
2. Lead identification: Selecting lead compounds with desirable properties from vast libraries of chemical compounds is a complex task. HTS methods often yield numerous hits, but most of them lack, potency, or desirable drug-like attributes such as solubility and non-toxicity.
3. Lead optimization: Lead compounds identified through screening often require optimization to enhance their efficacy, selectivity, pharmacokinetics, and safety profile. Traditional optimization methods involve iterative synthesis and testing, which are both time-consuming and costly.
4. Preclinical research: Evaluating the safety, efficacy, and pharmacokinetics of lead compounds in animal models is a critical step. However, predicting human outcomes based on animal studies can be challenging, and preclinical trials may not always accurately reflect human responses.

14.3 MACHINE LEARNING IN DRUG DISCOVERY

AI, particularly machine learning (ML), has experienced a significant shift from theoretical research to practical applications including drug discovery [18]. This increase can be linked to two main factors. First, the availability of vast amounts of biological data across various databases has provided a rich resource for training and testing ML models. Second, the widespread accessibility of advanced computer hardware has greatly expedited parallel processing, particularly in computationally intensive tasks. The entire spectrum of drug discovery including clinical trials, has therefore witnessed a profound integration of ML algorithms. By integrating ML-based computational approaches, researchers tries to overcome the challenges faced in the drug discovery process as highlighted in Section 14.2. From target identification [19] to understanding target-disease associations [20], from drug candidate selection [21] to protein structure predictions [22], and from compound design and optimization [23] to elucidating disease mechanisms [24], ML has emerged as a powerful tool driving innovation across the drug discovery pipeline. ML algorithms can analyze diverse data types, including genomic, proteomic, and clinical data, to uncover hidden patterns, predict biological interactions, and optimize therapeutic properties. This data-driven approach accelerates the identification of promising drug candidates and streamlines preclinical and clinical trial workflows. We illustrate the various applications of ML across various stages of the drug discovery pipeline in Figure 14.1. In drug discovery, ML techniques are broadly categorized into two types: supervised learning and unsupervised learning. Supervised learning entails training a model on datasets where the input-output relationships are already known, enabling the model to make predictions for new, unseen inputs. This can be useful for tasks such as predicting drug-target interactions and classifying molecules based on their properties. Conversely, unsupervised learning uncovers underlying patterns or structures within the input data, making it valuable for tasks like discovering new chemical scaffolds or clustering molecules with similar characteristics. In drug discovery, the initial step involves selecting a molecular target and validating its role in the disease. Due the abundance of biological data available today, including human genetic information and various omics data [25], ML methods have been utilized in various aspects of target identification and validation. For instance, Conversely, Jeon [19] utilized genomic data to train a support vector machine (SVM) classifier, aiming to categorize proteins as either drug targets or non-drug targets across various types of cancer. Moreover, ML have been employed to predict drug effects specific to different cancers. For instance, Iorio et al. [26] conducted screenings of cancer cell lines with anticancer drugs and applied ML algorithms to pinpoint molecular characteristics that could forecast drug responses. Another crucial aspect for drug developers is assessing the likelihood of successfully targeting a given protein. ML techniques have been employed to predict druggable targets based on physicochemical properties derived from protein sequences. The methods, such as SVMs or deep learning models like stacked autoencoders, help narrow down the search space by identifying targets likely to bind drugs [27]. To find potential drugs, scientists screen many compounds virtually and experimentally. They refine and adjust these compounds to make them better at targeting specific proteins and safer for use in the body. Another important application of ML in drug discovery is biomarker discovery [28]. It involves identifying biological markers that are predictive of

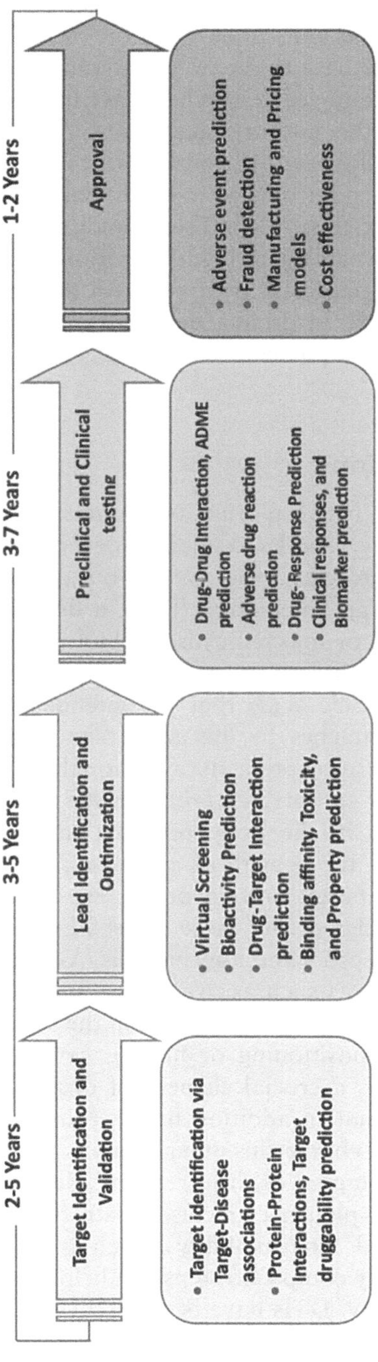

Figure 14.1 Applications of ML in drug discovery and development.

disease onset, progression, or response to treatment. Biomarkers can be various types of data, including genetic, genomic, proteomic, or imaging data, that provide insights into underlying biological processes. ML algorithms can analyze these data to uncover patterns between biomarkers and clinical outcomes. For example, Researchers have utilized ML on multi-omics data to gain deeper insights into drug responses in patients with rheumatoid arthritis [29]. Additionally, new ML frameworks, including gradient boosted regression trees, have been introduced to create polygenic risk scores that are used to predict complex traits [30]. These predictive models help improve clinical success rates by enabling early identification of patients who are most likely to benefit from a particular treatment. All these advancements underscore the potential of ML in driving more personalized and effective drug discovery and development pipeline.

14.3.1 DTI prediction

Prediction of interaction between drugs and targets has a very important role to play in drug discovery. It seeks to uncover new compounds for biological targets also known as proteins and is carried out during the early phases of the process. In drug target interaction (DTI), a drug is any chemical compound that when taken or injected causes a biological response in a living body to cure or prevent disease symptoms. On the other hand, targets are substances made of nucleic acids that are intended to be modified. DTI occurs when a drug attaches to the active site of a target by creating temporary bonds hence disrupting the functionality of the target protein. This is accomplished by stopping certain enzymes from engaging with specific catalytic processes in the body resulting in the resolved metabolic imbalances and curbing the growth of a disease. The interactions of most medications with their target protein or nucleic acid reveal their efficacy against the disease associated with those targets. Examples of target protein classes are enzymes, receptors and ion channels. As a result, finding DTI is a critical foundation in areas such as drug development, drug repositioning, side effect prediction, etc., drastically reducing the scope of candidate medicines searches. Drug repositioning or finding new targets for existing or discarded medications is a crucial element of drug development. The key point to remember is that in addition to the primary therapeutic targets, most medications bind to numerous other proteins also which can be advantages in some cases. The goal of drug repositioning is to find new clinical applications for current pharmaceuticals. Existing medications have previous tests for safety and bioavailability which is a clear benefit. Hence, skipping some previously completed steps can help to speed up the development process significantly. DTIs have been discovered in wet lab tests. The enormous difference between known and unknown interaction pairs has sparked attention in DTI prediction. Traditional prediction procedures have been limited by time and money costs, therefore newly proposed computational approaches can prove to be effective at predicting probable interactions possibilities. Drug screening is a method used to identify chemical compounds that may interact with particular targets linked to a disease. It involves testing large libraries of compounds to identify those that exhibit desired biological activity, such as binding to a target protein or modulating a biological pathway. Drug screening is carried out in early phase of drug discovery which primarily depends on costly traditional wet-lab experiments incurring huge time and resources [27]. Moreover, situation becomes more critical when the screened drugs are later discovered to have unsatisfactory efficacy, unfulfilled properties and toxic side-effects eventually leading to development failure [31]. DTI prediction is therefore critical for pharmacological research and development and can significantly aid in the screening of new drug candidates [32]. It guides drug screening by identifying potential drug-target interactions, facilitating the selection of candidate compounds for experimental validation. In a DTI, a drug (or a ligand) is a chemical molecule which upon entering inside a living body produces an intended therapeutic outcome by targeting proteins of interest. Targets, on the other hand, are substances, often nucleic acids, intended for modification. The majority of target molecules in drug discovery are proteins, predominantly categorized into four key families: Enzymes, G protein-coupled receptors (GPCRs), ion channels, and nuclear receptors. These four families represent 44% of all known targets. Notably, 70% of the drugs currently in development are specifically designed to interact with these protein families. An interaction occurs when a drug links (or binds) to the active site of a target, forming temporary bonds that disrupt the target protein function. This interference can inhibit enzymes from participating in specific catalytic processes, leading to the restoration of metabolic balance and the suppression of disease growth.

Besides recognizing the DTIs, it is also vital to predict the binding strength, referred to as DTBA prediction, to fully understand the potential efficacy of the drugs. DTBA prediction quantitatively measures the strength of the interaction between a drug and its target that offers valuable insights into the efficacy and potency of the candidate drug [33]. Binding affinity, or binding energy, represents the energy required to separate a drug from its target. A higher binding affinity indicates a stronger drug-target interaction, making it more difficult to separate and affecting both specificity and effectiveness. DTBA prediction plays a crucial role in drug repositioning by identifying potential new targets for existing drugs. Drug repositioning involves exploring new targets for the existing or abandoned medications. This approach can significantly reduce the time, cost, and risk associated with drug development, as the safety profiles of the drugs are already well established [34, 35].

14.4 COMPUTATIONAL APPROACHES TO DTI PREDICTION

In this section, we provide an overview of computational approaches to DTI predictions. The computational strategies for the prediction of DTIs can be broadly divided into ligand-based, docking-based, and chemogenomic approaches.

14.4.1 Ligand-based techniques

Ligand-based approaches to DTI prediction rely on the information derived from known ligands that interact with specific protein targets. These methods use the chemical and biological data of these ligands to predict interactions for new, untested compounds. This approach is particularly useful when the structure of the target protein is not available, making structure-based methods infeasible [36]. The rationale behind ligand-based techniques is that identical compounds bind to identical biological targets and have identical features [37]. It starts with a single molecule or a group of chemicals known to be effective against the target and is further guided by the structure-activity relationships. By comparing the chemical structure of new compounds to known ligands, predictions are made about their potential interactions with the target protein. However, there are certain drawbacks to this strategy. Because the protein sequence information is not employed in the prediction process, discovering new interactions reduces the connection across the identified ligand and protein families, which can impact the accuracy of predictions. Additionally, the reliability of prediction results from ligand-based methods can diminish when there is a lack of sufficient known ligands or when the novel compounds are structurally dissimilar to existing ligands [38].

14.4.2 Docking-based techniques

The docking-based approach, uses the 3D structure of the proteins and chemical compounds to determine the possibilities of interaction between them [39]. The goal is to predict the preferred orientation of the ligand where it binds to the target. The docking algorithm predicts the possible orientations (poses) of the ligand within the binding site of the target. This involves placing the ligand in various positions and orientations within the active site. Each pose is evaluated using scoring functions that estimate the binding affinity based on factors such as hydrogen bonding, hydrophobic interactions, van der Waals forces, and electrostatic interactions. The scoring function ranks the poses, predicting which ligand poses are most likely to be biologically relevant [40]. However, the accuracy of docking predictions heavily relies on the quality of the target protein and ligand 3D structures. Inaccurate structures can lead to incorrect predictions. Moreover, this method cannot be applied to proteins with unknown 3D structures such as the membrane proteins [41].

14.4.3 Chemogenomic techniques

The chemogenomic approaches are the ML-based methods that use drug and protein information together to anticipate interactions. To infer probable interactions, a shared subspace is created by unifying the biochemical space of drugs and the genome space of targets. The main benefit of this method is that it utilizes a significant amount of biological data that is freely accessible from public repositories [42]. Chemogenomic approaches are roughly divided into similarity-based, network-based methods and feature-based methods. Figure 14.2 illustrates a branch diagram of the computational methods used for DTI prediction. Among chemogenomic approaches, feature-based methods have received significant attention due to their robust predictive performance. These approaches generally utilize the chemical and biological attributes of drugs and targets and employ various ML techniques to predict interactions. The flowchart of the standard chemogenomic approaches for drug-target interaction prediction is shown in Figure 14.3.

14.4.3.1 Similarity-based methods

The "guilt-by-association" assumption is a fundamental principle behind similarity-based methods which suggest that similar drugs often target similar biological entities, and vice versa. This assumption forms the basis of computational approaches where the similarity among drugs or targets is quantified using various similarity or distance measures. These measures

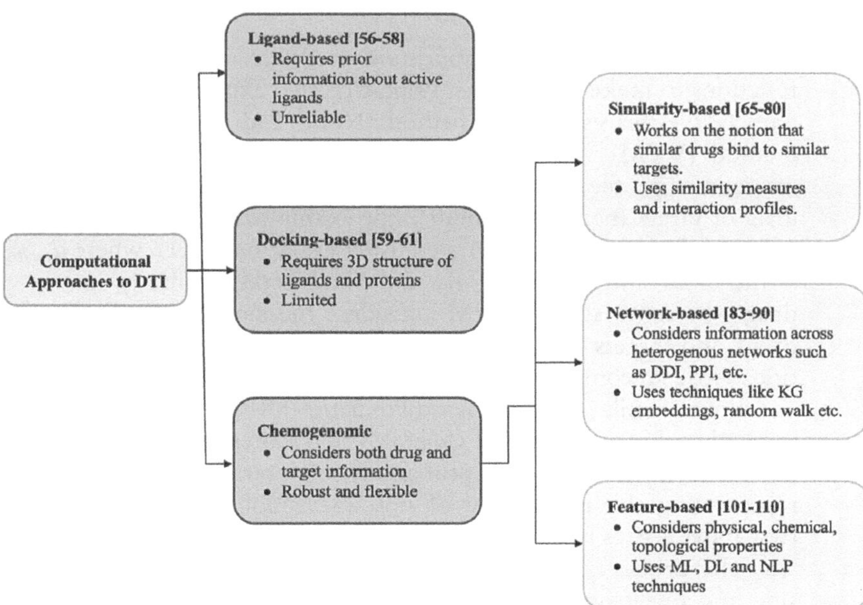

Figure 14.2 Computational approaches to DTI prediction.

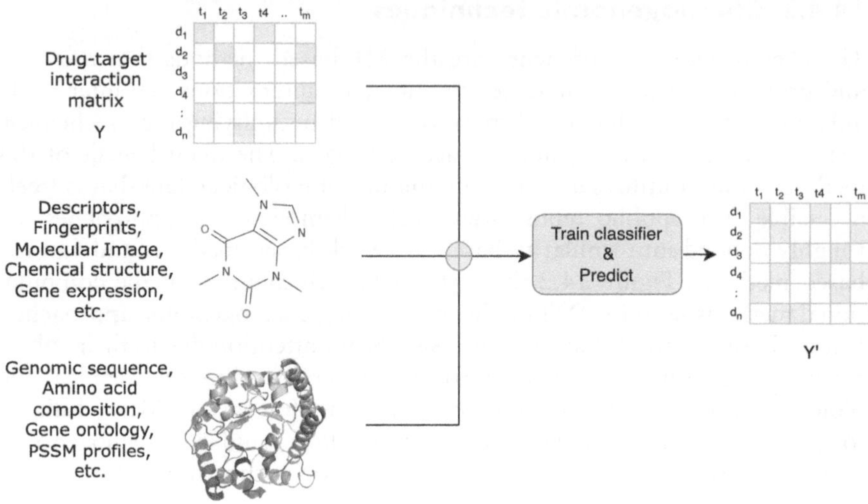

Figure 14.3 Flowchart of a standard chemogenomic approach for drug-target interaction prediction.

facilitate the construction of similarity matrices, which in turn define several types of kernel functions. Various similarity or distance functions used in these methods are Euclidean distance, Jaccard score, Tanimoto score, and Cosine similarity. Similarity-based methods can further be subdivided into neighborhood, bipartite and matrix factorization methods.

1. Neighborhood-based: Neighborhood methods use simple similarity functions to make predictions. Primarily, two exploratory approaches namely the nearest profile method (NPN) and the weighted profile method (WPM) were proposed [42]. The NPN method infers the interaction profile of a new drug or target based on its most similar drug or target (nearest neighbor). For example, the interaction profile $X(d_i)$ of drug d_i can be calculated using Equation (14.1), where d_{nearest} is the most similar drug to d_i, and Sim_d is the similarity matrix of drugs. In contrast, the WPM considers the similarities of all other drugs and targets and adopts a weighted average to make its predictions [43]. To compute weighted profile for d_i Equation (14.2) is given as follows. Similarity Rank-based Predictor (SRP) [44] is another novel method in this category that generates two scores for each drug-target pair: one representing the probability of interaction and the other representing the probability of non-interaction. The ratio of these two above scores is taken to generate interaction likelihood score. This way SRP produces two interaction likelihood score, one from the drug side and one from the target side. The final prediction score is the average of both the interaction likelihood score. In recent years,

researchers proposed novel similarity-based methods that incorporate the pharmacological similarity of drugs and the genomic similarity of targets

$$X(d_i) = \mathrm{Sim}_d(d_i, d_{\mathrm{nearest}}) \times X(d_{\mathrm{nearest}}) \tag{14.1}$$

with the topological properties of a multipartite network of existing drugs and targets [38, 45]. Instead of calculating only chemical structure similarity between drugs and sequence similarity between genes, Perlman et al. [46] introduced an approach called SITAR that uses novel multiple measures (e.g., gene expression, gene ontology, etc.) to compute drug-drug and gene-gene similarity measures, respectively. The method integrates drug-drug and gene-gene similarities into classification features. To enhance prediction accuracy, they employed forward selection and backward elimination feature selection techniques to identify the most relevant features.

$$X(d_i) = \frac{\sum_{j=1}^{n} \mathrm{Sim}_d(d_i, d_j) \times X(d_i)}{\sum_{j=1}^{n} \mathrm{Sim}_d(d_i, d_j)} \tag{14.2}$$

These selected features were then used in a logistic regression model for prediction. Zhang et al. [47] presented LPLNI which calculated linear neighborhood similarity between drugs using various fingerprints such as PubChem, MACCS, EState, Interaction profiles, etc., and used label propagation for predicting unobserved interactions between ligands and targets.

2. Bipartite local models: The network of DTIs can be structured as a bipartite network. Based on the successful application of local models to train and predict protein-protein interactions and regulatory networks [48, 49], Bleakley introduced the concept of local models to analyze the bipartite network of DTIs. This approach transforms the task of edge prediction into a binary classification task, where the goal is to predict the presence or absence of interactions (labels) between drugs and targets. They employed SVM [50] to train two local models: one based on drug chemical similarity and the other on target sequence similarity. This method generates two set of predictions: one from the drug side, indicating the set of interacting proteins, and the other from the target side, indicating the set of interacting drugs. The final prediction for each drug-target pair is obtained by averaging two set of predictions [51]. Researchers have demonstrated that a simple ML approach that use only the interaction network as its source of information, can accurately predict true interaction pairs. For example,

Laarhoven [45] proposed two models: RLS-avg and RLS-kron. RLS-avg employs a Regularized Least Squares (RLS) classifier with a Gaussian kernel applied to the interaction profiles of drugs and targets to generate predictions. In contrast, RLS-kron combines separate kernels for drugs and targets using the Kronecker product, which results in reduced runtime. Considering that BLM struggles to provide accurate predictions for new drug or target candidates, Mei et al. [52] introduced an improved version called BLM with neighbor-based interaction-profile inferring (BLM-NII). The NII procedure enhances the original BLM method by incorporating the ability to learn from neighbors. The model initially derives weighted interactions for the new candidate from the interaction profiles of its neighbors. These inferred interactions are then used as label information to train the model, thereby improving prediction accuracy for new candidates. Nascimento et al. [53] extended the KronRLS method by proposing the MKL model, which builds multiple kernels for drugs and targets based on heterogeneous information, rather than relying solely on interaction profiles. This approach utilizes L2 regularization, allowing it to handle large datasets without the need for subsampling.

3. Matrix factorization method: Matrix factorization algorithms, which are widely used in recommendation systems to identify probable user-item interactions, can also be used to predict DTIs [54–56]. In this context, DTI prediction is viewed as a matrix completion task where the goal is detecting missing interactions between drugs and targets. This method involves splitting the interaction matrix into two lower-dimensional matrices which upon multiplication resemble the original interaction matrix, indicating possible interactions. This factorization captures the latent properties of drugs and targets for facilitating accurate prediction of unobserved interactions. Gonen proposed Kernelized Bayesian Matrix Factorization with Twin Kernels (KBMF2K) [54], introducing matrix factorization for DTI prediction. KBMF2K employs two kernel matrices: one based on chemical similarity between drugs and the other on genomic similarity between targets. The chemical similarity between drug compounds is calculated using SIMCOMP [57], which represents drug compounds as graphs and computes a similarity score based on the size of common substructures between two graphs. For target proteins, sequence similarities are determined using a normalized version of the Smith–Waterman score [58]. This method integrates a Bayesian probabilistic framework with matrix factorization and binary classification to address the prediction problem by leveraging comprehensive similarity information. Building upon KBMF2K, Cobanoglu et al. [56] incorporated a probabilistic framework into matrix factorization with active learning. The objective is to eliminate the reliance on predefined drug and target similarity matrices, enabling the model to be

applied to larger datasets with a greater number of DTI pairs. Zheng et al. [59] introduced Multiple Similarities Collaborative Matrix Factorization (MSCMF), an extension of weighted low-rank approximation. Unlike methods that use a single similarity measure for drugs and targets, MSCMF incorporates multiple similarity matrices for both, enhancing the accuracy of DTI predictions. The method estimates two low-rank matrices and optimizes the weights of the similarity matrices using an alternating least squares algorithm to improve predictive performance. Based on a study by Tenenbaum et al. [60] indicating that data typically lies on or near a low-dimensional and non-linear manifold, Ezzat et al. [61] presented two matrix factorization methods: Graph Regularized Matrix Factorization (GRMF) and Weighted Graph Regularized Matrix Factorization (WGRMF). Recognizing that non-interacting edges in the DTI network represent unknown or missing interactions, they developed a preprocessing step to improve predictions for new drugs and new targets. This step, known as WKNKN, enhances predictions by transforming all zeros in the original drug-target matrix into interaction likelihood values based on close neighbors. Unlike KBMF2K which uses kernel regularization, GRMF and WGRMF employ graph regularization to prevent overfitting to increase the robustness and accuracy of the predictions. Contrary to these, Liu et al. [62] proposed neighborhood regularized logistic matrix factorization (NRLMF) in which logistic matrix factorization is integrated with neighborhood regularization method. The method employs the properties of drugs and targets using two latent vectors within a shared low-dimensional space. For each drug-target pair, the interaction probability is modeled using a logistic function with neighborhood regularization that combines the drug-specific and target-specific latent vectors.

14.4.3.2 Network-based methods

Incorporating diverse data sources, such as drug-disease associations, drug-drug interactions, protein-protein interactions, etc., along with chemical and genomic data, can also enhance the accuracy of DTI prediction and offer new perspectives on drug repositioning. Various computational methods have been developed to integrate these heterogeneous data sources for DTI prediction. Network-based approach involves merging heterogeneous information via a network diffusion process and using the resulting diffusion distributions to calculate DTI prediction scores. Luo et al. [63] presented DTINet that combines various types of data, such as information about drugs, proteins, diseases, and side-effects, to make predictions about how drugs interact with proteins. To obtain a condensed representation of features, DTINet combines dimensionality reduction methods like Diffusion component analysis (DCA) [64] with a network diffusion model such as random walk with restart (RWR). It then identifies the best mapping from drug space to protein space, ensuring that the projected feature vectors of drugs are similar to their known interacting targets. This process allows DTINet to predict new interactions for drugs by ranking potential target candidates based on their proximity to the projected feature vector of the drug. Chen et al. [65] introduced a novel approach called the molecular associations network (MAN) for predicting DTIs. MAN incorporates information on miRNA, lncRNA, protein, drug, and disease and nine distinct relationships between pairs of molecules. By analyzing this network, each molecule is assigned a feature vector based on its interactions with other molecules, by using the deep walk network embedding method. This innovative method represents the first attempt to predict DTIs comprehensively from a complex heterogeneous network, providing insights at the cellular level. In a similar method, You et al. [66] also emphasize the importance of other biomolecules in predicting DTIs. For this, the researchers constructed a heterogeneous multi-molecular information network which integrates known associations among diseases, proteins, drugs, lncRNAs (long non-coding RNAs), and miRNAs (microRNAs) from multiple databases, with nodes representing the biomolecules and edges representing their interactions. LINE (Large-scale Information Network Embedding) [67] method is employed to extract association information between drugs, proteins, and other nodes in the network. This involves mapping tightly connected nodes to similar locations in a low-dimensional vector space, capturing the information of drugs and proteins based on their relationships with other biomolecules. Subsequently, the method integrates this information with attribute information such as protein sequences and drug molecular fingerprints to represent known drug-protein interaction pairs comprehensively. Finally, a random forest classifier is used to train the model on this integrated data to enable the prediction of new DTIs based on the learned patterns. Moving a step further in integrating diverse drug-related and protein-related information, Xuan et al. [68] proposed DTIP, which encodes and integrates multi-scale neighboring topologies, various similarities, and interactions related to drugs and proteins. The process begins with constructing a three-layer heterogeneous network to represent association among drug, protein, and disease nodes. To make the final predictions, they employed a convolutional neural network (CNN) to integrate the comprehensive information from the network. To enhance the integration of diverse information, An et al. [69] introduced a method called Network Embedding framework in Multiplex networks (NEDTP). This approach leverages linking information from various nodes (drugs, proteins, diseases, and side-effects) within 15 networks to construct feature vectors for drugs and targets. Initially, a similarity network is created, and the random walk algorithm is applied to extract features by simulating paths through the network. These features are then merged to obtain comprehensive representations for both the entities. Finally, the feature are used to predict DTIs using the gradient boosting decision tree (GBDT) model. Recognizing the importance of effectively integrating information from heterogeneous networks, various graph convolution operations have significantly improved performance in numerous network-related prediction tasks [70, 71]. Wan et al. [72] introduced an end-to-end technique called NeoDTI, which integrates data from omics networks using multiple message passing and aggregation operations. They devised a scheme to retain the topology-related features in the node embeddings. Recent years have seen a fast growth of ML models based on knowledge graphs (KG). Thafar et al. [73] proposed DTi2vec, which leverages the similarity between drugs and targets to enhance the DTI network. This method first applies the K-nearest neighbors (KNN) algorithm to retain the top-k similar nodes for both drugs and targets. Next, a random walk using node2vec is performed on the augmented network to learn embeddings for the drugs and targets. These embeddings are then fed into a boosting model for classification. Mohammad et al. [74] introduced TriModel, a knowledge graph (KG) encompassing various biological entities associated with drugs and targets. Subsequently, the model was trained to acquire effective vector representations for drugs and targets within this knowledge graph. Based on the similar notion, Wang et al. [75] introduced a novel KG-based DL approach wherein they gathered 59,204 drug-target pairs from the DrugBank database [76]. They utilized DistMult [77] embedding strategy to build a knowledge graph of DTPs for generating embeddings. These vectors were then inputted into a Conv-Conv module to extract additional features of DTPs. Subsequently, a fully connected neural network was designed to predict potential DTIs based on the extracted features. These studies indicate that the application of network-based methods in drug repurposing is an area of growing interest. The approach holds the potential to uncover novel drug-target associations and elucidate underlying mechanisms of drug action.

14.4.3.3 Feature-based methods

The majority of ML methods used for DTI prediction fall into this category, including SVM, tree-based approaches, and other kernel-based algorithms. Typically, the input for these methods consists of drug-target pairs expressed as fixed-length vectors. Drugs and proteins are transformed into descriptors based on their chemical properties, and the integration of individual features from both drugs and targets forms a 1D array which is used as input for these approaches. Most researchers predict DTIs focused on fingerprint-based structural information of drugs. For example, Wan et al. [78] developed a model for DTI prediction that leverages the structural properties of drugs and the evolutionary properties of proteins using a rotation forest classifier as the final predictor. The structural properties of drugs are captured through structural key fingerprints, while PSSM is used to quantify the evolutionary information of target proteins. The researchers compared their method with other methods and demonstrated superior performance.

To solve the data imbalance problem of the benchmark dataset, they randomly selected instances from the non-interacting pairs as negative samples. Researchers have developed several methods to extract meaningful features from PSSM profiles of target proteins. For instance, Wang et al. [79] employed stacked autoencoders to effectively extract meaningful features from PSSM profiles and combined these with drug feature vectors for model classification. Wang et al. [80] utilized Legendre moments to extract features from PSSM profiles and combined them with drug fingerprint information to generate a feature vector. This feature vector for each drug-target pair was then compressed using sparse principal component analysis [81] before being input into a long short-term memory network for classification. In addition to using the PSSM matrix for protein representation, other features are also employed to capture heterogeneous information. For example, Mahmud et al. [82] proposed iDTi-CSsmoteB and suggested incorporating sequence information about proteins, such as amphiphilic pseudo amino acid composition (AM-PseAAC) and dipeptide amino acid composition (DP-AAC), along with evolutionary data. They addressed the issue of data imbalance by using SMOTE (Synthetic minority oversampling technique) to oversample the minority instances, demonstrating better performance compared to random sampling. Later in 2020, Mahmud et al. proposed pdti-EssB [83], which integrated multiple types of protein information, including evolutionary, sequence, and structural features. This included the PSSM-Bigram, PseAAC, and SPIDER2 for protein sequence encoding, alongside substructural fingerprints for drug encoding. Hansan et al. [84] introduced PreDTIs, a method designed to address both the curse of dimensionality and data imbalance in DTI prediction. PreDTIs utilizes PsePSSM, DC, and PseAAC for target encoding, and MACCS substructure keys for drug encoding. To tackle imbalance and select relevant features, the method incorporates the FastCUS and MoIFS algorithms, respectively. FastCUS addresses imbalance by removing majority class samples that are similar to minority class samples and retaining those that are more distinct, thereby preserving valuable information. MoIFS modifies an incremental feature selection [85] approach to eliminate noisy and redundant features. Recently, Khojasteh et al. [86] proposed SRX-DTI, a method that combines multiple features with a data imbalance technique. They integrated over nine types of features for encoding targets and used FP2-fingerprints for encoding drugs. In addition to using standard datasets, they demonstrated the performance of SRX-DTI on a binding affinity dataset as well, highlighting its effectiveness in diverse scenarios.

Ensemble models have also shown promising performance in DTI prediction. Sharma et al. [87] introduced a framework employing bagging-based ensemble learning to enhance classifier diversity. Drug features were generated using the Rcpi package [88], while target features were obtained from the PROFEAT [89]. To address class imbalance, they utilized an active learning approach. Peng et al. [90] proposed a methodical approach considering ML models build on multiple fingerprints and descriptors. The study revealed that out of all the models developed, Morgan-PSSM-SVM outperformed. A case study on data curated from ChembL database was also conducted to validate the findings. DL has gained popularity as a result of its superior performance in a variety of fields including speech recognition and image recognition. DL approaches to DTI prediction appear to address some difficulties by reducing feature information loss. The majority of approaches based has one key step of extracting relevant features from the raw data. For instance, Xu et al. [91] proposed a method to transform SMILES into a lower-dimensional vector using an encoder-decoder architecture based on Gated Recurrent Units (GRU). In their approach, a multi-layered GRU network maps the input molecule into a continuous feature vector of fixed dimensionality. This feature vector is then decoded back to the original molecule by another deep GRU network. The continuous encoding vector is designed to capture comprehensive and detailed information, sufficient to reconstruct the original molecule and predict its chemical properties. This method emphasizes the importance of representation learning in accurately encoding the SMILES of drugs for effective prediction and analysis. Three types of attributes i.e. biological, topological and physicochemical of drugs and targets are typically employed to generate feature vectors. Neural networks variants such as Deep Belief Network (DBN), Multi-Layer Perceptron (MLP), Convolutional Neural Network (CNN) and Long Short Term Memory (LSTM) were employed to create DTI prediction systems in recently published articles. As CNNs are known to have explainability and interpretability though filters and feature maps, Tsubaki et al. [92] extracted features from SMILES using CNN for ligands. Graph neural network (GNN) is used on AA sequences for target encodings. N-gram techniques is used to encode the amino acid sequences into n-grams. Instead of using substructure fingerprints such as PubChem and MACCS available through packages and web servers, GNN has gained popularity to learn them through graph of the molecule by extracting and mapping substructure present in the molecule in new dimensional space. The handling of text-based representations of molecules has become a subject of considerable scientific interest due to advancements in NLP approaches. NLP approaches for DTI prediction have seen significant growth and improvement with ever increasing amount of information offered by the publicly accessible databases rich in text-based biochemical knowledge [93]. SMILE notations and amino acid sequences are the most commonly utilized text-based representations for ligands and proteins respectively. For instance, k-mers were successfully applied on SMILE strings for DTI task. Word embedding, a NLP technique of significant importance maps words into a vector of real numbers keeping their context and syntax intact with reference to the document. Word embeddings based on frequency such as count-vector, TF-IDF and co-occurrence vector that are based on predictions such as word2vec have acquire great deal of attention. Inspired by unsupervised representation learning methods like Word2vec, Zhang et al. [94] introduced SPVec, a novel approach for automatically transforming raw data such as SMILES strings and protein sequences into lower-dimensional informative vectors. This method addresses the issues of sparsity and bit collisions associated with manually extracted features. SPVec demonstrated superior performance compared to AAC and MACCS on independent test sets. Zheng et al. [95] introduced DTI-BERT, a method that utilizes pre-trained Bidirectional Encoder Representations from Transformers (BERT) for encoding protein sequences and employs Discrete Wavelet Transform for generating drug fingerprints. The resulting vectors from both processes are concatenated and then fed into a feature extraction module, which includes batch normalization and dense layers, to make predictions. Gao et al. [96] suggested using GCN and gene ontology annotations for AA to identify learnable features from the SMILE strings and protein sequences. They generated the joint interaction space for DTI pairs by concatenating the ligand and protein spaces within an end-to-end learning framework that incorporates both LSTM and graph CNN. Moreover, studies demonstrated that domains and motifs work in unison just as well as the entire protein sequence [97].

14.4.4 Computational approaches to DTBA prediction

Computational methods for predicting DTIs have traditionally focused on binary classification to determine if a given drug-target pair interacts. However, protein-ligand interactions exist on a spectrum of binding strength values, known as binding affinity, and predicting these values remains a significant challenge. To address this, researchers have developed various methods, leveraging the availability of binding affinity data in several databases. We provide a brief summary of DTI- and DTBA-based methods in Table 14.1. Inspired by the successful application of ML and DL techniques in the binary classification of DTIs, researchers are now applying these methods to predict binding affinity as well. Öztürk et al. [101] presented DeepDTA employing two CNN blocks each for drug and target to learn representations from the raw protein sequences and SMILES strings. To encode protein sequences and SMILES strings, label encoding is used which prepare the data in the form that is expected by the CNN. They demonstrated the performance on Kinase binding affinity datasets against KronRLS and SimBoost algorithms. Based on observations from DeepDTA, it was found that the CNN-based modules were less effective at modeling proteins compared to SMILES in the affinity prediction task. This was attributed to the loss of biologically important short subsequences during the modeling process. To address this issue, Öztürk et al. [98] presented WideDTA, which employs word-level encoding instead of character-level encoding for representing entities from raw data. For SMILES, WideDTA

Table 14.1 A brief description about some of the DTI and DTBA methods in literature

Task	*Dataset*	*Feature*	*Imbalance strategy*	*Methods*	*Reference*
IP	Enzymes, GPCR, IC, NR	PSSM, Substructural Fingerprints	Random selection	Rotation Forest	[78]
IP	Enzymes, GPCR, IC, NR	AM-PseAAC, DP-AAC, fingerprints	SMOTE	Rotation Forest	[82]
IP	Enzymes, GPCR, IC, NR	PSSM, Substructural Fingerprints	Random selection	Legendre Moments, Rotation Forest	[80]
IP	Enzymes, GPCR, IC, NR	DC, PseAAC, MACCS	Under sampling	LightGBM	[84]
IP and BA	Davis, Enzymes, GPCR, IC, NR	FP2, AAC, DPC, GCPC, GTPC, and others	One-SVM-US	Forward Feature Selection, Random Forest	[86]
IP	ChEMBL, BindingDB	Descriptors, Fingerprints, PSSM	SMOTE	PCA, GBDT, KNN, SVM, DT, Bagging	[90]
IP	Human and C. elegans	SMILES, Amino acid sequences	NA	CNN, GNN	[92]
BA	Davis, KIBA	SMILES, Amino acid sequences	NA	K-mers, CNN	[98]
BA	Davis, KIBA	SMILES, Amino acid sequences	NA	CNN, LSTM	[99]
BA	Davis, KIBA	SMILES, Amino acid sequences	NA	CNN, LSTM, Attention mechanism	[100]

uses Maximum Common Substructures (LMCS) and k-mers, while for target proteins, it employs k-mers along with Domains and Motifs (PDM). To enhance prediction performance, Zhao et al. [102] introduced AttentionDTA, highlighting the significance of attention mechanism to focus on the most relevant subsequences of both drugs and proteins. By applying 1D-CNN to extract detailed information from drug and protein sequences, the model uses attention mechanisms to ensure that the representations of drugs and proteins mutually adapt, emphasizing the most important subsequences for accurate affinity prediction. In a similar approach, Abbasi et al. [99] presented the Deep-CDA model, which employs a combination of CNN and LSTM networks to achieve enhanced representations of proteins and drugs. DeepCDA uses a two-sided attention mechanism and enhances generalization through a domain adaptation technique. Yuan et al. [100] highlighted the significance of feature aggregation and the complexities of encoder networks in affinity prediction, which can lead to information loss and increased model size. They proposed FusionDTA, which employs a multi-head linear attention mechanism instead of the traditional pooling method. The process starts with encoding inputs into continuous distributed representations using a pre-trained transformer. This is adopted as one-hot encoding fails to capture context information from large unsupervised biological corpora. The basic block of the encoder network consists of LSTM layers. To capture both local and global dependencies, a two-layer bidirectional LSTM is applied to the learned embeddings. Inspired by the success of similarity-based method in DTI, Shim et al. [103] presented similarity-based model SimCNN-DTA using 2D CNN approach on the outer product of column vectors of Tanimoto similarity matrix and Smith-Waterman similarity [58] matrix for the drugs and targets. However, these methods rely on supervised ML using known labels. To develop a model that can learn features from the input with minimal or no label information, Zhao et al. [104] proposed a semi-supervised model called GANsDTA, based on generative adversarial networks (GANs). In this approach, the generator first creates fake samples according to a given noise distribution. These fake samples, along with real samples from available datasets, are then fed into the discriminator network. The task of the discriminator is to distinguish between real and fake sequences of proteins and SMILES of compounds. It does this by mapping the input into a feature space using a local feature extractor, which aids in sample classification. Through the training of the GANs, a local feature extractor is developed within the discriminator that effectively represents the characteristics of the input protein or SMILES sequence. The model includes two GANs, one for each entity (proteins and compounds), for feature extraction, and a CNN model for regression. Zeng et al. [105] pointed out that existing approaches often neglect the relationships between the atoms in drug molecules during encoding, and merely concatenate the drug-target pairs. Their proposed method addresses this by employing a relation-aware self-attention block to effectively capture atomic relationships, and uses multi-head attention to improve upon the direct concatenation of drug and target features. Nyugen et al. [106] argued that representing drugs as strings is not a correct way to model molecules. To address this, they proposed GraphDTA, a new model that represents molecules as graphs. GraphDTA leverages various GNN variants, such as GAT, GIN, and GCN, to predict drug-target affinity. This approach significantly outperforms competing DL methods. As previous studies relied on single sources of information and did not use binding affinity and neighborhood information as direct features, Tanoori et al. [107] proposed a non-structure-based method that utilizes multiple information sources. This method combines various similarity measures for drug-drug and protein-protein similarities, integrating neighborhood information and binding affinities. Thafar et al. [108] introduced the concept of depicting the DTBA problem as a graph-based task in Affinity2vec. This model constructs a weighted network by integrating three graphs: the binding affinity graph, the target-target similarity graph, and the drug-drug similarity graph. Many studies focus solely on extracting sequence information, which often lacks rich features. To address this, Pu et al. [100] introduced DeepFusionDTA, a two-stage DNN ensemble model that incorporates spatial features to integrate various data from drug and target spaces. DeepFusionDTA utilizes both sequence and structural information to create a fusion feature map of candidate protein and drug pairs through multiple DL-based modules. By leveraging the strengths of different algorithms for efficient feature abstraction and regression calculation, this method achieves outstanding results.

CONFLICT OF INTEREST

The authors have no competing interests to declare that are relevant to the content of this article.

REFERENCES

1. Y. Xu, X. Liu, X. Cao, C. Huang, E. Liu, S. Qian, X. Liu, Y. Wu, F. Dong, C.W. Qiu, et al., Artificial intelligence: A powerful paradigm for scientific research. *The Innovation* 2(4) (2021).
2. N. Berdigaliyev and M. Aljofan, An overview of drug discovery and development. *Future Medicinal Chemistry* 12(10), 939–947 (2020).
3. A. Batta, B.S. Kalra, and R. Khirasaria, Trends in FDA drug approvals over last 2 decades: An observational study. *Journal of Family Medicine and Primary Care* 9(1), 105–114 (2020).
4. A. Carnero, High throughput screening in drug discovery. *Clinical and Translational Oncology* 8, 482–490 (2006).
5. S.J.Y. Macalino, V. Gosu, S. Hong, and S. Choi, Role of computer-aided drug design in modern drug discovery. *Archives of Pharmacal Research* 38, 1686–1701 (2015).
6. M. Aminpour, C. Montemagno, and J.A. Tuszynski, An overview of molecular modeling for drug discovery with specific illustrative examples of applications. *Molecules* 24(9), 1693 (2019).
7. D. Taylor, *The pharmaceutical industry and the future of drug development*, vol. 41. Royal Society of Chemistry, 2015. https://doi.org/10.1039/9781782622345
8. S. Sinha and D. Vohora, Drug discovery and development: An overview. *Pharmaceutical Medicine and Translational Clinical Research*, 19–32 (2018).
9. F. Ashall and A.M. Goate, Role of the β-amyloid precursor protein in Alzheimer's disease. *Trends in Biochemical Sciences* 19(1), 42–46 (1994).
10. J.R. Broach and J. Thorner, High-throughput screening for drug discovery. *Nature* 384(6604), 14–16 (1996).
11. W.P. Walters, M.T. Stahl, and M.A. Murcko, Virtual screening—An overview. *Drug Discovery Today* 3(4), 160–178 (1998).
12. M.P. Barcelos, S.Q. Gomes, L.B. Federico, I.A.G. Francischini, L.I.D.S. Hage-Melim, G.M. Silva, and C.H.T. de Paula da Silva, *Research topics in bioactivity, environment and energy: Experimental and theoretical tools*. Springer, 2022, pp. 481–500.

13. C. Isarankura-Na-Ayudhya, T. Naenna, C. Nantasenamat, and V. Prachayasittikul, A practical overview of quantitative structure-activity relationship. *EXCLIJournal* (2009).
14. I.L. Buxton, *Pharmacokinetics and pharmacodynamics. Goodman and Gilman's the pharmacologic basis of therapeutics*, 11th Ed. McGraw-Hill, 2006, pp. 1–52.
15. J.A. DiMasi, L. Feldman, A. Seckler, and A. Wilson, Trends in risks associated with new drug development: Success rates for investigational drugs. *Clinical Pharmacology & Therapeutics* 87(3), 272–277 (2010).
16. J.A. DiMasi, H.G. Grabowski, and R.W. Hansen, Innovation in the pharmaceutical industry: New estimates of R&D costs. *Journal of Health Economics* 47, 20–33 (2016).
17. C.H. Wong, K.W. Siah, and A.W. Lo, Estimation of clinical trial success rates and related parameters. *Biostatistics* 20(2), 273–286 (2019).
18. K.K. Mak, Y.H. Wong, and M.R. Pichika, Artificial intelligence in drug discovery and development. *Drug Discovery and Evaluation: Safety and Pharmacokinetic Assays*, 1–38 (2023).
19. J. Jeon, S. Nim, J. Teyra, A. Datti, J.L. Wrana, S.S. Sidhu, J. Moffat, and P.M. Kim, A systematic approach to identify novel cancer drug targets using machine learning, inhibitor design and high-throughput screening. *Genome Medicine* 6, 1–18 (2014).
20. E. Ferrero, I. Dunham, and P. Sanseau, In silico prediction of novel therapeutic targets using gene–disease association data. *Journal of Translational Medicine* 15, 1–16 (2017).
21. D.M. Dambach, D. Misner, M. Brock, A. Fullerton, W. Proctor, J. Maher, D. Lee, K. Ford, and D. Diaz, Safety lead optimization and candidate identification: Integrating new technologies into decision-making. *Chemical Research in Toxicology* 29(4), 452–472 (2016).
22. B. Kuhlman and P. Bradley, Advances in protein structure prediction and design. *Nature Reviews Molecular Cell Biology* 20(11), 681–697 (2019).
23. S. Riniker, Y. Wang, J.L. Jenkins, and G.A. Landrum, Using information from historical high-throughput screens to predict active compounds. *Journal of Chemical Information and Modeling* 54(7), 1880–1891 (2014).
24. W.J. Godinez, I. Hossain, S.E. Lazic, J.W. Davies, and X. Zhang, A multi-scale convolutional neural network for phenotyping high-content cellular images. *Bioinformatics* 33(13), 2010–2019 (2017).
25. P. Mamoshina, M. Volosnikova, I.V. Ozerov, E. Putin, E. Skibina, F. Cortese, and A. Zhavoronkov, Machine learning on human muscle transcriptomic data for biomarker discovery and tissue-specific drug target identification. *Frontiers in Genetics* 9, 242 (2018).
26. F. Iorio, T.A. Knijnenburg, D.J. Vis, G.R. Bignell, M.P. Menden, M. Schubert, N. Aben, E. Gonçalves, S. Barthorpe, H. Lightfoot, et al., A landscape of pharmacogenomic interactions in cancer. *Cell* 166(3), 740–754 (2016).
27. R. Chen, X. Liu, S. Jin, J. Lin, and J. Liu, Machine learning for drug-target interaction prediction. *Molecules* 23(9), 2208 (2018).
28. J. Wang, G.J. Tan, L.N. Han, Y.Y. Bai, M. He, and H.B. Liu, Novel biomarkers for cardiovascular risk prediction. *Journal of Geriatric Cardiology: JGC* 14(2), 135 (2017).
29. S. Tasaki, K. Suzuki, Y. Kassai, M. Takeshita, A. Murota, Y. Kondo, T. Ando, Y. Nakayama, Y. Okuzono, M. Takiguchi, et al., Multi-omics monitoring of drug response in rheumatoid arthritis in pursuit of molecular remission. *Nature Communications* 9(1), 2755 (2018).
30. G. Paré, S. Mao, and W.Q. Deng, A machine-learning heuristic to improve gene score prediction of polygenic traits. *Scientific Reports* 7(1), 12665 (2017).

31. S.M. Paul, D.S. Mytelka, C.T. Dunwiddie, C.C. Persinger, B.H. Munos, S.R. Lindborg, and A.L. Schacht, How to improve R&D productivity: The pharmaceutical industry's grand challenge. *Nature Reviews Drug discovery* 9(3), 203–214 (2010).
32. Z. He, J. Zhang, X.H. Shi, L.L. Hu, X. Kong, Y.D. Cai, and K.C. Chou, Predicting drug-target interaction networks based on functional groups and biological features. *PloS One* 5(3), e9603 (2010).
33. M. Wen, Z. Zhang, S. Niu, H. Sha, R. Yang, Y. Yun, and H. Lu, Deep-learning based drug–target interaction prediction. *Journal of Proteome Research* 16(4), 1401–1409 (2017).
34. A. Cichonska, J. Rousu, and T. Aittokallio, Identification of drug candidates and repurposing opportunities through compound–target interaction networks. *Expert Opinion on Drug Discovery* 10(12), 1333–1345 (2015).
35. T.T. Ashburn and K.B. Thor, Drug repositioning: Identifying and developing new uses for existing drugs. *Nature Reviews Drug discovery* 3(8), 673–683 (2004).
36. M.J. Keiser, B.L. Roth, B.N. Armbruster, P. Ernsberger, J.J. Irwin, and B.K. Shoichet, Relating protein pharmacology by ligand chemistry. *Nature Biotechnology* 25(2), 197–206 (2007).
37. M.A. Johnson and G.M. Maggiora, *Concepts and applications of molecular similarity*. Wiley, 1990, p. 22.
38. L. Jacob and J.P. Vert, Protein-ligand interaction prediction: An improved chemogenomics approach. *Bioinformatics* 24(19), 2149–2156 (2008).
39. H. Li, Z. Gao, L. Kang, H. Zhang, K. Yang, K. Yu, X. Luo, W. Zhu, K. Chen, J. Shen, et al., TarFisDock: A web server for identifying drug targets with docking approach. *Nucleic Acids Research* 34(suppl 2), W219–W224 (2006).
40. G. Pujadas, M. Vaque, A. Ardevol, C. Blade, M. Salvado, M. Blay, J. Fernandez-Larrea, and L. Arola, Protein-ligand docking: A review of recent advances and future perspectives. *Current Pharmaceutical Analysis* 4(1), 1–19 (2008).
41. A.C. Cheng, R.G. Coleman, K.T. Smyth, Q. Cao, P. Soulard, D.R. Caffrey, A.C. Salzberg, and E.S. Huang, Structure-based maximal affinity model predicts small-molecule druggability. *Nature Biotechnology* 25(1), 71–75 (2007).
42. Y. Yamanishi, M. Araki, A. Gutteridge, W. Honda, and M. Kanehisa, Prediction of drug–target interaction networks from the integration of chemical and genomic spaces. *Bioinformatics* 24(13), i232–i240 (2008).
43. T. Van Laarhoven and E. Marchiori, Predicting drug-target interactions for new drug compounds using a weighted nearest neighbor profile. *PloS One* 8(6), e66952 (2013).
44. J.Y. Shi and S.M. Yiu, SRP: A concise non-parametric similarity-rank-based model for predicting drug-target interactions, in *Proceedings of the IEEE International Conference on Bioinformatics and Biomedicine (BIBM)*. IEEE, 2015, pp. 1636–1641.
45. T. Van Laarhoven, S.B. Nabuurs, and E. Marchiori, Gaussian interaction profile kernels for predicting drug–target interaction. *Bioinformatics* 27(21), 3036–3043 (2011).
46. L. Perlman, A. Gottlieb, N. Atias, E. Ruppin, and R. Sharan, Combining drug and gene similarity measures for drug-target elucidation. *Journal of Computational Biology* 18(2), 133–145 (2011).
47. W. Zhang, Y. Chen, and D. Li, Drug-target interaction prediction through label propagation with linear neighborhood information. *Molecules* 22(12), 2056 (2017).
48. K. Bleakley, G. Biau, and J.P. Vert, Supervised reconstruction of biological networks with local models. *Bioinformatics* 23(13), i57–i65 (2007).

49. F. Mordelet and J.P. Vert, Sirene: Supervised inference of regulatory networks. *Bioinformatics* 24(16), i76–i82 (2008).
50. H. Xue, Q. Yang, and S. Chen, *The top ten algorithms in data mining*. Chapman and Hall/CRC, 2009, pp. 51–74.
51. K. Bleakley and Y. Yamanishi, Supervised prediction of drug–target interactions using bipartite local models. *Bioinformatics* 25(18), 2397–2403 (2009).
52. J.P. Mei, C.K. Kwoh, P. Yang, X.L. Li, and J. Zheng, Drug–target interaction prediction by learning from local information and neighbors. *Bioinformatics* 29(2), 238–245 (2013).
53. A.C. Nascimento, R.B. Prudêncio, and I.G. Costa, A multiple kernel learning algorithm for drug-target interaction prediction. *BMC Bioinformatics* 17, 1–16 (2016).
54. M. Gönen, Predicting drug–target interactions from chemical and genomic kernels using Bayesian matrix factorization. *Bioinformatics* 28(18), 2304–2310 (2012).
55. W. Dai, X. Liu, Y. Gao, L. Chen, J. Song, D. Chen, K. Gao, Y. Jiang, Y. Yang, J. Chen, et al., Matrix factorization-based prediction of novel drug indications by integrating genomic space. *Computational and Mathematical Methods in Medicine* 2015 275045 (2015).
56. M.C. Cobanoglu, C. Liu, F. Hu, Z.N. Oltvai, and I. Bahar, Predicting drug–target interactions using probabilistic matrix factorization. *Journal of Chemical Information and Modeling* 53(12), 3399–3409 (2013).
57. M. Hattori, Y. Okuno, S. Goto, and M. Kanehisa, Development of a chemical structure comparison method for integrated analysis of chemical and genomic information in the metabolic pathways. *Journal of the American Chemical Society* 125(39), 11853–11865 (2003).
58. T.F. Smith and M.S. Waterman, Identification of common molecular subsequences. *Journal of Molecular Biology* 147(1), 195–197 (1981).
59. X. Zheng, H. Ding, H. Mamitsuka, and S. Zhu, Collaborative matrix factorization with multiple similarities for predicting drug-target interactions, in *Proceedings of the 19th ACM SIGKDD International Conference on Knowledge Discovery and Data Mining*, 2013, pp. 1025–1033.
60. J.B. Tenenbaum, V.D. Silva, and J.C. Langford, A global geometric framework for nonlinear dimensionality reduction. *Science* 290(5500), 2319–2323 (2000).
61. A. Ezzat, P. Zhao, M. Wu, X.L. Li, and C.K. Kwoh, Drug-target interaction prediction with graph regularized matrix factorization. *IEEE/ACM Transactions on Computational Biology and Bioinformatics* 14(3), 646–656 (2016).
62. Y. Liu, M. Wu, C. Miao, P. Zhao, and X.L. Li, Neighborhood regularized logistic matrix factorization for drug-target interaction prediction. *PLoS Computational Biology* 12(2), e1004760 (2016).
63. Y. Luo, X. Zhao, J. Zhou, J. Yang, Y. Zhang, W. Kuang, J. Peng, L. Chen, and J. Zeng, A network integration approach for drug-target interaction prediction and computational drug repositioning from heterogeneous information. *Nature Communications* 8(1), 573 (2017).
64. H. Cho, B. Berger, and J. Peng, Diffusion component analysis: Unraveling functional topology in biological networks, in *Proceedings of the International Conference on Research in Computational Molecular Biology*. Springer, 2015, pp. 62–64.
65. Z.H. Chen, Z.H. You, Z.H. Guo, H.C. Yi, G.X. Luo, and Y.B. Wang, Prediction of drug–target interactions from multi-molecular network based on deep walk embedding model. *Frontiers in Bioengineering and Biotechnology* 8, 338 (2020).

66. B.Y. Ji, Z.H. You, H.J. Jiang, Z.H. Guo, and K. Zheng, Prediction of drug-target interactions from multi-molecular network based on line network representation method. *Journal of Translational Medicine* 18, 1–11 (2020).
67. J. Tang, M. Qu, M. Wang, M. Zhang, J. Yan, and Q. Mei, Line: Large-scale information network embedding, in *Proceedings of the 24th International Conference on World Wide Web*, 2015, pp. 1067–1077.
68. P. Xuan, Y. Zhang, H. Cui, T. Zhang, M. Guo, and T. Nakaguchi, Integrating multi-scale neighbouring topologies and cross-modal similarities for drug–protein interaction prediction. *Briefings in Bioinformatics* 22(5), bbab119 (2021).
69. Q. An and L. Yu, A heterogeneous network embedding framework for predicting similarity-based drug-target interactions. *Briefings in Bioinformatics* 22(6), bbab275 (2021).
70. J. Gilmer, S.S. Schoenholz, P.F. Riley, O. Vinyals, and G.E. Dahl, Neural message passing for quantum chemistry, in *Proceedings of the International Conference on Machine Learning (PMLR'17)*, 2017, pp. 1263–1272.
71. W. Hamilton, Z. Ying, and J. Leskovec, Inductive representation learning on large graphs. *Advances in Neural Information Processing Systems* 30 (2017).
72. F. Wan, L. Hong, A. Xiao, T. Jiang, and J. Zeng, NeoDTI: Neural integration of neighbor information from a heterogeneous network for discovering new drug–target interactions. *Bioinformatics* 35(1), 104–111 (2019).
73. M.A. Thafar, R.S. Olayan, S. Albaradei, V.B. Bajic, T. Gojobori, M. Essack, and X. Gao, DTi2Vec: Drug–target interaction prediction using network embedding and ensemble learning. *Journal of Cheminformatics* 13, 1–18 (2021).
74. S.K. Mohamed, V. Nováček, and A. Nounu, Discovering protein drug targets using knowledge graph embeddings. *Bioinformatics* 36(2), 603–610 (2020).
75. S. Wang, Z. Du, M. Ding, A. Rodriguez-Paton, and T. Song, KG-DTI: A knowledge graph based deep learning method for drug-target interaction predictions and Alzheimer's disease drug repositions. *Applied Intelligence* 52(1), 846–857 (2022).
76. D.S. Wishart, C. Knox, A.C. Guo, D. Cheng, S. Shrivastava, D. Tzur, B. Gautam, and M. Hassanali, Drugbank: A knowledgebase for drugs, drug actions and drug targets. *Nucleic Acids Research* 36(suppl 1), D901–D906 (2008).
77. B. Yang, W.T. Yih, X. He, J. Gao, and L. Deng, Embedding entities and relations for learning and inference in knowledge bases. arXiv preprint arXiv:1412.6575 (2014).
78. L. Wang, Z.H. You, X. Chen, X. Yan, G. Liu, and W. Zhang, RFDT: A rotation forest-based predictor for predicting drug-target interactions using drug structure and protein sequence information. *Current Protein and Peptide Science* 19(5), 445–454 (2018).
79. L. Wang, Z.H. You, X. Chen, S.X. Xia, F. Liu, X. Yan, Y. Zhou, and K.J. Song, A computational-based method for predicting drug–target interactions by using stacked autoencoder deep neural network. *Journal of Computational Biology* 25(3), 361–373 (2018).
80. Y.B. Wang, Z.H. You, S. Yang, H.C. Yi, Z.H. Chen, and K. Zheng, A deep learning-based method for drug-target interaction prediction based on long short-term memory neural network. *BMC Medical Informatics and Decision Making* 20, 1–9 (2020).
81. H. Zou, T. Hastie, and R. Tibshirani, Sparse principal component analysis. *Journal of Computational and Graphical Statistics* 15(2), 265–286 (2006).
82. S.H. Mahmud, W. Chen, H. Jahan, Y. Liu, N.I. Sujan, and S. Ahmed, iDTi-CSsmoteB: Identification of drug–target interaction based on drug chemical structure and protein sequence using XGBoost with over-sampling technique smote. *IEEE Access* 7, 48699–48714 (2019).

83. S.H. Mahmud, W. Chen, H. Meng, H. Jahan, Y. Liu, and S.M. Hasan, Prediction of drug-target interaction based on protein features using undersampling and feature selection techniques with boosting. *Analytical Biochemistry* 589, 113507 (2020).
84. S.H. Mahmud, W. Chen, Y. Liu, M.A. Awal, K. Ahmed, M.H. Rahman, and M.A. Moni, Predtis: Prediction of drug–target interactions based on multiple feature information using gradient boosting framework with data balancing and feature selection techniques. *Briefings in Bioinformatics* 22(5), bbab046 (2021).
85. H. Liu and R. Setiono, Incremental feature selection. *Applied Intelligence* 9, 217–230 (1998).
86. H. Khojasteh, J. Pirgazi, and A. Ghanbari Sorkhi, Improving prediction of drug-target interactions based on fusing multiple features with data balancing and feature selection techniques. *Plos One* 18(8), e0288173 (2023).
87. A. Sharma and R. Rani, BE-DTI': Ensemble framework for drug target interaction prediction using dimensionality reduction and active learning. *Computer Methods and Programs in Biomedicine* 165, 151–162 (2018).
88. D.S. Cao, N. Xiao, Q.S. Xu, and A.F. Chen, Rcpi: R/bioconductor package to generate various descriptors of proteins, compounds and their interactions. *Bioinformatics* 31(2), 279–281 (2015).
89. Z.R. Li, H.H. Lin, L. Han, L. Jiang, X. Chen, and Y.Z. Chen, Profeat: A web server for computing structural and physicochemical features of proteins and peptides from amino acid sequence. *Nucleic Acids Research* 34(suppl 2), W32–W37 (2006).
90. Y. Peng, J. Wang, Z. Wu, L. Zheng, B. Wang, G. Liu, W. Li, and Y. Tang, MPSM-DTI: Prediction of drug–target interaction via machine learning based on the chemical structure and protein sequence. *Digital Discovery* 1(2), 115–126 (2022).
91. Z. Xu, S. Wang, F. Zhu, and J. Huang, Seq2seq fingerprint: An unsupervised deep molecular embedding for drug discovery, in *Proceedings of the 8th ACM International Conference on Bioinformatics, Computational Biology, and Health Informatics*, 2017, pp. 285–294.
92. M. Tsubaki, K. Tomii, and J. Sese, Compound–protein interaction prediction with end-to-end learning of neural networks for graphs and sequences. *Bioinformatics* 35(2), 309–318 (2019).
93. H. Öztürk, A. Ozgür, P. Schwaller, T. Laino, and E. Ozkirimli, Exploring chemical space using natural language processing methodologies for drug discovery. *Drug Discovery Today* 25(4), 689–705 (2020).
94. Y.F. Zhang, X. Wang, A.C. Kaushik, Y. Chu, X. Shan, M.Z. Zhao, Q. Xu, and D.Q. Wei, SPVec: A word2vec-inspired feature representation method for drug-target interaction prediction. *Frontiers in Chemistry* 7, 895 (2020).
95. J. Zheng, X. Xiao, and W.R. Qiu, DTI-BERT: Identifying drug-target interactions in cellular networking based on BERT and deep learning method. *Frontiers in Genetics* 13, 859188 (2022).
96. K.Y. Gao, A. Fokoue, H. Luo, A. Iyengar, S. Dey, and P. Zhang, Interpretable drug target prediction using deep neural representation, in *Proceedings of the International Joint Conferences on Artificial Intelligence*, 2018, pp. 3371–3377.
97. P. Greenside, M. Hillenmeyer, and A. Kundaje, Prediction of protein-ligand interactions from paired protein sequence motifs and ligand substructures, in *Proceedings of the Pacific 27th Symposium on Biocomputing*. World Scientific, 2018, pp. 20–31.
98. H. Öztürk, E. Ozkirimli, and A. Ozgür, Widedta: Prediction of drug-target binding affinity. arXiv preprint arXiv:1902.04166 (2019).

99. K. Abbasi, P. Razzaghi, A. Poso, M. Amanlou, J.B. Ghasemi, and A. Masoudi-Nejad, DeepCDA: Deep cross-domain compound–protein affinity prediction through LSTM and convolutional neural networks. *Bioinformatics* 36 (17), 4633–4642 (2020).
100. Y. Pu, J. Li, J. Tang, and F. Guo, DeepFusionDTA: Drug-target binding affinity prediction with information fusion and hybrid deep-learning ensemble model. *IEEE/ACM Transactions on Computational Biology and Bioinformatics* 19(5), 2760–2769 (2021).
101. H. Öztürk, A. Ozgür, and E. Ozkirimli, DeepDTA: Deep drug–target binding affinity prediction. *Bioinformatics* 34(17), i821–i829 (2018).
102. Q. Zhao, F. Xiao, M. Yang, Y. Li, and J. Wang, AttentionDTA: Prediction of drug–target binding affinity using attention model, in *Proceedings of the IEEE International Conference on Bioinformatics and Biomedicine (BIBM)*, IEEE, 2019, pp. 64–69.
103. J. Shim, Z.Y. Hong, I. Sohn, and C. Hwang, Prediction of drug–target binding affinity using similarity-based convolutional neural network. *Scientific Reports* 11(1), 4416 (2021).
104. L. Zhao, J. Wang, L. Pang, Y. Liu, and J. Zhang, GANsDTA: Predicting drug-target binding affinity using GANs. *Frontiers in Genetics* 10, 1243 (2020).
105. Y. Zeng, X. Chen, Y. Luo, X. Li, and D. Peng, Deep drug-target binding affinity prediction with multiple attention blocks. *Briefings in Bioinformatics* 22(5), bbab117 (2021).
106. T. Nguyen, H. Le, T.P. Quinn, T. Nguyen, T.D. Le, and S. Venkatesh, GraphDTA: Predicting drug–target binding affinity with graph neural networks. *Bioinformatics* 37(8), 1140–1147 (2021).
107. B. Tanoori, M.Z. Jahromi, and E.G. Mansoori, Drug-target continuous binding affinity prediction using multiple sources of information. *Expert Systems with Applications* 186, 115810 (2021).
108. M.A. Thafar, M. Alshahrani, S. Albaradei, T. Gojobori, M. Essack, and X. Gao, Affinity2vec: Drug-target binding affinity prediction through representation learning, graph mining, and machine learning. *Scientific Reports* 12(1), 4751 (2022).

Chapter 15

Enhanced detection of epileptic seizure using supervised and unsupervised machine learning algorithms

Sonia Juneja

15.1 INTRODUCTION

Involuntary movements of an individual due to aberrant electrical signals in brain causes a neurological condition known as epilepsy. It is typified by frequent and spontaneous seizures World Health Organization (WHO) [1] has also raised its concern by publishing a report stating that around 1% of the world's population is suffering from epilepsy and hence it can be considered as one of the most prevalent neurological conditions. The recurrent seizures that occurs in epilepsy, vary in frequency and severity. Based on the brain area involved in abnormal activity, the seizures can be broadly categorized as focal seizures (originating in a specific region of the brain) and generalized seizures (affecting both cerebral hemispheres) [2]. The sudden occurrence of seizures has proven to be a threat to security of patient suffering from epilepsy. Early and accurate diagnosis is crucial for effective treatment and management of the condition. EEG recordings, neuroimaging data, and patient history must all be carefully examined in order to provide an accurate diagnosis of epilepsy. For management and treatment of epileptic seizures to be successful, early and precise detection is essential.

The abnormal and excessive neuronal activity in the brain may originate due to genetic factors, structural anomalies, metabolic issues, or some unidentified reasons. Typical indications that can be observed during epilepsy are seizures, altered consciousness, sensory disruptions, and involuntary muscle contractions. Treatment approaches [3] can be effectively applied only after proper classification and characterization of seizures. Machine learning (ML) has emerged as a significant asset in medical diagnostics, offering improved accuracy, speed, and efficiency in the diagnosis of epilepsy [4]. Conventional diagnosis methods primarily rely on neurologists manually interpreting EEG patterns, which is a laborious process based on individual perception of person involved. The emergence of ML has revolutionized the detection process by facilitating the automated analysis of EEG data, resulting in notable enhancements in the accuracy of seizure detection systems and improving their operational efficiency.

DOI: 10.1201/9781003634560-15

To examine the applicability of various supervised and unsupervised ML algorithms for the detection of epileptic seizures, the chapter is divided into multiple sections. Section 15.1 gives a brief introduction to the concept involved followed by the steps involved seizure diagnosis process. It also addresses the examination involved in extraction of features of EEG signals, and challenges involved. Section 15.3 briefs about the different classification methods based of ML and corresponding performance metrics required to validate the efficiency of algorithms involved. An exhaustive literature review underscores the advancements made in the subject area. Future research avenues and hybrid methodologies are discussed to present a comprehensive viewpoint.

15.2 EPILEPTIC SEIZURE DIAGNOSIS

A seizure is a brief episode of aberrant brain electrical activity that can alter awareness, movement, and behavior. A seizure has four phases namely the prodromal stage during which behavioral, emotional, or cognitive symptoms could manifest, the aural phase, which is defined by changed perceptions or feelings, the ictal phase, which is the actual seizure, and the postictal phase, which is the final stage and can linger anywhere from a few seconds to several hours or days. The four phases of a seizure are shown in Figure 15.1. Broadly seizures can be differentiated into two categories viz epileptic seizures and non-epileptic seizures. Both epileptic and non-epileptic seizures can sometimes appear similar with physical symptoms like jerking movements or loss of consciousness, but there are few key differences as listed in Table 15.1 on the basis of which one can differentiate.

The most used technique for identifying seizures is electroencephalogram (EEG) monitoring of brain activity signals. Interictal activity, or signals recorded in between epileptic seizures, and ictal activity, or abnormal activity recorded during an epileptic seizure, are the two types of activity found in the EEG recordings of patients with epileptic seizures [5]. Interictal and ictal EEG signals, with the exception of postictal states, are taken into consideration in order to concentrate on the identification of epileptic seizures. An ictal activity's EEG signature is made up of a continuous discharge of polymorphic waveforms with varying amplitude and frequency, whereas an interictal activity's signature consists of sporadic transient waveforms [6].

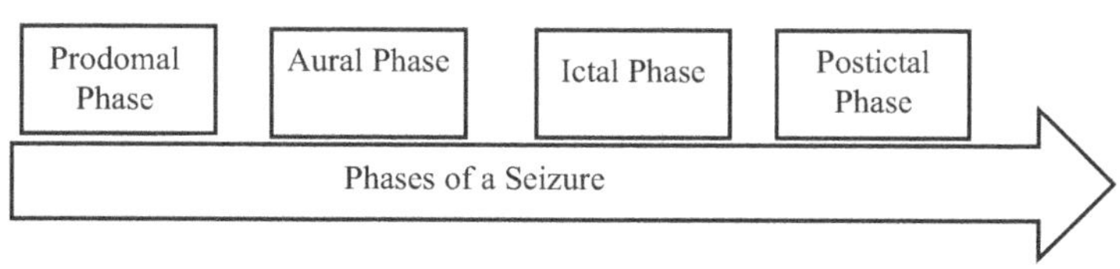

Figure 15.1 Phases of a seizure.

Table 15.1 Criteria to differentiate between epileptic seizures and non-epileptic seizures

Criteria	*Epileptic seizures*	*Non-epileptic seizures*
Cause	Epileptic seizures occurs due to abnormal electrical activity in the brain.	Non-epileptic seizures are often linked to psychological stress or trauma.
Brain activity	Abnormal electrical activity are observed in EEG.	Normal brain wave patterns are observed in EEG.
Triggering factors	Epileptic seizures can be triggered by various factors like stress, lack of sleep, flashing lights, or specific stimuli.	Non-epileptic seizures can be triggered by emotional stress, trauma, or psychological triggers.
Duration	Epileptic seizure can last for smaller duration.	Non-epileptic seizures may sometimes last longer than epileptic seizures.
Treatment	Epileptic seizures are typically treated with anti-seizure medications.	Non-epileptic seizures often require psychological therapies to address underlying emotional issues.

Traditional EEG recording methods come in two variations: scalp/no invasive EEG and invasive EEG. In order to perform surgery to implant electrodes in the brain, invasive EEG recording is required. The user must connect a number of electrodes to a monitoring equipment via numerous wires in order to perform a scalp EEG. As a result, patients must endure the discomfort of having to attach several electrodes or introduce something into their bodies. Additionally, a skilled medical professional performs the intricate setup for the scalp EEG, and studies are frequently carried out in hospitals. In addition to the conventional EEG-based method, other methods for detecting epileptic seizures include blood pressure, respiration, perspiration, heart rate, eye (lid) movement, and arterial oxygenation (SpO2) [7]. Physiology signals such as electrooculography (EOG), electrocardiography (ECG), electromyography (EMG), electrodermal activity (EDA), mobility, audio/video recording, and multimodality sensing techniques can be used to record these activities [7, 8]. The diagnosis of epilepsy involves multiple steps, including:

- **Clinical history and physical examination:** Physicians evaluate patient-reported seizure descriptions, family history, and possible triggers [9].
- **Electroencephalogram (EEG):** EEG records brain wave patterns and helps identify epileptic abnormalities. However, the interpretation of EEG signals requires expertise [10].
- **Neuroimaging:** Magnetic resonance imaging (MRI) and computed tomography (CT) scans help detect structural brain abnormalities that may contribute to epilepsy [11].
- **Laboratory tests:** Blood tests may be conducted to identify metabolic or genetic factors associated with epilepsy [12]. Despite these diagnostic tools, misdiagnosis rates remain high due to the complexity of seizure manifestations and the limitations of traditional methods [13].

15.2.1 EEG data for seizure detection

EEG is a non-invasive technique used to record electrical activity in the brain. The signals are typically represented as time-series data, characterized by amplitude fluctuations across various frequency bands. Key frequency bands include delta (0.5–4 Hz), theta (4–8 Hz), alpha (8–13 Hz), beta (13–30 Hz), and gamma (>30 Hz). EEG is a key diagnostic tool for epilepsy as it captures electrical activity in the brain using electrodes placed on the scalp. The steps involved in Seizure detection is presented in a flow diagram as shown in Figure 15.2.

Each step involved in analysis of EEG data for seizure detection typically is given below:

1. **Signal acquisition:** EEG signals are recorded from multiple electrodes over a period of time. Seizure detection requires continuous monitoring to capture abnormal brain activity [14]. Tiny excitatory post-synaptic potentials generated by pyramidal neurons in the brain's cortical layers add up to electric potential changes on the order of tens of μV that reach the scalp, which are detected by EEG. As a result, the potentials that are detected represent neural activity and can be utilized to investigate a variety of brain functions.
2. **Signal preprocessing:** Raw EEG data is often contaminated with noise, including muscle artifacts and environmental interference. Thermal noise,

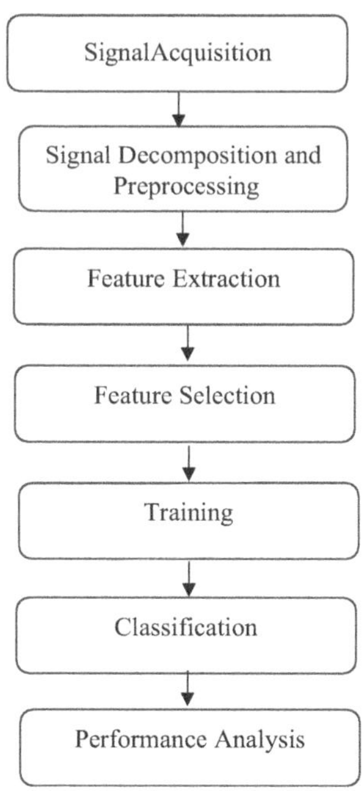

Figure 15.2 Steps in seizure detection using EEG data.

flicker noise, power line interference (PLI), and electrode offset voltage are the main types of interference that make measuring EEG difficult. The EEG is a common non-stationary time-varying signal with a micro-volt amplitude. Wavelet transform, wavelet entropy, frequency-domain and time-domain analysis, and the improved multi-scale entropy algorithm are prominent techniques for analyzing and processing EEG signals. Techniques such as bandpass filtering and independent component analysis (ICA) are applied to remove noise and enhance signal quality. Data preprocessing involves the transformation of raw data into a format that is more conducive to subsequent analysis and comprehensible for the user. The different processes involved in preprocessing are essential resulting in improved quality of EEG signals are listed below. These steps are applied prior to application of ML algorithms:

a. Filtering: Band pass filters and notch filters are applied to restrict a certain band of frequencies and allow a definite band of frequencies. The application of these filters can significantly reduce noise and interruptions.
b. Normalization: To ensure consistency among the voluminous data, it is required to standardizing the amplitudes of signals. Normalization improves the efficiency of ML model as all features contribute equally in the learning process.
c. Segmentation: As the duration of seizure is small, it is required to spilt the EEG data into small epochs. Each segment represents a distinct state of brain. It also minimizes computational demands. Techniques such as overlapping and non-overlapping windows are employed for segmentation.

3. **Feature extraction:** EEG recordings can be analyzed based on different features expressed in different domains. Each domain is used to extract a different set of features identifying specific characteristics. Time domain features are characteristics of a signal that are extracted from its time domain representation like mean, variance, and skewness. Frequency domain features like power spectral density and wavelet coefficients are extracted using frequency domain representations. Other features like entropy, fractal dimensions, and Lyapunov exponents are characterized as non-linear features.

   The extraction of EEG features is conducted using constrained independent component analysis. Techniques for feature selection, including Principal Component Analysis (PCA) and Recursive Feature Elimination (RFE), are employed to minimize dimensionality and enhance model efficacy. Significant statistical and spectral features are derived from EEG signals, encompassing wavelet coefficients, power spectral density, and entropy metrics. These features are instrumental in distinguishing between seizure and non-seizure occurrences

4. **Seizure classification:** After the preprocessing of EEG data and the extraction of significant features, the role of classifiers comes into picture.

Utilizing the identified features, the classification process differentiates between abnormal and normal brain activity. Keeping in view inherent complexity of EEG data, traditional approaches for seizure detection are less effective and involves more computational time. In contrast, ML algorithms such as support vector machines (SVM), artificial neural networks (ANN), and K Nearest Neighbors (KNN) networks present a more effective solution, enabling the classification of EEG segments as either normal or epileptic. Notably, deep learning models like CNN have shown remarkable accuracy in automated seizure detection due to their ability to process large volumes of data.

5. **Clinical validation and deployment:** AI-driven seizure detection systems [15] are validated through extensive EEG datasets and incorporated into clinical workflows to support neurologists in their decision-making processes. To evaluate the performance of classification models in seizure detection, several standard metrics as shown in Eqs. (15.1)–(15.5) are used:

$$\text{Accuracy} = \frac{\text{TP} + \text{TN}}{\text{TP} + \text{TN} + \text{FP} + \text{FN}} \tag{15.1}$$

The term accuracy can be expressed as the ratio of the number of EEG signals accurately classified to the total number of EEG signals, where TP is True Positives, TN is True Negatives, FP is False Positives, and FN is False Negatives.

$$\text{Precision} = \frac{\text{TP}}{\text{TP} + \text{FP}} \tag{15.2}$$

Precision is expressed as ratio of True Positives to the total number of actual ictal signals.

$$\text{Specificity} = \frac{\text{TN}}{\text{TP} + \text{TN}} \tag{15.3}$$

Specificity is presented as the ratio of True Negatives to the total number of actual ictal signals.

$$\text{Recall (Sensitivity)} = \frac{\text{TP}}{\text{TP} + \text{FN}} \tag{15.4}$$

Sensitivity is evaluated as the ratio of True Positives to the total number of actual ictal signals

$$\text{F1} - \text{score} = 2 * \frac{\text{Precision} * \text{Recall}}{\text{Precision} + \text{Recall}} \tag{15.5}$$

15.2.2 Challenges in EEG data analysis

- Noise and artifacts: Electroencephalogram (EEG) signals frequently suffer from interference caused by muscle activity, eye movements, and external electrical influences. To effectively manage these artifacts, it is necessary to employ sophisticated filtering and denoising methods, including Independent Component Analysis (ICA) and wavelet thresholding.
- High dimensionality: EEG data is characterized by its extensive and intricate nature, consisting of numerous channels and elevated sampling frequencies. To address the challenges posed by this complexity, dimensionality reduction methods such as Principal Component Analysis (PCA) or t-SNE are crucial.
- Inter-subject variability: The differences in seizure manifestations across individuals can hinder the applicability of ML models. To alleviate this challenge, techniques such as transfer learning and domain adaptation have been suggested.

Authors [16, 17] presented his work to review various EEG preprocessing techniques presented in the published research work so as to identify the applicability of suitable data preprocessing technique to specific application.

15.3 MACHINE LEARNING ALGORITHMS FOR EPILEPTIC SEIZURE DETECTION

15.3.1 Historical background

ML has emerge as a considerable technique for automating the detection of seizures, imparting stronger accuracy, performance, and scalability. Through ML techniques, computational models can process sizable quantities of EEG information, discern complicated patterns, and appropriately classify activities as either seizures or non-seizures [18]. The effectiveness of ML algorithms for the detection of seizures using EEG indicators is extensively influenced by the progress made in both supervised and unsupervised learning algorithms. Supervised learning procedures make use of categorized EEG datasets to develop classifiers, inclusive of support Vector Machines (SVM), synthetic Neural Networks (ANN), and Convolutional Neural Networks (CNN). Furthermore, the combination of deep learning methodologies, specifically recurrent neural networks (RNNs) and Long Short-Term memory (LSTM) networks, has significantly stepped forward the efficacy of seizure detection structures. These models are adept at capturing temporal relationships inside EEG data, rendering them mainly appropriate for the evaluation of time series data analysis [19]. Unsupervised learning based techniques, inclusive of clustering techniques and autoencoders, perceive anomalies in EEG indicators independently of pre-categorized seizure activities.

Significant advancements have been made in EEG based seizure detection; however, numerous challenging situations persist. The variability in EEG signals amongst distinct patients, the presence of noise from artifacts, and the scarcity of labeled datasets restrict the advent of incredibly dependable models. Overcoming these boundaries necessitates ongoing improvements in feature extraction strategies, version interpretability, and strategies for real-time implementation. This literature review offers an in depth examination of algorithms gaining knowledge of strategies applied in EEG-based seizure detection [20]. It delves into critical algorithms, recent tendencies, and modern-day challenges, offering treasured insights for future research perspectives. The objective is to aid researchers and clinicians in formulating extra effective, precise, and scalable answers for seizure detection.

15.3.2 Supervised machine learning approaches

Supervised learning, a class of ML, which employs labeled datasets to educate models, where the target labels are distinctly described. The model validates its knowledge by evaluating its predictions toward the actual results from the training dataset. Over time, it refines its overall performance to minimize errors and improve accuracy. The prime objective of supervised learning is to make correct predictions while confronted with new or previously unseen data, commonly known as testing data. As an instance, a model skilled to categorize certain objects will leverage its obtained understanding to properly classify new times into established classes, although they have not been encountered earlier. Supervised learning encompasses various forms, including classification, which organizes data into predefined categories, and regression, which forecasts future values, establishing it as a vital technique in artificial intelligence and supervised data mining. A supervised learning algorithm [21] can work on a dataset consisting of input features along with their corresponding target output labels. A supervised learning algorithm workflow requires:

1. Training dataset: A training dataset which include input records (capabilities) and matching output statistics (labels or goal variables) is given to the model.
2. Learning procedure: By analyzing the training dataset, the algorithm discovers the connections among the output labels and the input attributes. That is achieved by way of minimizing the discrepancy among the version's predictions and the real labels via modifying the model's parameters.
3. Testing data: To assess the accuracy and performance of trained model, testing dataset is used.
4. Optimization algorithms: After testing phase, the model's performance is enhanced with the aid of adjusting model parameters and balancing bias and variance with techniques known as optimization algorithms.

This guarantees that the model optimized performance while performing on unseen/test data. Supervised mastering has practical applications in risk assessment, image categorization, fraud detection, spam mail filtering, and many more. The following subsection describes numerous supervised learning techniques that may be used to detect epileptic seizures.

15.3.2.1 Support vector machines (SVMs)

Support Vector Machines (SVM) belongs to a class of supervised learning algorithms which are notably utilized for both classification and regression purposes. The fundamental operation in SVMs includes figuring out the optimal hyperplane that maximizes the margin among distinct classes within the feature space. This feature enables SVM to handle high-dimensional data and situations where separation is non-linear, activated through kernel features including radial basis feature (RBF) or polynomial kernels. Inside the realm modern seizure detection, SVMs have been widely employed to differentiate electroencephalogram (EEG) waveforms into seizure (ictal) and non-seizure (interictal) states. Given the inherent complexity and high of modern EEG records, SVMs are the best choice of researchers keeping in mind performance in processing complex information. The implementation involves preprocessing the EEG signals to extract dominant features (e.g., time-domain, frequency-domain, or wavelet-based features), followed by training the SVM model through labeled data. Once trained, the model is capable of be classifying new EEG recordings into seizure or non-seizure categories.

Several research have illustrated the efficacy of Support Vector Machines (SVMs) to detect seizures. As an instance, Tzallas et al. [22] utilized SVMs time-frequency evaluation with non-linear characteristic extraction, achieving an accuracy exceeding 90% on benchmark datasets in classifying epileptic EEG data. Relatively, Sharma et al. [23] applied SVMs version to utilize wavelet-based features for the automated detection of seizures and its applicability in real time scenarios. Zhang et al. [24] confirmed the applicability of SVMs to accurately classify EEG signals as either seizure or non-seizure, emphasizing the critical role of feature selection in enhancing model performance.

15.3.2.2 Artificial neural networks

The primary and most versatile type of neural network is an artificial neural network (ANN). It consists of an output layer, an input layer, and one or more hidden layers. Every node in one layer has a weight for every node in the subsequent layer since each layer is fully connected to the one before it. One particular kind of neural network that is intended for processing images or other spatial data is the convolutional neural network (CNN). It contains one or more convolutional layers that extract features or patterns from the input data by applying filters or kernels. A feature map or activation map is created as the filters move over the input data. Convolutional neural networks (CNNs), are increasingly used in seizure detection by analyzing electroencephalogram (EEG) signals, allowing for automated identification of seizure patterns within brain activity data, which can be significantly more accurate and efficient than traditional manual analysis by clinicians; essentially, the neural network "learns" to recognize the distinct electrical patterns associated with a seizure from the EEG data, enabling real-time detection and potential interventions. Shoebi and Guttag [25] pioneered the use of deep learning for seizure detection, employing Convolutional Neural Networks (CNNs) to automatically extract features from EEG data. Their work laid the foundation for modern deep learning applications in this field.

15.3.2.3 Ensemble techniques

In ML, ensemble methods are strategies that integrate several models to increase overall robustness, accuracy, and performance. Ensemble approaches improve generalization on unseen data by utilizing the strengths of multiple models rather than depending on a single model. Common ensemble techniques include:

1. Bagging (bootstrap aggregating): Trains multiple models independently on different subsets of the data (sampled with replacement) and averages their predictions. Example: Random Forests.
2. Boosting: Sequentially trains models, where each subsequent model focuses on correcting the errors of the previous one. Examples: AdaBoost, Gradient Boosting, and XGBoost.
3. Stacking: Combines predictions from multiple models using a meta-model (e.g., a linear regression or neural network) to produce the final output.
4. Voting: Aggregates predictions from multiple models through majority voting (for classification) or averaging (for regression).

Ensemble methods are widely used because they reduce overfitting, handle complex datasets effectively, and often achieve state-of-the-art performance in competitions and real-world applications. Brophy et al. [26] explored the use of Random Forests and Gradient Boosting Machines for seizure classification. Their findings underscored the importance of ensemble learning in handling imbalanced datasets.

15.3.3 Unsupervised ultra-modern strategies

By using clustering, dimensionality reduction, and anomaly detection to recognize seizure patterns on its own, unsupervised ML presents a viable substitute that eliminates the requirement for human annotations and deals with the intrinsic complexity of EEG signals. Different strategies have evolved in this emerging discipline, ranging from sophisticated deep learning mechanisms to traditional clustering techniques. Unsupervised learning deals with unlabeled data, with an aim to identify hidden patterns or anomalies. The training model has only input parameter values and evolves the similar clusters/groups or patterns on its own. The target data is unlabeled. The task can be a challenging one, but it can also be very rewarding, as it can reveal undiscovered insights into the data that would not be predicted from a labeled dataset. In seizure detection, unsupervised methods are particularly valuable due to the scarcity of labeled seizure data. Different unsupervised algorithms used for seizure detection are elaborated in following subsections.

15.3.3.1 Clustering techniques

Clustering methodologies, including K-means, hierarchical clustering, and DBSCAN (Density Based Spatial Clustering of Applications with Noise), allows the grouping of similar EEG patterns without the requirement of predefined labels. These techniques are judgmental in differentiating seizure patterns from typical brain activity by identifying anomalies in EEG signal patterns. Research conducted by Charupanit et al. [27] implemented hierarchical clustering to examine high frequency oscillations present in EEG signals to notify the occurrence of seizure and hence its detection. These approaches are especially effective in identifying rare or novel seizure patterns within extensive datasets. Variants like fuzzy c-means clustering have also been investigated for enhanced adaptability. Alotaiby et al. [28] implemented K-means clustering to differentiate EEG data into seizure and non-seizure events, showcasing the efficacy of unsupervised techniques in contexts with limited labeled data. Furthermore, Hunyadi et al. [29] introduced a hierarchical clustering framework that yielded encouraging outcomes in the detection of rare seizure patterns.

15.3.3.2 Auto encoder based methods

More recent studies are focused on advancements in deep learning to improve the robustness of unsupervised algorithms. Autoencoder-based methods have been particularly influential, offering powerful tools for feature extraction and anomaly detection. AE is an unsupervised ML model for which the input is the same as output. Input is compressed to a latent-space representation, and then the output is obtained from the representation. Therefore, in AE, the compression and decompression functions are coupled with the neural network. AE consists of three parts, i.e., encoder, code, and decoder. AE networks are most commonly used for feature extraction or dimensionality reduction in the brain signal processing. As the first research in this section, Rajaguru et al. [30] separately surveyed the multilayer AE (MAE) and expectation-maximization with principal component analysis (EMPCA) methods to diminish the representation dimensions and then employed the GA for classification. They obtained an average classification accuracy of 93.78% when MAEs were applied for dimensionality reduction and combined with GA as classifier. In another work, it was proposed to design an automated system based on AEs for the diagnosis of epilepsy using the EEG signals [31]. Chandola et al. [32] provided a comprehensive review of anomaly detection techniques, emphasizing their applicability to EEG data for identifying outliers indicative of seizures. Taken together, these studies highlight the diverse landscape of unsupervised ML in EEG-based seizure detection. While classical clustering remains a viable approach for simpler applications, the integration of deep learning, as evidenced by autoencoders, VAEs, and transformers, represents a pivotal advancement toward scalable and more accurate seizure detection models. These emerging methods hold potential for alleviating clinical burdens, yet further research is needed to standardize evaluation protocols, ensure cross-dataset generalizability, and enhance real-world clinical adoption.

15.3.4 Comparative analyses and key findings

Supervised and unsupervised ML algorithms have proven to be a verified set of methodologies as far as seizure detection is concerned. Within the context related to seizure detection, both supervised and unsupervised ML algorithms offer advantages and demanding situations too. However, it has been observed through available literature that supervised algorithms usually achieves superior accuracy in comparison to unsupervised strategies. Unsupervised approaches offer superior flexibility and robustness while dealing with unlabeled datasets. Supervised approaches, in particular deep learning frameworks such as Convolutional Neural Networks (CNNs) and Long Short Term Memory networks (LSTMs), have a tendency to generate higher accuracy because of their ability to learn from classified datasets. Nonetheless, their effectiveness is significantly encouraged via the availability of labeled electroencephalogram (EEG) data. Conversely, unsupervised strategies, which includes clustering and autoencoders, are useful in scenarios in which classified statistics is restrained, although they'll exhibit decreased accuracy in figuring out seizure events. Supervised models may suffer from the issue of overfitting when trained on small datasets, while unsupervised models can produce effective generalization across various EEG datasets by identifying intrinsic patterns rather than relying on specific predefined labels. Additionally, deep learning-based supervised models necessitate substantial computational resources for training, whereas unsupervised models [33], particularly those based on clustering, are less computationally demanding and more appropriate for real-time applications. Deep learning based neural networks utilized in supervised learning are often regarded as "black-box" models. Techniques such as Principal Component Analysis (PCA) and Independent Component Analysis (ICA)

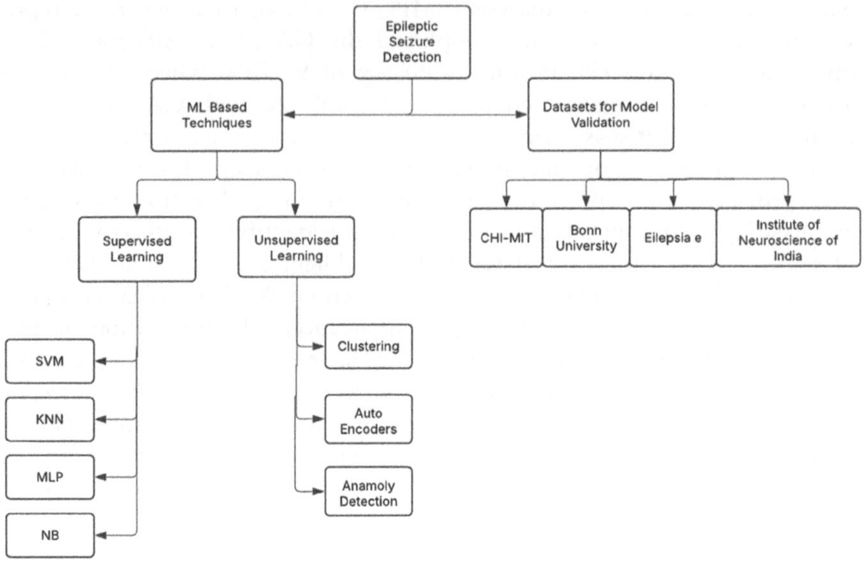

Figure 15.3 Taxonomy of epileptic seizure detection system.

in the unsupervised category provide improved interpretability by emphasizing critical features of seizure-related EEG activity, thus offering valuable clinical insights. The emerging contemporary hybrid procedures, which combine the strengths of both supervised and unsupervised paradigms, gives a promising field for researchers to work upon. It is important to mention that unsupervised methods necessitate meticulous hyperparameter tuning and can be sensitive to additive noise. Future investigations are in process to combine unsupervised approach with domain knowledge to strengthen robustness and interpretability. The general findings have been summarized in a block diagram as shown in Figure 15.3.

15.4 FUTURE RESEARCH DIRECTIONS

15.4.1 Challenges and Gaps

The main disparity that has been observed is that methods that are primarily employed for the detection of seizures in generalized epilepsy can be applied exclusively to petit mal epilepsy. As per the available literature, there is little information available on the identification of petit mal epilepsy also known as absence seizures. Absence seizures often exhibit a spike-wave discharge pattern of 3 Hz per second and are commonly undetected in children due to their brief duration, typically lasting 30 seconds. There hasn't been a lot of research on ML methods used just to identify absence seizures [34].

The creation of a gadget that is easy to use at home and less frightening than an electroencephalogram could present a significant potential. Normally, children with absence seizures show mild signs or symptoms of absence or abnormal behavior, such as staring blankly at the wall or not understanding a word someone says. A device should be made after testing the algorithms for the detection process with less chance of false positives so that the absence seizures can be detected and monitored at home by parents or guardians.

15.4.2 Explainability and interpretability

As ML models become increasingly complex, ensuring their interpretability is crucial for gaining trust in clinical applications. Techniques such as SHAP and LIME can provide insights into model decision-making processes. Future efforts should focus on developing domain-specific explainability frameworks tailored to seizure detection.

15.4.3 Integration with neuromorphic computing

Emerging technologies, such as neuromorphic chips, hold promise for real-time seizure detection with low power consumption. Research should focus on adapting ML algorithms to these platforms. This includes exploring spiking neural networks (SNNs) and edge-computing frameworks.

REFERENCES

1. World Health Organization (2023). *Epilepsy: Key facts*. World Health Organization.
2. Fisher, R.S., et al. (2017). "Operational classification of seizure types by the International League against Epilepsy." *Epilepsia* 58(4): 522–530.
3. Shinnar, S., et al. (2000). "Treatment of newly diagnosed pediatric epilepsy: A community-based study." *JAMA Pediatrics* 153(12): 1267–1271.
4. Rasheed, K., et al. (2020). "Machine learning for predicting epileptic seizures using EEG signals: A review." *IEEE Reviews in Biomedical Engineering* 14: 139–155.
5. Tzallas A.T., et al. (2012). "Automated epileptic seizure detection methods: A review study." In *Epilepsy-Histological, Electroencephalographic and Psychological Aspects*, edited by Dejan Stevanovic. InTech, pp. 75–98. doi:10.5772/31597
6. McGrogan, N. (1999). *Neural Network Detection of Epileptic Seizures in the Electroencephalogra*. Department of Engineering Science Probationary Research Transfer Report, Oxford University.
7. Van de Vel, A., et al. (2016). "Non-EEG seizure detection systems and potential SUDEP prevention: State of the art: Review and update." *Seizure* 41: 141–153. doi:10.1016/j.seizure.2016.07.012
8. Ramgopal, S., et al. (2014). "Seizure detection, seizure prediction, and closed-loop warning systems in epilepsy." *Epilepsy & Behavior* 37: 291–307. doi:10.1016/j.yebeh.2014.06.023

9. Engel, J. *Seizures and Epilepsy*. Oxford University Press, 2013.
10. Gloss, D., et al. (2014). "The role of high-frequency oscillations in epilepsy surgery planning." *Cochrane Database of Systematic Reviews*. doi:10.1002/14651858.CD010235.pub2
11. Bernasconi, A., et al. (2011). "Advances in MRI for 'cryptogenic' epilepsies." *Nature Reviews Neurology* 7: 99–108.
12. Scheffer, I.E., et al. (2017). "ILAE classification of the epilepsies: Position paper of the ILAE Commission for Classification and Terminology." *Epilepsia* 58(4): 512–521.
13. Beniczky, S., et al. (2021). "Automated seizure detection using wearable devices." *Epilepsia* 62(3): 632–646.
14. Acharya, U.R., et al. (2018). "Deep convolutional neural network for automated detection of epileptic EEG signals." *IEEE Transactions on Neural Systems* 100: 270–278.
15. Salim, S., et al. (2019). "A review of machine learning approaches for epileptic seizure prediction review on preprocessing of EEG signal" In *14th International Conference on Computer Engineering and Systems (ICCES)*, Cairo, Egypt, pp. 239–244. doi:10.1109/ICCES48960.2019.9068190
16. Truong, N.D., et al. (2018). "Convolutional neural networks for seizure prediction using intracranial and scalp EEG." *NeuroImage*. 105: 104–111.
17. Craik, A., et al. (2019). "Deep learning for electroencephalogram (EEG) classification tasks: a review." *Journal of Neural Engineering* 16(3). doi:10.1088/1741-2552/ab0ab5
18. Suveetha Dhanaselvam, P., & Nadia Chellam, C. (2023). "A review on preprocessing of EEG signal." In *Proceedings of the International Conference on Bio Signals, Images, and Instrumentation (ICBSII)*, Chennai, India, pp. 1–7. doi:10.1109/ICBSII58188.2023.10181071
19. Kiral-Kornek, I., et al. (2018 January). "Epileptic seizure prediction using big data and deep learning: Toward a mobile system." *EBioMedicine* 27: 103–111. doi:10.1016/j.ebiom.2017.11.032. PMID: 29262989; PMCID: PMC5828366.
20. Adeli, H., & Ghosh-Dastidar, S. (2010). *Automated EEG-Based Diagnosis of Neurological Disorders: Inventing the Future of Neurology* (1st ed.). CRC Press. doi:10.1201/9781439815328
21. Yuan, Y., et al. (2019). "A Multi-View Deep Learning Framework for EEG Seizure Detection." *IEEE Journal of Biomedical and Health Informatics*, 23(1): 83–94
22. Tzallas, A.T., Tsipouras, M.G., & Fotiadis, D.I. (2009). "Epileptic seizure detection in EEGs using time-frequency analysis." *IEEE Transactions on Information Technology in Biomedicine* 13(5): 703–710.
23. Sharma, R., Pachori, R.B., & Acharya, U.R. (2017). "An integrated index for the identification of focal electroencephalogram signals using discrete wavelet transform and entropy measures." *Entropy* 19(8): 380.
24. Zhang, Z., Parhi, K.K., & Netoff, T.I. (2013). "Discrimination of seizure and non-seizure EEG signals using SVMs." *IEEE Transactions on Biomedical Engineering* 60(4): 1063–1070.
25. Shoebi, A.H., & Guttag, J.V. (2009). "Application of machine learning to epileptic seizure detection." In *Proceedings of the ACM Conference on Bioinformatics, Computational Biology, and Health Informatics*, pp. 527–534.
26. Brophy, E., Reilly, R.B., & Lalor, E.C. (2017). "Exploring ensemble machine learning techniques for EEG classification in epilepsy." *IEEE Transactions on Neural Systems and Rehabilitation Engineering* 25(7): 1018–1025.
27. Charupanit, K., et al. (2018). "Automated detection of high frequency oscillations in human scalp electroencephalogram." In *Proceedings of the 40th Annual International Conference of the IEEE Engineering in Medicine and Biology Society (EMBC)*, Honolulu, HI, pp. 3116–3119, doi:10.1109/EMBC.2018.8513033

28. Alotaiby, T.N., Alshebeili, S.A., Alshawi, T., Ahmad, I., & Abd El-Samie, F.E. (2014). "Eeg seizure detection and prediction algorithms: A survey." *EURASIP Journal on Advances in Signal Processing* 2014: 1–21.
29. Hunyadi, B., Tousseyn, S., Dupont, P., Huffel, S., Paesschen, W., & de Vos, M. (2014). "Automatic selection of epileptic independent fMRI components." In *Proceedings of the 36th Annual International Conference of the IEEE Engineering in Medicine and Biology Society (EMBC'14)*. doi:10.1109/EMBC.2014.6944464
30. Rajaguru, H., & Prabhakar, S.K. (2018). "Multilayer autoencoders and EM-PCA with genetic algorithm for epilepsy classification from EEG." In *Proceedings of the 2018 Second International Conference on Electronics, Communication and Aerospace Technology (ICECA)*, Coimbatore, India. New York: Institute of Electrical and Electronics Engineers (IEEE), pp. 353–358.
31. Sharathappriyaa, V., Gautham, S., & Lavanya, R. (2018). "Auto-encoder based automated epilepsy diagnosis." In *Proceedings of the International Conference on Advances in Computing, Communications and Informatics (ICACCI)*, Bangalore, India. New York: Institute of Electrical and Electronics Engineers (IEEE), pp. 976–982.
32. Chandola, V., Banerjee, A., & Kumar, V. (2009). "Anomaly detection: A survey." *ACM Computing Surveys* 41(3): 58p., Article 15. doi:10.1145/1541880.1541882
33. Tsiouris, K.M., et al. (2018). "Unsupervised detection of epileptic seizures from EEG signals: A channel-specific analysis of long-term recordings." In *Proceedings of the IEEE EMBS International Conference on Biomedical & Health Informatics*, pp. 92–95. doi:10.1109/BHI.2018.8333377
34. Moeller, F., LeVan, P., Muhle, H., Stephani, U., Dubeau, F., Siniatchkin, M., & Gotman, J. (2010). "Absence seizures: Individual patterns revealed by EEG-fMRI." *Epilepsia* 51: 2000–2010.

Chapter 16

Network setup model over a private blockchain network dealing with security issues

Priyanka Tyagi, Mohit Mittal, Latha Banda, and Ashwani Kumar

16.1 INTRODUCTION

Over the last few years, blockchain technology has gained popularity and is frequently linked to developments in distributed networks [1]. Satoshi Nakamoto, the creator of the open-source P2P digital currency system Bitcoin, is behind this amazing technology [2]. Haber and Stornetta [3] created the concept of digital time-stamping electronic documents. After that, the time-stamped documents are kept in a decentralised network integrated with Proof-of-Work (PoW) [4, 5], starting the Nakamoto consensus process. Collaboration Blockchain algorithms have extensive applications, particularly in identity management. Creating and maintaining digital identities have become popular as most people live online. Anyone can distinguish between various entities and digitally confirm their identity using digital identification. The majority of the data in identity management systems today is controlled by a central authority, which gives them access to and control over all data. It leads to serious security problems, concerns about confidentiality, and the ease with which black hat hackers can deploy honeypots. Incidents like the Equifax attack [6] are an excellent example of the fact that the identities owned by the central system are not always safe and secure. The Self-Sovereign-Identity (SSI) model helps establish trust, a significant issue with most identity management systems. The user has total control over their data due to SSI, including portability, access, and control, as shown in Figure 16.1. Through the use of a cryptographic public key, users can safeguard the secrecy of their data using the key exchange mechanism, as employed by SSI [7]. Considering mobile devices are an integral part of everyone's life, SSI users may manage their digital data on any cloud-based platform and their phones.

The scenario shows how our system would work and outperform existing systems.

 DOI: 10.1201/9781003634560-16

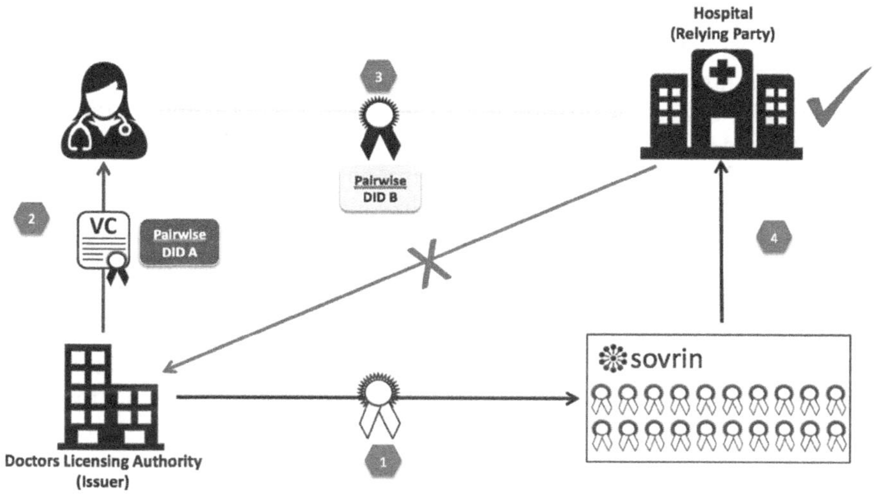

Figure 16.1 Self-sovereign identity.

16.2 EXISTING WORK

Al-Bassam [8] is the man behind the SCPKI framework, a system with foundations of Ethereum and IPFS (InterPlanetary File System), which supplies it with identity management capabilities. Unlike our system implementation, which depends on Hyperledger Indy, it does not look after crucial management functions and critical recovery. Also [8], the storage management of PII users on the Ethereum and IPFS networks is led by this. It is particularly suited for public claims such as organisational certification, which has trouble with personal identity management. Faísca and Rogado [9] developed a system on the Namecoin blockchain [10], which uses WebID [11] and IPFS as well. It is a decentralised model to control and authenticate identity. The blockchain was used to manage public keys and store them in the profile address of the WebID. Each WebID address is mapped to a WebID profile data stored on IFPS. In order to create an identity management system, our implementation system depends on DID and authorised distributed ledger. OpenBadges [12], Civic [13] and UPort [14] are some of the eminent projects. OpenBadges manages and verifies digital badges that may be achievements or qualifications. The badges are stored in JSON-LD, having specific components like attributes, which are later used to verify the user making claims. Unlike our implementation, OpenBadges uses distributed ledgers to store identifier attributes, mainly focussing on managing tokens.

Blockcert is an open standard for blockchain credentials based on SSI implementation. It uses the Bitcoin public blockchain to carry out the verification process of documents such as official documents and certifications provided by any organisation, and our system is designed to distribute it for the management of identities, thereby following consensus. Also, it includes eminent features like zero-knowledge proof. ShoCard is an organisation that developed a system to provide verifiable credentials by mapping its cryptographic credentials with the users' fingerprints. It is accomplished on the Bitcoin blockchain. Users can use their app on their mobile devices to provide their identities for verification at places like airports. UPort is a way for users to register their identity on the Ethereum blockchain. It uses the SSI framework to map public keys and store them on a decentralised system like IPFS. It provides methods to assign unique IDs to its users, who can share specific parts of their identity like that in Indy. It is possible to write intelligent contracts on uPort since it is deployed on the Ethereum blockchain. Civic is an identity management service system on the Ethereum blockchain with an incentive mechanism. Civic is used to create, consume and verify the users' identities. The Civic ecosystem comprises the Civic servers and its app. Unlike the Indy system, this is not an open-source initiative.

All these platforms could be used depending on their nature and the services they provide. However, Hyperledger Indy is an open-source project used to build identity management systems, and it also supports verifiable credentials, DID, and anonymous credentials. Indy was the best choice for our implementation.

16.3 WORKING MODEL

The working model comprises three main parts:

1. Blockchain nodes development
2. Hyperledger network setup
3. DApp development

PHASE I: BLOCKCHAIN NODES DEVELOPMENT

In the first part, we will set up Blockchain nodes on any cloud platform and use Google Cloud Platform virtual machines. We have created five nodes and established a consensus mechanism amongst them. Four nodes manage the transactions and decentralised identity stored in them in the form of metadata; hence, we have named them indy nodes, while the last node manages the rights to read and write to the ledger of all the other nodes, named indy explorer.

PHASE 2: HYPERLEDGER NETWORK SETUP

In this step, we have set up Hyperledger Indy by installing several packages onto the virtual machine nodes we created in the first phase. Hyperledger Indy is a decentralised identity manager that manages and stores the identity in a distributed ledger. This ledger is set up by installing all the relevant packages and establishing a TLS and consensus mechanism amongst all the nodes so that they can interact with each other in a secure manner governed by cryptographical means. Setting up Indy on Indy nodes and Ursa and Aries on Explorer nodes is challenging since every package has to be installed and initiated sequentially or adequately, which would result in hours of debugging.

Finally, there would be wallet creation at these nodes, with access to members such as Issuer, Holder, and Inspector provided by the Indy network. The fundamental architectural analysis of Indy, Aries and Ursa is depicted in Figures 16.1 and 16.2.

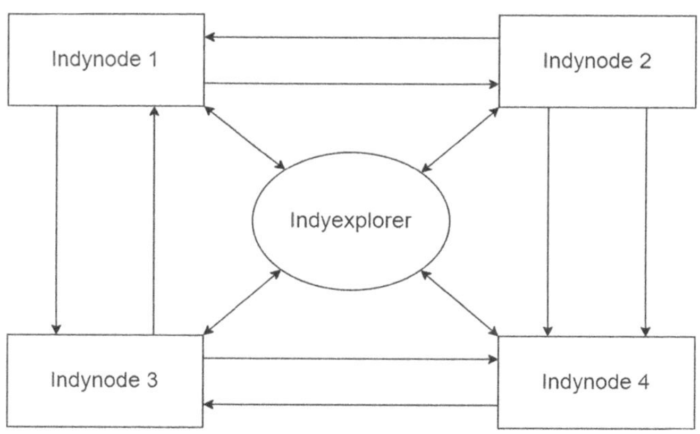

Figure 16.2 Node setup flow.

PHASE 3: DAPP DEVELOPMENT

The last stage of the development phase is to build a VON network to display the running status of the nodes and metadata in Figure 16.3. The network is containerised via docker and deployed on the port for live access to all the users or viewers.

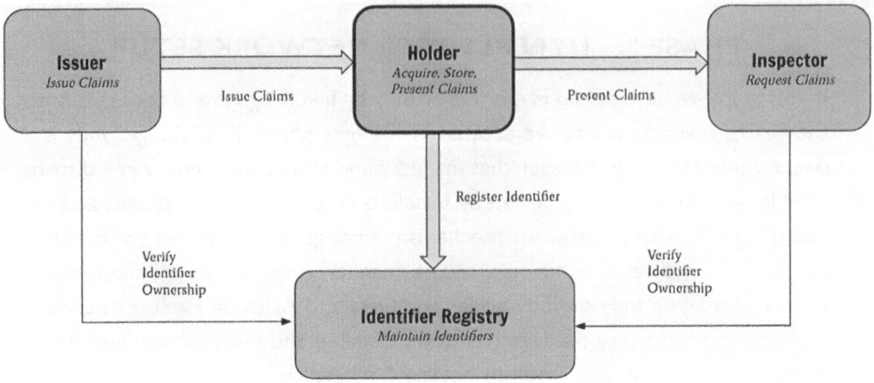

Figure 16.3 Basic work-flow.

16.3.1 Network model architecture

The SSI architecture is based upon Distributed Ledger Technology (DLT), making the system independent from control over the ledger by a single authority. Public blockchains allow any entity to access data but not alter them due to the immutability of blockchain [15]. In a private blockchain, access to this ledger lies only with competent parties with authorisation, and this copy of the ledger is hosted by the entities, thereby establishing complete trust.

All the pre-existing identity management systems are based on the architecture in which the service provider was at the centre, making it user-centric (Figure 16.4).

Figure 16.5 shows the interactivity between different actors of the system. The claim issuer is liable for issuing the identity proof by mentioning definite features of the identity holder. This issued identity provided to the user could be verified via any relying party that needs to verify the user employing documents issued by the issuing authority with details pertinent to the user. The relying party must have some trust in the claim issuer to verify or trust the documents issued by it. The architecture based on the distributed ledger. Here, blockchain technology is the substitute for the registration department in the central identity system [16]. This task performed by the blockchain (identifier registry) is associated with the pairing of both identification and authentication of the utiliser. The verifiable claims and the identifiers are maintained by the user directly. Asymmetric cryptography maps the identifier to a specific user by an authentication mechanism. By coupling the public key with the identifier on the distributed ledger, it would be accessible to anyone on the network. The authentic identity is stored in the database, usually not on the blockchain network (IPFS), which is also decentralised in functioning and controlled by the user. It is done to ensure data privacy. The relying party or the claim verifier can differentiate between the available and

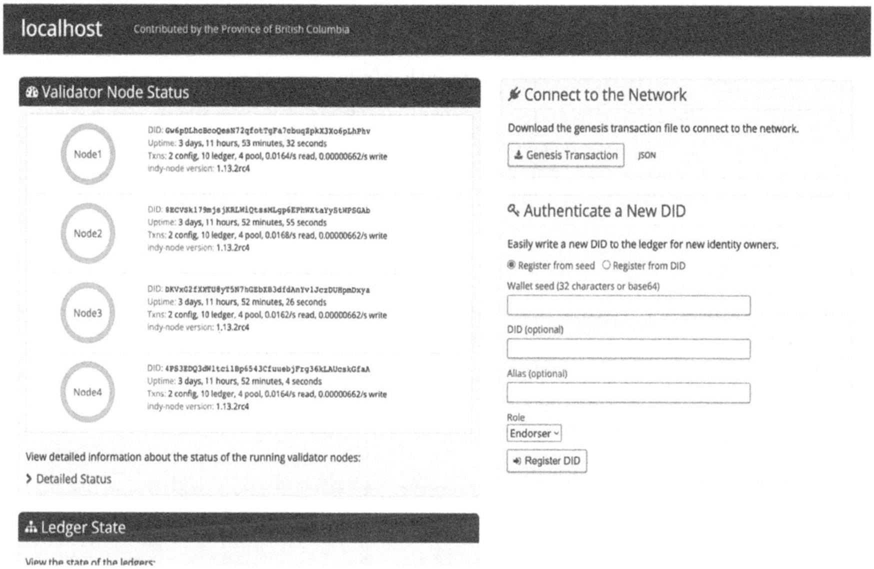

Figure 16.4 VON network.

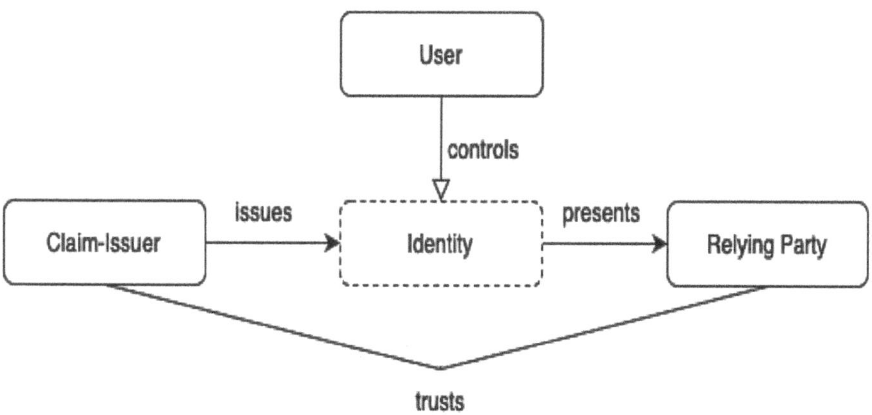

Figure 16.5 Self sovereign identity actors.

claim identifiers. After validating the user with an authentication method, the claim could be verified and accepted or rejected based on verification (Figure 16.6).

The Hyperledger Consortium [17] is a comprehensive plan governed by the Linux Foundation. Hyperledger-Fabric [17, 18], Hyperledger Ursa [17, 19], Hyperledger-Aries [17], and Hyperledger-Indy are some of the distributed ledgers technologies (DLT) that are incorporated in this hyperledger. Hyperledger Indy is a distributed open-source ledger [20]. Since it is a

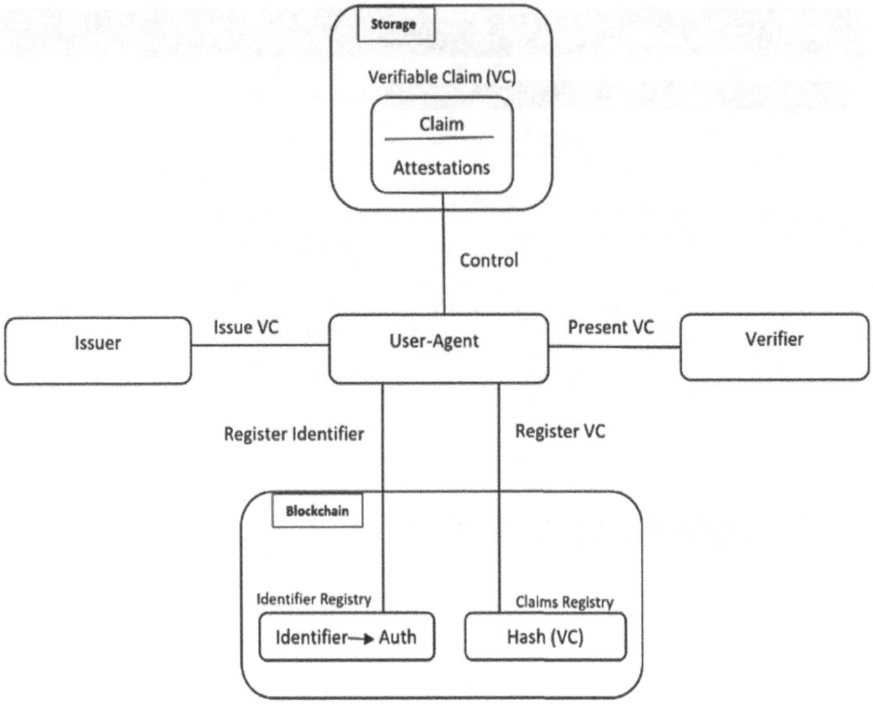

Figure 16.6 Self-sovereign identity architecture.

permission-natured DLT, it was used for decentralised identity. Indy is a specimen of the project by the Sovrin Foundation; therefore, it governs and manages it. Hyperledger Indy is associated with many technologies that are as follows.

DID is an identifier unique all over the globe and similar to a universally unique identifier (UUID). It makes it redundant for any centralised authority to change the ledger, such as updating, registering, or revoking the identifiers. Each DID is associated with a public and private key, where the private key is used for document creation, and the public key is used for verifying the signature.

Sample DID Document

```
{
  "@context": "https://w3id.org/did/v1",
  "id": "did:example:123456789abcdefghi",
  "authentication": [{
   //authentication of did:...
   "id": "did:example:123456789abcdefghi#keys-1",
   "type": "RsaVerificationKey2018",
   "controller": "did:example:123456789abcdefghi",
```

```
    "publicKeyPem": "———BEGIN PUBLIC KEY...END PUBLIC
    KEY———\r\n"
  }],
  "Service": [{
    // returns Verifiable Credentials accompanied with the DID
    "type": "VerifiableCredentialService",
    "service endpoint": "https://example.com/vc/"
  }]}
```

W3C developed Verifiable Credentials. A verifiable credential depicts the physical credential combined with a cryptographical digital signature, making it resilient to alteration. The owner of the credentials can foster and dispense documents to the verifiers for verification via digital means. It establishes their ownership. It is a part of Zero Knowledge Proof (ZKP) [21]. These credentials let the holder verify it is the claim with the verifier. It lets the holder present only a particular claim that needs to be verified, allowing the user's or holder's privacy to be maintained. Some of the implementations of ZKP are U-Prove by Microsoft [22] and Identity Mixer (Idemix) by IBM[22].

The essential components of the indy architecture are *agents*, *wallets*, and *validator nodes* [23]. The validator nodes are connected under the enforcement of consensus protocol and Redundant Byzantine Fault Tolerance (RBFT) [24]. The indy nodes represent the validator nodes. Indy nodes represent validator nodes. The Indy Explorer functions as the agent; it uses their combined possession of wallets and transactions to write or access data. The indy nodes run the Plenum consensus algorithm [25].

16.4 NETWORK MODEL TESTING

This type of testing usually involves the presence of hardware and software that performs the system's performance [26]. This testing involves sending requests to the nodes, increasing the network load and rating the performance based on observation. The client uses mechanisms to increase the workload on the Hyperledger Blockchain system. Some examples of clients are intelligent contracts, anchor peers, endorsers, orderers, state databases, etc. This client increases the system load by initiating the transactions to the endorsing peers through automated scripting (Figure 16.7).

An interface between them allows the client and SUT to test the network's performance under load. The observer node is a type of client which records and manages the status of the onboarded transaction again with the help of an automated script. These observer nodes are mostly generally more than one. The SUT kind of system does not need any APIs or interfaces to read from the nodes of the developed system. Since the nodes are independent devices running and communicating with each other, the load is distributed, which is called sharding.

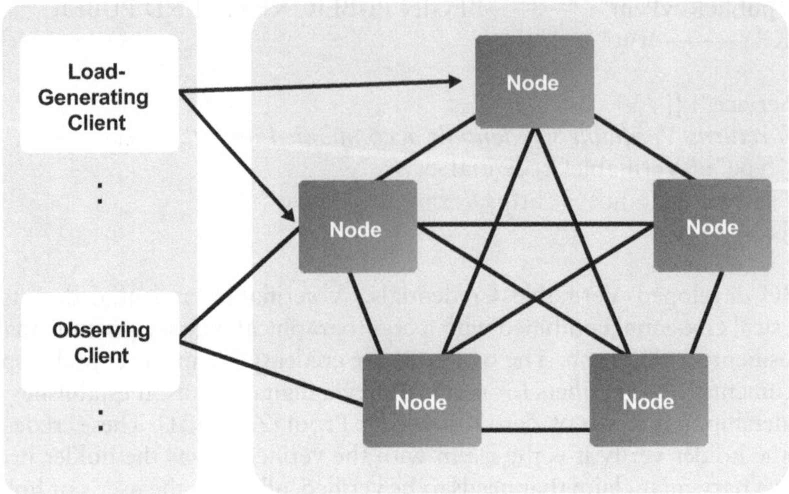

Figure 16.7 Configuration for blockchain performance evaluation.

16.4.1 Test cases

Test case ID	4.1
Test case name	Valid VM Setup
Test case description	The test case is to verify the functionality of the VM
Steps	1. Open the GCP to navigate to VM Instances. 2. Check whether it is running or not.
Expected results	1. The page should be displayed running. 2. The IP addresses of the nodes should be static; otherwise, when they are stopped, the consensus will break.
Actual results	As expected

Test case ID	4.2
Test case name	Performance Test
Test case description	This test is to verify the performance of the nodes of Hyperledger
Steps	The client uses okmechanisms to increase the workload on the Hyperledger Blockchain system. Some examples of clients are intelligent contracts, anchor peers, endorsers, orderers, state databases, etc.
Expected results	The node should be able to process the scan and display the results in a reasonable amount of time.
Actual results	As expected

16.5 RESULT LAYOUT OF SYSTEM

In the first part, we will set up Blockchain nodes on any cloud platform. Here, we used Google Cloud Platform virtual machines. We have created five nodes and established a consensus mechanism amongst them. Four nodes manage the transactions and decentralised identity stored in them in the form of metadata; hence, we have named them indy nodes, while the last node manages the rights to read and write to the ledger of all the other nodes, hence named indy explorer.

In this step (Figure 16.8), we have set up Hyperledger Indy by installing several packages onto the virtual machine nodes we created in the first phase. Hyperledger Indy is a decentralised identity manager that manages and stores the identity in a distributed ledger [27]. This ledger is set up by installing all the relevant packages and establishing a TLS and consensus mechanism amongst all the nodes so that they can interact with each other in a secure manner governed by cryptographical means. Setting up Indy on Indy nodes and Ursa and Aries on Explorer nodes is challenging since every package has to be installed and initiated sequentially or adequately, which would result in hours of debugging. Finally, there would be wallet creation at these nodes, with access to members such as Issuer, Holder, and Inspector provided by the Indy network (Figures 16.9 and 16.10).

The last stage of the development phase is to build a VON network to display the running status of the nodes and metadata. The network is containerised via docker and deployed on the port for live access to all the

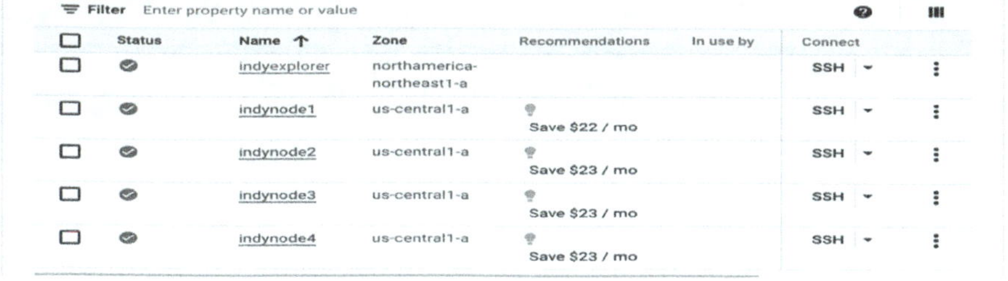
VM instances
CREATE INSTANCE
IMPORT VM
REFRESH
OPERATIONS
INSTANCES
INSTANCE SCHEDULES
4 instances could be resized to save you up to an estimated $91 per month. Learn more
DISMISS ALL
VM instances are highly configurable virtual machines for running workloads on Google infrastructure. Learn more
Filter Enter property name or value
Status
Name
Zone
Recommendations
In use by
Connect
indyexplorer
northamerica-northeast1-a
SSH
indynode1
us-central1-a
Save $22 / mo
SSH
indynode2
us-central1-a
Save $23 / mo
SSH
indynode3
us-central1-a
Save $23 / mo
SSH
indynode4
us-central1-a
Save $23 / mo
SSH

Figure 16.8 VM instances implemented and running live on GCP.

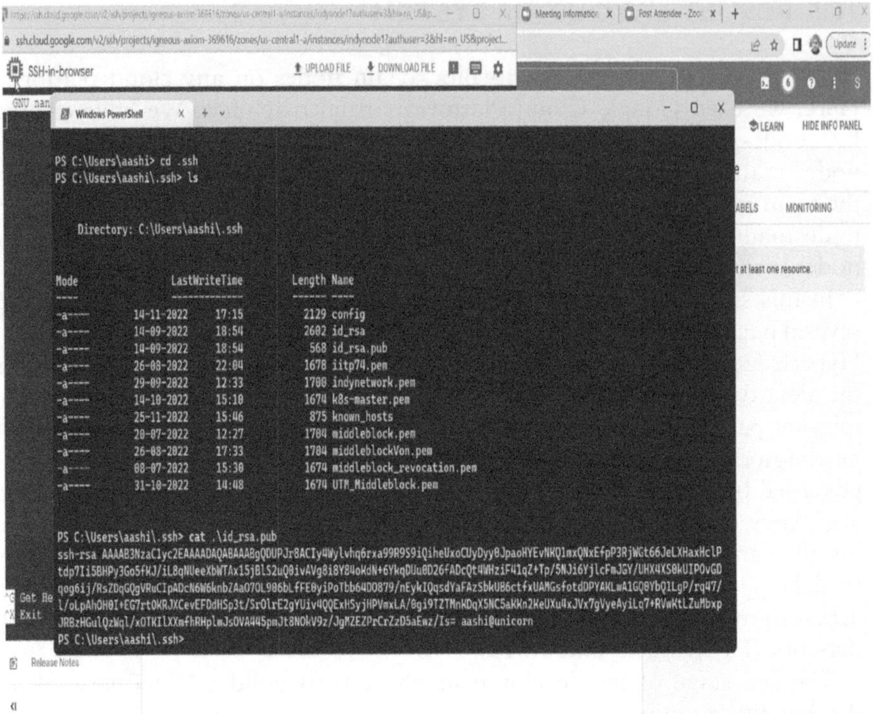

Figure 16.9 Public key used for SSH connection.

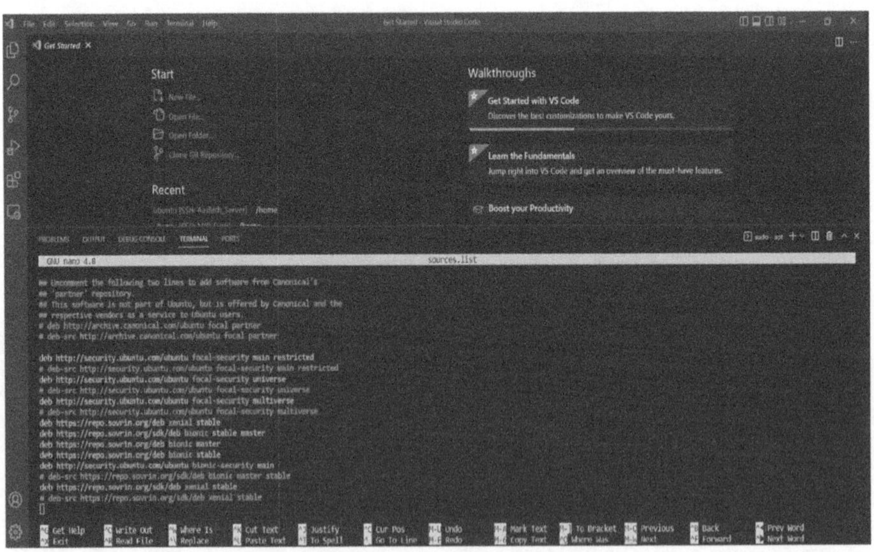

Figure 16.10 Setting up nodes.

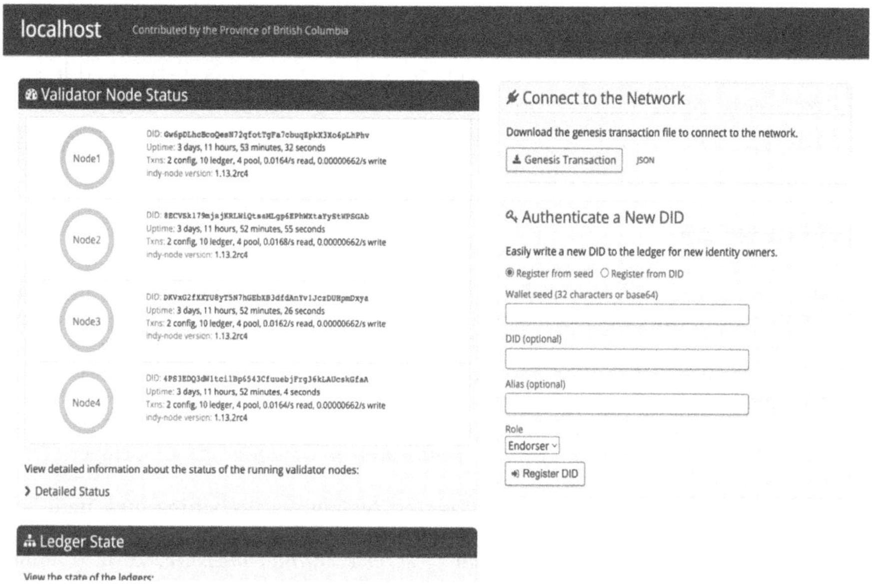

Figure 16.11 Live website showing nodes.

users or viewers. The modular approach towards developing and deploying complex software projects is quite beneficial. It works very efficiently, so we will use it to make this project successful.

All the Participants will be included in completing every phase. However, in general work, distribution will occur based on the experience of working on a particular Tech—Stack, eagerness to learn a particular technology, etc. (Figure 16.11).

16.6 CONCLUSION

Due to increased digital interactions and data analysis, Self-Sovereign Identities have become popular. It ensures that the users have more control and privacy over their sensitive data and more user-centric disabling management by centralised entities. Therefore, trustworthy models that provide users with several benefits, such as control and confidentiality, must be introduced. Blockchain technology should be widely adapted to achieve this goal; therefore, this paper provides an architectural analysis of self-sovereign identity using distributed ledgers so that this model can be widely adopted for issuing and maintaining identities. Till now, our implementation consists of five nodes. Among them is one full node; others are light nodes, a bare minimum requirement for working the system and pool generation. They follow consensus and other attributes associated with any advanced blockchain systems.

In the future, we will extend our model by mining more nodes in our network and allowing transactions. This system could be made public for other developers, serving them as a platform to read and write on this distributed ledger. Unlike many other blockchains, this platform could also be used to collect monetary incentives.

REFERENCES

1. Gayvoronskaya Meinel, *Schnjakin*. Blockchain: Hype oder innovation, 2018, ISBN: 978-3-86956-394-7 [Online]. Available: https://publishup.uni-potsdam.de/opus4-ubp/frontdoor/deliver/index/docId/10314/file/tbhpi113.pdf
2. S. Nakamoto, *Bitcoin: A peer-to-peer electronic cash system*, 2008 [Online]. Available: https://bitcoin.org/bitcoin.pdf
3. S. Haber and W.S. Stornetta, "How to time-stamp a digital document," in: *Conference on the Theory and Application of Cryptography*. Springer, 1990, pp. 437–455.
4. C. Dwork and M. Naor, "Pricing via processing or combatting junk mail," in: *Annual International Cryptology Conference*. Springer, 1992, pp. 139–147.
5. A. Back, et al., *Hashcash-a denial of service counter-measure*, 2002 [Online]. Available: http://www.hashcash.org/papers/hashcash.pdf
6. Globalnews.ca, *Equifax breach: total number of Canadians impacted by cyber attack passes 19,000 – National*, 2024 [Online]. Available: https://globalnews.ca/news/3886756/equifax-canada-data-breach [Accessed: 12 July 2024].
7. R. C. Merkle, "Secure communications over insecure channels," *Communications of the ACM*, vol. 21, no. 4, pp. 294–299, 1978.
8. M. Al-Bassam, "SCPKI: A smart contract-based PKI and identity system," in *Proceedings of the ACM Workshop on Blockchain, Cryptocurrencies and Contracts*, 2017, pp. 35–40.
9. J. G. Faísca and J. Q. Rogado, "Decentralised semantic identity," in *Proceedings of the 12th International Conference on Semantic Systems*, 2016, pp. 177–180.
10. Namecoin, 2024 [Online]. Available: https://namecoin.org [Accessed: 12 July 2024].
11. WebID specifications, 2024 [Online]. Available: https://www.w3.org/2005/Incubator/webid/spec [Accessed: 12 July 2024].
12. Open badges homepage, 2024 [Online]. Available: https://openbadges.org [Accessed: 12 July 2024].
13. "Civic Identity Verification | Secure & Protect Identities," *Civic*, 2024 [Online]. Available: https://www.civic.com [Accessed: 12 July 2024].
14. uPort.me, 2024 [Online]. Available: https://www.uport.me [Accessed: 12 July 2024].
15. M. Vukolic, "Eventually returning to strong consistency," *IEEE Data Engineering Bulletin*, vol. 39, no. 1), pp. 39–44, 2016.
16. Christopher Allen. "The path to self-sovereign identity," *Life with Alacrity*, pp. 214–220, 2016.
17. Home – Hyperledger, 2024 [Online]. Available: https://www.hyperledger.org [Accessed: 12 July 2024]
18. Hyperledger, *Hyperledger fabric*, 2024 [Online]. Available: https://www.hyperledger.org/projects/fabric [Accessed: 12 July 2024].
19. W. Li, H. Guo, M. Nejad, and C. -C. Shen, "Privacy-preserving traffic management: A blockchain and zero-knowledge proof inspired approach," *IEEE Access*, vol. 8, pp. 181733–181743, 2020. doi:10.1109/ACCESS.2020.3028189

20. P. Dunphy and F. A. Petitcolas, "A first look at identity management schemes on the blockchain," ArXiv Prepr. ArXiv180103294, 2018.
21. U. Feige, A. Fiat, and A. Shamir, "Zero-knowledge proofs of identity," *Journal of Cryptology*, vol. 1, no. 2, pp. 77–94, 1988.
22. "U-Prove," *Microsoft Research*, 2024 [Online]. Available: https://www.microsoft.com/en-us/research/project/u-prove [Accessed: 12 July 2024].
23. R. Soltani, U. T. Nguyen, and A. An, "A new approach to client onboarding using self-sovereign identity and distributed ledger," in *2018 IEEE International Conference on Internet of Things (iThings) and IEEE Green Computing and Communications (GreenCom) and IEEE Cyber, Physical and Social Computing (CPSCom) and IEEE Smart Data (SmartData)*, July 2018, IEEE, pp. 1129–1136.
24. P.-L. Aublin, S. B. Mokhtar, and V. Quéma, "Rbft: Redundant byzantine fault tolerance," in *Proceedings of the IEEE 33rd International Conference on Distributed Computing Systems (ICDCS)*, 2013, pp. 297–306.
25. M.S. Ferdous, M.J.M. Chowdhury, M.A. Hoque, and A. Colman, "Blockchain consensus algorithms: A survey," arXiv preprint arXiv:2001.07091, 2020.
26. Blockcerts, "Blockchain credentials," *Blockcerts*, 2024 [Online]. Available: http://blockcerts.org [Accessed: 12 July 2024].
27. ShoCard, *Secure enterprise identity authentication*, 2024 [Online]. Available: https://shocard.com [Accessed: 12 July 2024].

Index

Pages in *italics* refer to figures and pages in **bold** refer to tables.